Occupational Exposure Assessment for Air Contaminants

Occupational Exposure Assessment for Air Contaminants

Gurumurthy Ramachandran

Taylor & Francis
Taylor & Francis Group
Boca Raton London New York Singapore

A CRC title, part of the Taylor & Francis imprint, a member of the Taylor & Francis Group, the academic division of T&F Informa plc.

Published in 2005 by
CRC Press
Taylor & Francis Group
6000 Broken Sound Parkway NW, Suite 300
Boca Raton, FL 33487-2742

Printed in the United States of America on acid-free paper
10 9 8 7 6 5 4 3 2 1

International Standard Book Number-10: 1-5667-0609-2 (Hardcover)
International Standard Book Number-13: 978-1-5667-0609-4 (Hardcover)

Library of Congress Cataloging-in-Publication Data

Catalog record is available from the Library of Congress

T&F informa

Taylor & Francis Group
is the Academic Division of T&F Informa plc.

Visit the Taylor & Francis Web site at
http://www.taylorandfrancis.com

and the CRC Press Web site at
http://www.crcpress.com

Abstract

Exposure assessment is a key responsibility for most practicing occupational hygienists and forms the basis for a required course in most graduate programs in industrial hygiene. Over the last three decades, significant progress has been made, not only in the technology of measuring air contaminants, but also in the statistical descriptions of exposure distributions and exposure assessment strategies. This book addresses the various aspects of occupational exposure assessment for air contaminants as a coherent body of knowledge.

The first few sections of the book describe the process of obtaining a number that represents the value of exposure to an air contaminant (gas, vapor, or aerosol) and the science and technology underlying this process. This necessarily involves a discussion of the physical properties of the contaminants and the way in which measurement technologies take advantage of these properties. Respiratory tract deposition of aerosols is treated in sufficient depth. Concepts of measurement uncertainty and error and the propagation of error in physical measurements are also addressed. The last section describes sources of variability in exposures, including a discussion of between- and within-worker variability, the statistics of exposure distributions, and exposure assessment strategies for routine monitoring as well as occupational epidemiology.

This integrated approach is intended for use in a graduate or upper-level undergraduate course on occupational exposure assessment to airborne contaminants. The book targets students and practitioners in occupational hygiene and other environmental health disciplines.

Author

Gurumurthy Ramachandran is associate professor in the Division of Environmental Health Sciences of the School of Public Health at the University of Minnesota. Dr. Ramachandran has a Bachelor's degree in electrical engineering from the Indian Institute of Technology, Mumbai, a Master's degree in environmental engineering from the Virginia Institute of Technology, and a Ph.D. from the University of North Carolina, Chapel Hill. He is a Certified Industrial Hygienist (CIH).

Preface

I have been teaching a graduate course on occupational exposure assessment for air contaminants for almost a decade now. Occupational hygiene has lacked a book that addressed all aspects of exposure assessment for air contaminants as a coherent body of knowledge. This is despite the fact that exposure assessment is a key responsibility for most practicing occupational hygienists and forms the basis for a required course in most graduate programs in industrial hygiene. Although there are several books available on the measurement of air contaminants, they deal solely with the description of the technology involved in monitoring air contaminants (again focusing only on gases and vapors or only on aerosols). Some of the books, although excellent reference books, are not suitable as textbooks for teaching. A good example is *Air Sampling for Evaluation of Atmospheric Contaminants*, published by the American Council of Governmental Industrial Hygienists (ACGIH) and updated every few years. Several excellent textbooks are available for teaching aerosol science, e.g., those by Hinds (1999) and Vincent (1995). However, they do not address gas and vapor monitoring. Another limitation of these books is that they fail to cover the context in which exposures are measured, the design of exposure assessment strategies, and the statistical interpretation of exposure measurements. Only one book (Mulhausen and Damiano, 1998), to my knowledge, deals with this important topic. I continue to recommend this excellent reference book to students. However, it does not describe the different schools of thought regarding exposure assessment strategies. It also does not describe the actual measurement methods.

I wrote this book with the intention of addressing all of these important themes in one textbook. It is intended for use in a graduate or upper-level undergraduate course on occupational exposure assessment to airborne contaminants. It targets students and practitioners in occupational hygiene and other environmental health disciplines. The book covers not only the technological aspects of measuring air contaminants — gases, vapors, and aerosols — but also the occupational hygiene framework within which such measurements take place. Hence, it includes a solid treatment of exposure assessment strategies and statistics.

The book is divided into four broad sections: (1) a short introduction that describes the framework for studying air pollutants in occupational environments, (2) properties and measurement of gases and vapors, (3) properties and measurement of aerosols, and (4) sources of variability in exposures and exposure assessment strategies. The first chapter provides the context of exposure in the continuum between contaminant sources and the final biologically relevant dose.

Given that the focus is only on the measurement of exposures and not the measurement of dose, Section II and Section III deal with the measurement of air contaminants — gases, vapors, and aerosols. This portion of the book deals with the process of obtaining a number that represents the value of exposure to a contaminant, and the science and technology underlying this process. This necessarily involves a discussion of the physical properties of the contaminants and the way in which measurement technologies take advantage of these properties. Section II (Chapter 2 to Chapter 8) deals with the properties and measurements of gases and vapors, whereas Section III (Chapter 9 to Chapter 14) deals with the properties and measurements of aerosols. Numerous worked examples are presented in these chapters illustrating important concepts, e.g., ideal gas law calculations, calculating gas and vapor concentrations using different measurement methods, airflow monitoring, estimating size distributions from aerosol instrument measurements, and estimating respiratory deposition — to name a few. I have tried to address topics that I felt were the most important from an occupational exposure assessment perspective. Some topics have been given greater emphasis than others. For example, light scattering instruments get a more in-depth treatment than electrostatic classifiers. I have also omitted discussing research instruments or methods that are not widely used by practitioners (e.g., diffusion chargers). A crucial chapter is Chapter 4, which discusses the important concepts of measurement uncertainty and error and the propagation of error in physical measurements. Section IV (Chapter 15 to Chapter 18) discusses exposure assessment strategies for routine exposure monitoring as well as for occupational epidemiology. Chapter 15 includes a discussion of exposure variability, between- and within-worker variability, the statistics of exposure distributions, the use of the lognormal distribution, and exposure misclassification. Chapter 16 discusses similarly exposed groups (SEGs) and their exposure profiles for routine exposure monitoring, the use of occupational exposure limits for decision making regarding the acceptability of exposures of SEGs, and prioritizing SEGs based on exposure rankings. Chapter 17 describes the mathematical modeling of exposures. In many situations, sampling is impossible or expensive and difficult, or there may be so few actual measurements that they are of limited use. Assessing historical exposures for occupational epidemiology is such a scenario. Chapter 18 on retrospective exposure assessment discusses methods that combine measurements as well as mathematical modeling of exposures in a statistical framework.

Because this book provides a sweeping overview of exposure assessment to air contaminants, it precludes an advanced treatment of some topics. However, the book provides a framework for further study and research. I have provided sufficient references for the reader who is interested in researching some topics in greater depth.

I am grateful to a number of persons who have helped to make this book possible. The 2001–2003 classes for "Properties, Behavior, and Measurement of Air Contaminants" at the University of Minnesota provided valuable feedback on the approach used in various chapters. My colleagues Peter Raynor, Renee Anthony, Claudiu Lungu, and John Adgate were aggressive reviewers for various chapters, and their suggestions have strengthened this book. My father, Subrahmanya Gurumurthy, reviewed the entire book for grammar and construction. I thank all of them. Finally, I thank my wife, Candace, and daughter, Sandhya, who kept me so sufficiently distracted that I never lost my sense of perspective and balance.

Gurumurthy Ramachandran
Minneapolis

Table of Contents

Section I

Introduction

1 Framework for Occupational Exposure Assessment

1.1 INTRODUCTION

The occupational environment can be a source of significant risks to health due to a variety of potentially harmful agents workers can come in contact with. The role of the occupational hygienist is, therefore, to anticipate, recognize, evaluate, and control these health hazards. This concept is widely accepted as the paradigm of occupational hygiene. Although measurements of the contaminant concentrations play a crucial role in every component of this paradigm, this book primarily deals with the evaluation of health hazards through measurement of the exposure of workers to these hazards. Additionally, while a worker may be exposed to harmful agents through various routes — inhalation, ingestion, or dermal contact — this book focuses on the inhalation route. The respiratory tract offers the greatest amount of contact between the human body and the environment, and a vast majority of existing occupational health standards are based on this exposure route.

1.2 FRAMEWORK FOR OCCUPATIONAL EXPOSURE ASSESSMENT

1.2.1 Exposure Evaluation

Figure 1.1 shows a schematic context in which occupational exposure assessment is conducted. The work environment may contain several sources of contaminant generation. The amount of contaminants generated depends on the processes occurring in the workplace, as well as the physical and chemical properties of the contaminant, e.g., its vapor pressure. Once airborne, the contaminant gets dispersed through the environment by air movement. The amount of the contaminant in a unit volume of air is called the *concentration* of the contaminant and is typically expressed in units of mass of contaminant per cubic meter of air. However, it can also be expressed in terms of other metrics, e.g., parts per million, or number of particles per cubic meter. The dispersal of the contaminant is again dependent on the contaminant properties. For example, large particles generated in a grinding process may not travel far before they settle out by gravity, whereas smaller particles generated in a combustion source may be well dispersed. Workers moving through this environment performing various tasks become exposed to these contaminants.

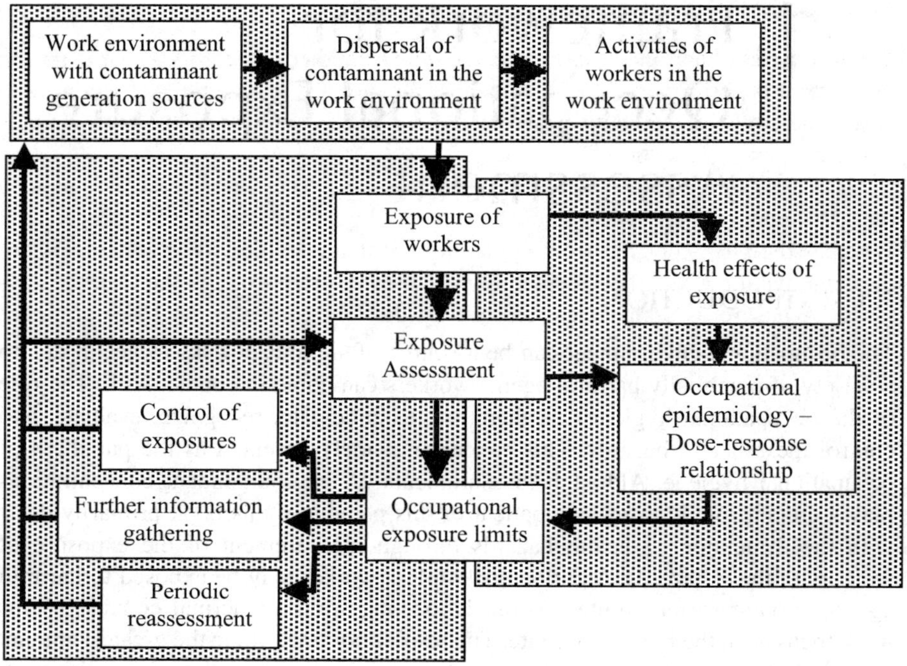

FIGURE 1.1 Context for occupational exposure assessment.

This exposure or human contact with contaminants leads to a dose that accumulates in the human body. These *exposures* and the resulting doses may result in adverse *health effects*. Exposure assessment is the process of evaluating these exposures. It may be carried out for a number of reasons, such as regulatory compliance, source characterization and evaluation of controls, and occupational epidemiology studies.

The lower left-hand block in Figure 1.1 shows the most common context in which exposure assessment is conducted: routine monitoring of worker exposures within a workplace. The strategy begins with a basic characterization of the workplace processes, controls, worker tasks, and contaminant properties. Based on this information, the workers are divided into several groups within which all workers have similar exposure profiles. Such groups are called *similar exposure groups* (SEGs). Next, the occupational hygienist (OH) determines the exposure profile of each SEG. By comparing these results with the occupational exposure limits (OELs), i.e., contaminant levels below which health effects are minimal, the OH decides whether the exposure is unacceptable, acceptable, or uncertain. If the exposure is unacceptable, control measures must be implemented to reduce it. Exposures are assessed again to determine the effectiveness of these control measures. If the exposure is acceptable, periodic reassessments are conducted to ensure that it continues to be acceptable. If the exposure is uncertain, then there is need for more information that could entail increased exposure measurements or information gathering about the processes, worker tasks, or contaminant properties. A detailed description of such routine monitoring strategies will be provided in Chapter 16.

1.2.2 Occupational Epidemiology

The lower right-hand block in Figure 1.1 shows another context in which exposure assessment is performed — occupational epidemiology, in which the objective is to determine a relationship between exposure and health outcome. This, in turn, leads to the development of OELs.

It is clear that both these contexts of performing exposure assessments, namely routine monitoring and occupational epidemiology, are linked and interdependent. Whereas the OELs derived from epidemiological studies provide a benchmark for decision making about the acceptability of an exposure profile by the OH, the day-to-day exposure assessment carried out by the OH could be the basis of future epidemiological studies. Occupational hygiene measurements may not always be suitable for epidemiological purposes and could bias any epidemiological study that uses these measurements. Caution needs to be exercised while using exposure data. For example, it is not sufficient to monitor the most highly exposed workers. An exposure profile of all worker categories, spanning a wide range from very low to very high exposures, is preferable. Such measurements, along with information about the plant processes, work practices, and job histories, will be invaluable for exposure reconstruction in future epidemiological studies.

1.2.3 Source Characterization and Evaluation of Controls

Measurements can be made to characterize the sources generating the contaminant. For example, leak detection is important to prevent accidental releases of unacceptable amounts of the contaminant into the workplace. It is also important to characterize all potential hazards in the workplace using screening measurements that identify concentrations of all the chemicals in the workplace, even those present in trace amounts. Although these measurements may not be considered as exposures, they are a very useful source of information about the chemical hazards in a workplace. If controls are installed to reduce exposures, air monitoring is crucial to test their adequacy. The controls could be a variety of things, ranging from ventilation systems to personal protective equipment to changing work practices. Each such control strategy can be evaluated using air monitoring.

1.2.4 Regulatory Purposes

Besides the routine monitoring carried out by the OHs at a workplace, regulatory agencies often require measurements of worker exposures to ensure that the health of the workers is protected in the work environment. This is referred to as *compliance monitoring*, and frequently involves making a small number of measurements of exposure of the workers at the greatest risk in a workplace. If these measurements are sufficiently below the legally mandated exposure limits, the exposures are said to be in compliance. Otherwise, the compliance officer issues a citation to the owner of the workplace, requiring that exposures be brought down to safe levels and periodic monitoring of worker exposures be carried out.

There are other reasons, as well, for making measurements of air concentrations in work places (Lynch, 1994), but these can also be viewed within the framework shown in Figure 1.1. These include validation of predictive physical exposure models, comparison of sampling methods, evaluation of contaminant sources, and investigation of complaints.

1.3 EXPOSURE VARIABILITY

Although a comprehensive exposure assessment that targets each worker would be ideal, it is often costly and impractical. Therefore, we need to develop an assessment scheme to sample a subset of the workers and measure their exposures. In any exposure assessment scheme, one has to account for the variability in the exposures of the workers. Occupational exposures vary significantly from day to day, from worker to worker, and from one group of workers to another. Even within a work shift, exposures vary from minute to minute. These variations result from changes in factors such as the generation rates of the contaminants, the levels of ventilation, and the activities of the workers, i.e., their tasks and work practices. This variability affects the number of samples needed to fully characterize these variations and the ability of the assessment scheme to compare different worker groups or compare exposures to an OEL.

One approach to deal with variability in worker exposures is to classify the workers into SEGs, which can be done by observing the similarity of tasks, work environments, and contaminants to which they are exposed. This approach is widely used for routine exposure monitoring as well as for occupational epidemiology. However, there is always a risk that exposures within the SEG are not sufficiently homogeneous.

Therefore, another approach proposes to first use sampling data to assess the variability of exposures and then divide the workers into SEGs. The overall variability in exposures can be divided into *within-worker variability* and *between-worker variability*. Within-worker variability arises due to changes in the exposure of a given worker from one day to the next and requires multiple measurements over time for the same worker. Between-worker variability arises due to the differences in the tasks and activity patterns of different workers. An SEG would be considered sufficiently homogeneous if the average exposures of 95% of the workers do not differ by more than a factor of two, i.e., the ratio of the 97.5th percentile to the 2.5th percentile is less than 2. Although this method poses a lower risk of misclassifying workers into SEGs, it requires measurements of more workers and multiple measurements of individual workers. Thus, it might be more reasonable to combine these approaches, and this technique is described in Chapter 15 and Chapter 16.

1.4 DEFINITION OF EXPOSURE

Exposure is the contact between a contaminant and a target that, in this context, is a worker. It is important to draw a distinction between measuring concentrations of air pollutants and measuring worker exposures to air pollutants. The workplace may have a number of processes being carried out simultaneously. Each process will have its own *microenvironment*, which may have a concentration that is different from the average workplace concentration. For example, the concentration near a source, such as a solvent bath, may be much higher than the average workplace concentration of that solvent. *Spatial inhomogeneity* also arises due to the location of sources and ventilation systems. In addition to the spatial variability in concentration, there is also *temporal variability* arising due to processes coming on and going off line and ventilation rates changing with time. While an individual worker moves around in this complex arena, the concentration of the air he or she breathes in at any point in time may be different from the average workplace concentration.

Even if the worker is stationary within a microenvironment, the concentration of the air pollutant he or she breathes in may be different from the average concentration in the microenvironment. This is especially true for airborne particles. However, for gases and vapors, the microenvironment concentration is a much closer approximation to the concentration of the air being breathed in by the worker.

It is useful to imagine an envelope of air surrounding the worker's head, from which the worker is inhaling. This envelope of air is called the *breathing zone* of the worker. The worker is exposed to the concentration of the air pollutants in this breathing zone. In some situations, even the breathing zone concentration may be inhomogeneous. Such situations may arise when there is a sharply defined plume arising from the source and going through the breathing zone, e.g., during welding. However, for most situations the breathing zone concentration is a reasonably good approximation of the concentration to which the worker is exposed.

If $C(t)$ is the concentration of a given pollutant that a worker is exposed to at any instant of time over an interval T, then the exposure over this time interval is defined as

$$E = \int_{t=0}^{T} C(t)\,\mathrm{d}t \tag{1.1}$$

This definition was recommended by the National Academy of Sciences (NAS, 1991). As can be seen, this definition of exposure has units of concentration-time, e.g., $\left(\frac{mg - hour}{m^3}\right)$ Thus, if the average concentration that the worker is exposed to in the ith microenvironment is C_i, and the time spent in that microenvironment is t_i, then the exposure is equal to

$$E = \sum_{i=1}^{N} C_i\, t_i \tag{1.2}$$

where the worker moves through N microenvironments, and $T = \sum_{i=1}^{N} t_i$.

In most cases, however, it has been customary to express exposure in terms of a time-weighted average concentration. Thus,

$$E = \frac{1}{T}\int_{t=0}^{T} C(t)\,\mathrm{d}t \tag{1.3}$$

Equation 1.3 captures the same information as Equation 1.1, except that the integral of the time-varying concentration is normalized by the total time. Hence, the units of exposure will be the same as that of concentration. Equation 1.2 will, therefore, be written as

$$E = \frac{\sum_{i=1}^{N} C_i t_i}{\sum_{i=1}^{N} t_i} = \frac{\sum_{i=1}^{N} C_i t_i}{T} = \sum_{i=1}^{N} C_i f_i \tag{1.4}$$

where f_i is the fraction of time spent by the worker in the ith microenvironment.

From the above discussion, we see that exposure is the intensity (i.e., the concentration) of the air pollutant at the interface between the environment and the worker for a specific contaminant over a specific time interval that has biological relevance. Figure 1.2 shows the relationships between the instantaneous exposure $C(t)$, the temporally averaged exposure C_{avg}, and the peak exposure C_{peak}. In the case of diseases caused by chronic exposures, a long-term time-weighted average might be appropriate, whereas for an acute effect, a short-term average of the order of a few minutes may be more relevant.

1.5 DEFINITION OF DOSE

A related but distinct concept is the dose of a given pollutant. For inhalation exposures, the dose is defined as the amount of the pollutant that causes an acute or chronic effect once it has entered the body, crossed the absorption barriers, and become biologically available. Figure 1.3 shows the relationships between sources, exposure pathways, exposures, and dose estimates. It is the cumulative amount of the harmful property that is delivered to the body over a period of time that drives the biological response. Thus, whereas there can be an exposure without a dose, there cannot be a dose without an exposure. The dose includes in its calculation (1) the exposure concentration, (2) the time period of the exposure, (3) the breathing rate of the individual (i.e., the contact rate), (4) the time-dependent retention of the contaminant in the body, and finally (5) the ability of the retained fraction in the body to cause a biological response that may be an acute or chronic health effect. We therefore need to know the exposure as well as the pharmacokinetics and pharmacodynamics of the pollutant in order to be able to estimate the dose. Dose is typically normalized to body weight or organ weight.

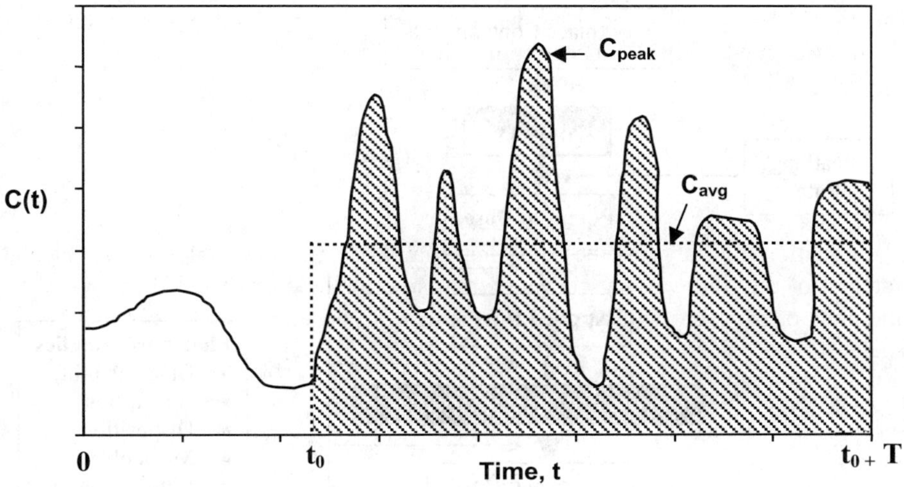

FIGURE 1.2 Exposure profile as a function of time. $C(t)$ is the instantaneous exposure, C_{avg} is the average exposure over a time interval T, and C_{peak} is the maximum instantaneous exposure over the time interval.

For a contaminant whose mass is the relevant harmful property, the unit is $\frac{\text{mass of contaminant}}{\text{kg of body weight}}$.

Let us consider a worker weighing 60 kg exposed to a concentration of 1 mg/m^3 over a typical work shift of 8 h every day. Let us assume that the worker breathes at the rate of 20 breaths l/min. Then the total volume of air inhaled over 8 h is 9.6 m^3. If only 50% of the contaminant is permanently retained by the body, the *normalized absorbed dose* per day is $1\frac{mg}{m^3} \times 9.6\frac{m^3}{day} \times \frac{1}{60kg} \times 0.5 = 0.08\frac{mg}{kg-day}$. If this worker were employed at this job for 5 years, 5 days a week for 48 weeks every year, then the absorbed dose at the end of 5 years will be $0.08\frac{mg}{kg-day} \times 5\frac{days}{week} \times 48\frac{weeks}{year} \times 5 years = 96\frac{mg}{kg}$.

In some cases when the fraction absorbed may be unknown, it is useful to define a *potential dose* that assumes 100% absorption. In the above example, the normalized potential dose per day would be $\left[1\frac{mg}{m^3} \times 9.6\frac{m^3}{day} \times \frac{1}{60kg}\right] = 0.16\frac{mg}{kg-day}$, and the potential dose at the end of 5 years would be 192 $\frac{mg}{kg}$.

We can now formally define potential dose over a time T as the mass of contaminant inhaled:

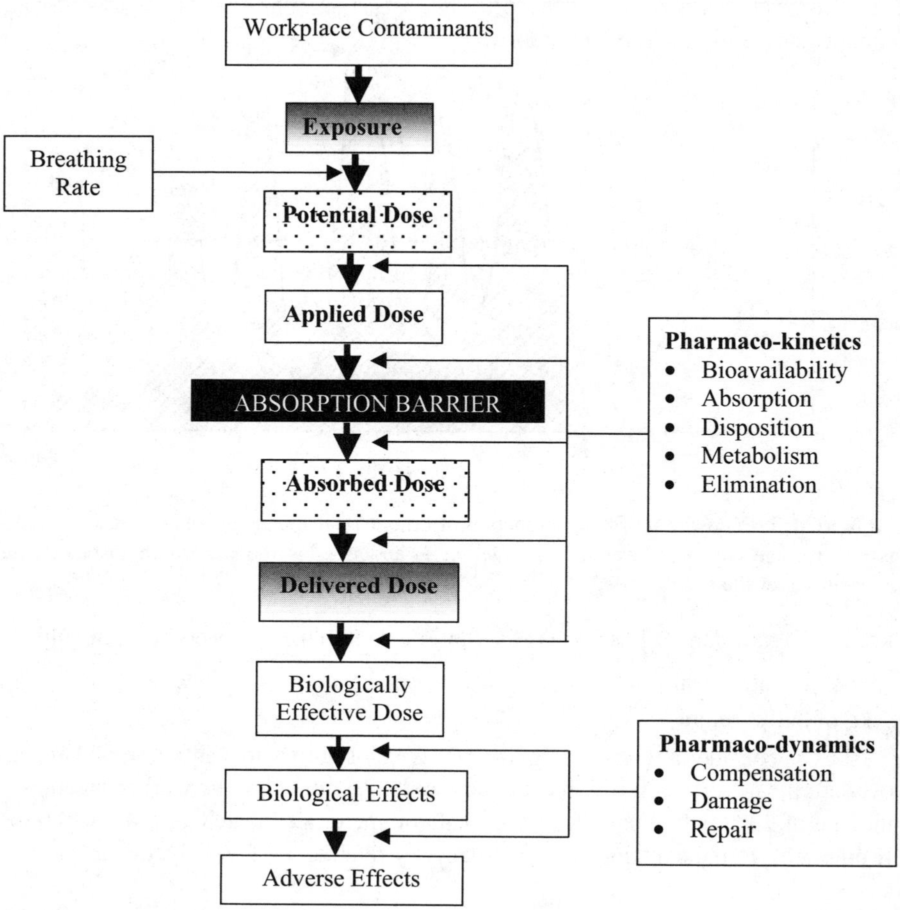

FIGURE 1.3 The relationship between exposure and dose. (Sexton et al., 1995.)

$$\textit{Potential Dose} = \int_{t=0}^{T} C(t) \times BR \, \mathrm{d}t \tag{1.5}$$

where *BR* is the breathing rate.

Only a fraction of the potential dose comes in contact with the respiratory tract. This fraction is the *applied dose.*

$$\textit{Applied Dose} = \alpha \int_{t=0}^{T} C(t) \times BR \, \mathrm{d}t \tag{1.6}$$

where α is the fraction of the potential dose that is available for absorption.

Now, we can define the *absorbed dose* as the amount of contaminant absorbed and available to undergo metabolism

$$D = \alpha \int_{t=0}^{T} C(t) \times BR \times f_{\text{abs}} \, \mathrm{d}t \tag{1.7}$$

where f_{abs} is the fraction of the contaminant that is absorbed (50% in the above example). Although the example uses simplified constant values for each of the factors, in reality all of the factors can be nonlinear and time-dependent. Only a fraction of this absorbed dose, called the *delivered dose*, reaches the tissue of interest. The portion of the delivered dose that reaches the sites of toxic action is called the *biologically effective dose*, and this causes the biological response.

To obtain an ideal understanding of the exposure–disease continuum, we need to be able to make measurements of exposure and each of the different types of doses in Figure 1.3. Alternatively, we should have a sufficient understanding of the pharmacokinetics and pharmacodynamics of the contaminant to be able to predict the doses from measurements of other parameters. As Figure 1.3 shows, the measurements of exposure and delivered dose are relatively straightforward, whereas those for potential and absorbed doses are more difficult, and those for applied and biologically relevant doses are usually impossible (Sexton et al., 1995). In this book we focus primarily on the measurement of exposure and not the measurement of dose. In recent years, the measurement of biological markers as a measure of internal dose has made rapid strides. However, a discussion of such biological markers is outside the scope of this book.

1.6 OVERVIEW OF THE BOOK

This chapter has defined exposure and dose, discussed the relevance of averaging time in defining exposures, described the context in which occupational exposure assessment occurs, and emphasized the central role of exposure variability in exposure assessment strategy. This discussion has set the stage for the rest of the book.

Given that we focus only on the measurement of exposures and not the measurement of dose, Section II and Section III of the book will deal with the measurement of air contaminants — gases, vapors, and aerosols. In essence, this portion of the book deals with the process of obtaining a number that represents the value of exposure to a contaminant and the science and technology underlying this process. This necessarily involves a discussion of the physical properties of the contaminant and how the measurement technologies take advantage of these properties. Section II (Chapter 2 to Chapter 8) deals with the properties and measurements of gases and vapors, while Section III (Chapter 9 to Chapter 14) deals with the properties and measurements of aerosols. Chapter 4 discusses the important concepts of measurement uncertainty and error and the propagation of error in physical measurements.

Section IV (Chapter 15 to Chapter 18) discusses exposure assessment strategies for routine exposure monitoring, as well as for occupational epidemiology. Chapter

15 includes a discussion of exposure variability, between-worker and within-worker variability, the statistics of exposure distributions, the use of the lognormal distribution, and exposure misclassification. Chapter 16 discusses SEGs and their exposure profiles for routine exposure monitoring, the use of OELs for decision making regarding the acceptability of exposures of SEGs, and prioritizing SEGs based on exposure rankings. In many situations, sampling is impossible or expensive and difficult, or there may be so few actual measurements that they are of limited use. Therefore, one has to characterize the exposures indirectly. Assessing historical exposures for occupational epidemiology is such a scenario. Mathematical modeling of exposures (Chapter 17) is an elegant solution in such situations, although many exposure models are not completely validated. Chapter 18 is based on retrospective exposure assessment and discusses methods that combine measurements as well as mathematical modeling of exposures in a statistical framework.

Section II

Properties and Measurement of Gases and Vapors

2 Properties of Gases and Vapors

2.1 THE IDEAL GAS LAW

A gas in equilibrium may be described by its macroscopic properties: volume V, pressure P, and temperature t. All other properties of the system can be determined if these properties are specified. The equation of state of this system is described by the functional relationship

$$V = m f\ (P, t) \tag{2.1}$$

where m is the mass of the gas present and $f(P, t)$ is some function of pressure and temperature.

The first quantitative data regarding the behavior of gases were reported by Robert Boyle in 1662. He showed that at any given temperature, the product of the pressure P exerted by a gas and its molar volume v is constant. In 1787, Jacques Charles observed that this constant is a function of temperature. Thus, the equation of state for one mole of a gas was determined to be

$$Pv = f\ (t) \tag{2.2}$$

It was found that $f(t)$ was approximately linear: $f(t) = a + bt$. The constants a and b were estimated from experimental data. In units of liters per mole and atmospheres, an expression for $f(t)$ was determined:

$$f(t) = 22.4140 + 0.082057\ t = 0.082057\ (273.16 + t) \tag{2.3}$$

where t is the temperature in degree Celsius (or Centigrade). This expression can be rewritten if a new temperature scale is adapted such that $T = 273.16 + t$°C. We then have, for one mole of a gas,

$$Pv = RT \tag{2.4}$$

where T is the absolute temperature and R is the universal gas constant whose numerical value depends on the choice of units. Table 2.1 gives the values of R in different sets of units.

Equation 2.4 can be alternatively expressed as

$$PV = n\mathrm{R}T \tag{2.5}$$

TABLE 2.1
Universal Gas Constant, R

Units	*R*
liter atmosphere/gram mole/degree kelvin	0.082057
liter mm Hg/gram mole/degree kelvin	62.4
m^3 Pa/gram mole/degree kelvin = joule/kg mole/degree kelvin	8.314

or

$$PV = \frac{m}{M} RT \tag{2.6}$$

or

$$P = \frac{\rho}{M} RT \tag{2.7}$$

where V is the total volume of the gas, n is the number of moles of the gas, m is the mass of the gas, M is its molecular weight, and ρ is its density.

Equation 2.5, Equation 2.6, and Equation 2.7 are different expressions of the equation of state of an ideal gas. Under normal atmospheric conditions, at sufficiently low pressure, which is the case in most workplace atmospheres, the behavior of most gas and vapor contaminants can be described by the ideal gas laws. From Equation 2.5, we can deduce

$$\frac{P_1 V_1}{T_1} = \frac{P_2 V_2}{T_2} \tag{2.8}$$

where the subscripts 1 and 2 refer to the values of pressure, volume, and temperature at two different conditions. This relationship is important for determining the properties of gases under various environmental or process conditions.

2.2 MOLAR VOLUME

One g-mol of an ideal gas at 0°C (273 K) and 1 atm pressure (101.325 kPa or 760 mm Hg) always occupies the same volume, 22.414 l. This can be derived by substituting $n = 1$ g-mol, $P = 101.325$ kPa, $T = 273.16$ K, and $R = 8.314$ J/g-mol/K in Equation 2.5 to obtain V. This is also seen in Equation 2.2 and Equation 2.3, with $P = 1$ atm and $t = 0$°C, in which the empirical function $f(t)$ reduces to the molar volume of 22.414 l.

2.3 STANDARD CONDITIONS FOR AIR SAMPLING

Air sampling can be conducted under different atmospheric conditions of temperature and pressure. The mass concentration of a pollutant (defined as mass of pollutant per unit volume of air) depends on the volume of air sampled, which in turn depends on the prevailing atmospheric conditions. In order to compare concentrations measured under different conditions, all gas volumes must be corrected to *standard conditions*.

In industrial hygiene air sampling, standard conditions are defined as 25°C (298 K) and 1 atm (760 mm Hg). Equation 2.8 can be used to calculate the molar volume for these conditions.

$$V_2 = V_1\left(\frac{P_1}{P_2}\right)\times\left(\frac{T_2}{T_1}\right) \tag{2.9}$$

$$= 22.414\left(\frac{760}{760}\right)\times\left(\frac{298}{273}\right)$$

$$= 24.45\ l$$

Air is a mixture of gases with 78% (by volume) nitrogen, 21% oxygen, and the remaining 1% being various trace gases such as argon, carbon dioxide, and water vapor. Its average molecular weight is ~29 g-mol. In some instances it may be useful to calculate the density of air at any temperature and pressure using Equation 2.7. At 25°C and 1 atm, the density of air is

$$\rho = \frac{PM}{RT} = \frac{101\ kPa\,x\,29\ g/mol}{8.314\ l\,kPa/mol/K \times 298\ K} = 1.18\ g/l = 1.18\ kg/m^3$$

2.4 MIXTURES OF IDEAL GASES

Let us assume that a container holds 2 g of hydrogen ($M = 2$) at 298 K and 1 atm, and 2 g of oxygen are added. The volume of the gas mixture will not be doubled by this addition. However, it will be doubled if 32 g ($M = 32$) of oxygen were added. This is an illustration of *Avogadro's hypothesis*, which states that equal volumes of gases at the same pressure and temperature contain equal number of molecules and therefore equal number of moles. The partial pressure of the ith species in a mixture of gases is given by

$$P_i V = n_i RT \tag{2.10}$$

Summing over all the N species in the mixture,

$$\left(P_1 + P_2 + \ldots + P_N\right)V = \left(n_1 + n_2 + \ldots + n_N\right)RT$$

Here, $P_i = x_i P$, and $x_i = n_i/n$ is the mole fraction of the *i*th species. Because the sum of all mole fractions is unity,

$$\sum_i P_i = P$$

that is, the total pressure of a mixture of ideal gases is given by the sum of the partial pressures of the individual species present. This is *Dalton's law.*

There is a counterpart to this law, called *Amagat's law,* which involves partial volumes. The partial volume v_i of a component of a gaseous mixture is the volume that component would occupy if it were by itself at the pressure and temperature of the mixture.

$$v_i = \frac{n_i RT}{P} \tag{2.11}$$

Because $\sum_i n_i = n$, it follows that $\sum_i v_i = V$, and $v_i = x_i V$.

This provides one basis for expressing the concentration of a contaminant. For a contaminant in air,

$$V = V_{\text{air}} + V_{\text{contaminant}}$$

The concentration of a contaminant can be expressed as a volume fraction:

$$c = \frac{V_{\text{contaminant}}}{V_{\text{contaminant}} + V_{\text{air}}} \approx \frac{V_{\text{contaminant}}}{V_{\text{air}}} \tag{2.12}$$

Typically, the volume of a contaminant is much smaller than the volume of air, and the concentration of the contaminant is expressed in parts per million (ppm) or parts per billion (ppb), i.e., volume of contaminant per million or billion volumes of air.

Consider a situation in which a sealed container is partially filled with a pure chemical in liquid form, and the rest of the container is filled with pure air. The liquid-phase chemical molecules that have sufficient kinetic energy escape the liquid and enter the headspace air. If the liquid's temperature and surface area remain constant, the rate of escape, i.e., evaporation, is constant. When the rate at which molecules leave the liquid surface is equal to the rate at which the molecules come back to the liquid surface, the system is at equilibrium, and the headspace air is saturated with chemical vapor. The partial pressure exerted by the gas-phase chemical molecules in the headspace at equilibrium is called the *vapor pressure, equilib-*

rium vapor pressure, or *saturation vapor pressure* (denoted by P_V) of a chemical. The P_V value of a chemical increases with the temperature of the system.

We know from Dalton's law that the *mole fraction* of a constituent in a mixture is equal to its partial pressure divided by the total pressure. The airborne concentration of the *i*th constituent in ppm is equal to its mole fraction multiplied by one million.

$$C(\text{in ppm}) = \frac{P_i}{P} \times 10^6 \tag{2.13}$$

If the partial pressure of the chemical is equal to its saturation vapor pressure, then the *saturation concentration* in air is given by

$$C_{sat}(\text{in ppm}) = \frac{P_V\ (\text{in mm Hg})}{760\ \text{mm Hg}} \times 10^6 \tag{2.14}$$

2.5 EXPRESSING GAS CONTAMINANT CONCENTRATION IN DIFFERENT WAYS

In many occupational situations, *mass concentration* of a pollutant is expressed as mg/m^3 (milligrams of pollutant gas per cubic meter of air). But, as discussed in the previous section, concentration can also be expressed as a volumetric ratio in ppm or ppb. The ideal gas law can be used to derive a useful relationship between these two ways of expressing concentration.

Let the concentration of a gas be m mg/m^3, i.e., there are m mg of the gas per cubic meter of air. From Equation 2.6, the volume (in liters) occupied by a mass m (in milligrams) of a gas is given by

$$V = \frac{m}{M}\frac{RT}{P} \times 10^{-3} \tag{2.15}$$

At $P = 760$ mm Hg and $T = 298$ K (25°C), with the molecular weight M in units of grams per mole, this becomes

$$V = \frac{m}{M} \times 24.45 \times 10^{-3}\ l = \frac{m}{M} \times 24.45 \times 10^{-6}\ \text{m}^3 \tag{2.16}$$

This is the volume of the gas per cubic meter of air. So, as a volume fraction, the gas concentration is

$$C = \frac{m}{M} \times 24.45 \times 10^{-6}\ \frac{m^3}{m^3} \tag{2.17}$$

Or, by expressing concentration in terms of volume parts of gas per million volume parts of air, we obtain

$$C\ (\text{ppm}) = \frac{m\ (\text{mg/m}^3)}{M} \times 24.45 \tag{2.18}$$

Equation 2.18 is widely used in industrial hygiene to convert concentrations between a mass metric and a volume metric.

2.6 KINETIC THEORY OF GASES

The kinetic theory of gases considers a gas as a collection of atoms and molecules and examines how the properties of a gas can be determined on the basis of the continual translational motion of its components. This molecular level description of the behavior of a gas offers ready interpretation of the ideal gas laws. The model on which the kinetic theory is based makes three assumptions:

1. The gas consists of individual particles, each of mass m, in continuous motion.
2. The particles have negligible size (their dimensions are much smaller than the average distance between them).
3. The particles do not interact except when they undergo elastic collisions.

The model considers the gas to contain a very large number of molecules. Avogadro's number, 6.023×10^{23}, gives the total number of molecules in one mole of a gas. Thus, at 25°C, the number of molecules per cubic meter of air can be calculated as $\frac{6.023 \times 10^{23}\,\text{molecules}}{24.45 \times 10^{-3}\,m^3} = 2.46 \times 10^{25}$ molecules. The molecules are negligibly small, perfect spheres that are in incessant motion. They travel in straight lines between collisions with each other. The molecules possess only kinetic energy, which is directly proportional to the absolute temperature. This energy is not lost in these collisions, but only exchanged between the colliding molecules, i.e., the collisions are elastic.

Let us consider a cubical box of volume V in which there is a molecule of mass m moving with a velocity u bouncing back and forth between the opposite, walls. When the molecule strikes the right side of the box (Figure 2.1), it reverses its direction. The change in its momentum is $mu - (-mu) = 2\ mu$. If the side of the container is of length L, then the frequency of such collisions is $\frac{u}{2L}$. The momentum change per second imparted to the wall is $\frac{mu^2}{L}$. The pressure or force per unit area becomes $P = \frac{mu^2}{L^3}$ or

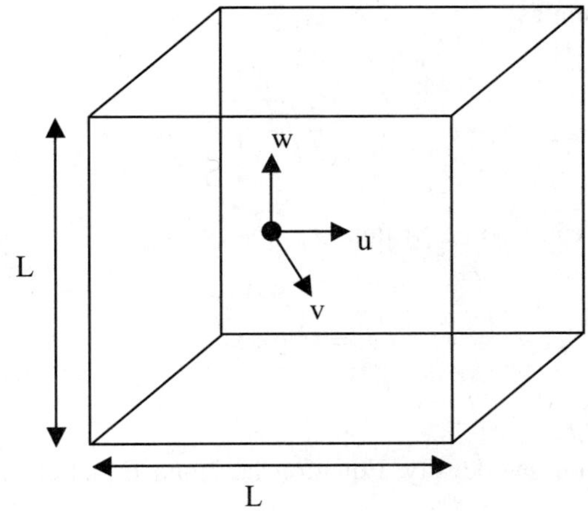

FIGURE 2.1 Velocity components of a molecule in a box.

$$P = \frac{m u^2}{V} \tag{2.19}$$

In the general case, u is the magnitude of the velocity along one of the Cartesian coordinate axes. The total velocity is given by the velocity vector c, which may be resolved into its components u, v, and w along the x, y, and z directions. Hence, $c^2 = u^2 + v^2 + w^2$. We assume, simplistically for the time being, that all molecules in the system have the same velocity c. Also, u, v, and w should be equal; otherwise, one direction would be preferred over another, and there would be an accumulation of particles in that direction, which is not true. Thus, $u^2 = \frac{c^2}{3}$, and Equation 2.19 can be rewritten as

$$P\,V = \frac{1}{3} m\,c^2 \tag{2.20}$$

For one mole, this becomes

$$P\,v = \frac{1}{3} M\,c^2 \tag{2.21}$$

where M is the molecular weight of the gas. This is similar to the ideal gas law for one mole given by Equation 2.4. Hence, the relationship between temperature and the molecular velocity is given by

$$RT = \frac{1}{3} M\,c^2 \tag{2.22}$$

which can be written as

$$c = \left(\frac{3RT}{M} \right)^{1/2} \tag{2.23}$$

Equation 2.21 can also be written as

$$P = \frac{1}{3} \rho \, c^2 \tag{2.24}$$

where $\rho = \frac{M}{v}$ is the gas density. Equation 2.22 and Equation 2.24 relate macroscopic properties of the gas, such as temperature and pressure, to a microscopic property, namely molecular velocity.

Clearly, the preceding treatment involves some simplifications. It is not realistic to assume that all molecules have the same velocity. In reality, the molecules of a gas have a distribution of velocities described by the Maxwell–Boltzmann distribution law. Therefore, the quantity c must really be some kind of an average.

For a system of molecules having kinetic energy due to its velocity the Maxwell–Boltzmann distribution gives the fraction of molecules $\frac{dN(u)}{N_0}$, having velocities between c and c + dc (in other words, the probability that an arbitrary molecule in the gas will have a velocity between c and c + dc):

$$\frac{dN(c)}{N_0} = \left(\frac{M}{2\pi RT} \right)^{3/2} \left[\exp\left(-\frac{M c^2}{2RT} \right) \right] 4\pi c^2 \, dc \tag{2.25}$$

where M is the molecular weight of the gas, and N_0 is the total number of molecules.

Equation 2.25 can now be used to calculate the average velocity $\bar{c}$ as

$$\bar{c} = \frac{1}{N_0} \int_0^\infty c \, dN = \int_0^\infty \left(\frac{M}{2\pi RT} \right)^{3/2} \left[\exp\left(-\frac{M c^2}{2RT} \right) \right] 4\pi c^3 \, dc = \left(\frac{8RT}{\pi M} \right)^{1/2} \tag{2.26}$$

Here, the integral $\int_0^\infty dN = N_0$, the total number of molecules. Similarly, the root-mean-square (rms) velocity of the molecules can be calculated as

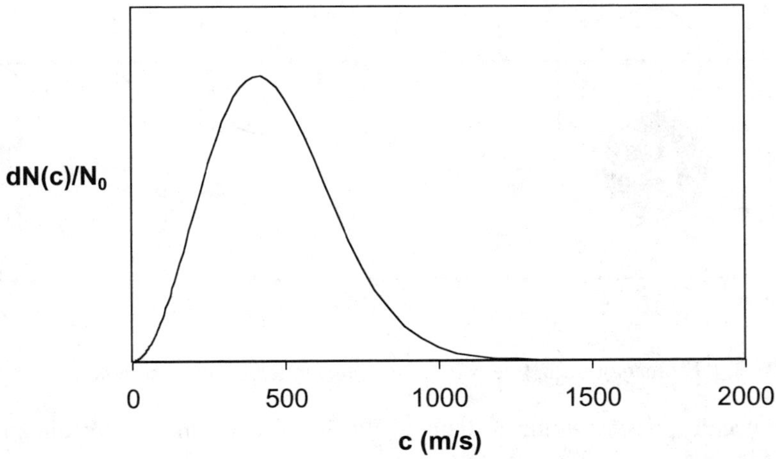

FIGURE 2.2 Maxwell–Boltzmann molecular velocity distribution for air molecules at 25°C.

$$c_{rms} = \frac{1}{N_0}\int_0^\infty c^2\, dN = \int_0^\infty \left(\frac{M}{2\pi RT}\right)^{3/2} \left[\exp\left(-\frac{M c^2}{2RT}\right)\right] 4\pi c^4\, dc = \left(\frac{3RT}{M}\right)^{1/2} \tag{2.27}$$

This is identical to Equation 2.23, and thus the assumption that all molecules have the same velocity leads to an expression for the velocity that is the same as the square root of the average of the squared velocities. This really is an expression of the fact that the molecules in a gas have the same average kinetic energy in both models.

Figure 2.2 shows this velocity distribution (Equation 2.25) for air molecules at 25°C. Note that in order to obtain the velocities in units of meters per second, we need to use $R = 8.314$ J/kgmol/K and $M = 0.029$ kg/mol. From Equation 2.25, we can see that the probability of having zero velocity is zero. That is, no molecule has a velocity of zero. The molecular velocities can be as high as 1300 m/sec. The average velocity as given by Equation 2.26 is calculated to be 466 m/sec, whereas the rms velocity as given by Equation 2.27 is 506 m/sec.

2.7 MEAN FREE PATH

As the kinetic theory assumes, all the molecules are in incessant motion and constantly in collision with one another. The mean free path λ of a molecule is the average distance traveled by it between collisions. A somewhat intuitive argument can be used to derive an expression for mean free path. We will assume a simple situation in which all the molecules in the system are identical, i.e., it is a pure gas and not a mixture of gases. As shown in Figure 2.3, we imagine a molecule of diameter d moving with an average velocity $\bar{c}$. As it moves, it will collide with

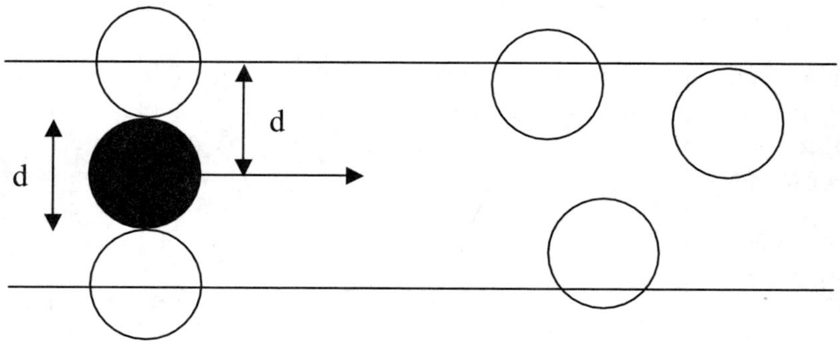

FIGURE 2.3 Estimating mean free path using collision frequency of a molecule.

any molecule present within a diameter of $2d$. The volume swept out in each second is thus $\pi d^2 \bar{c}$. If there are n' molecules per unit volume, then the average number of collisions per second is $\pi d^2 \bar{c} n'$. This intuitive argument has to be modified by a factor of $\sqrt{2}$, because the molecules are moving relative to each other, to give a collision frequency of $\sqrt{2}\,\pi d^2 \bar{c} n'$. The mean free path λ, then, is simply the mean velocity divided by the collision frequency so that

$$\lambda = \frac{\bar{c}}{\sqrt{2}\,\pi d^2 \bar{c} n'} = \frac{1}{\sqrt{2}\pi d^2 \; n'} \tag{2.28}$$

Several comments can be made regarding the mean free path. Because λ is inversely proportional to n', it implies that the mean free path is inversely proportional to the gas density, and therefore inversely proportional to the gas pressure (from Equation 2.7).

Example: What is the mean free path of an air molecule at 25°C?

$$d = 3.6 \times 10^{-10} \text{ m}$$

$$n' = 2.46 \times 10^{25} \text{ molecules/m}^3$$

$$\lambda = \frac{1}{\sqrt{2}\,\pi d^2 \; n'} = \frac{1}{\sqrt{2}\,\pi \left(3.6\times10^{-10}\right)^2 \left(2.46\times10^{25}\right)} = 7.06\times10^{-8} \text{ m} = 0.07 \text{ µm.}$$

2.8 TRANSPORT PHENOMENA

Transport phenomena refer to the spatial motion of some physical property. In this section, we will study two phenomena — diffusion and viscosity. In the case of diffusion, molecules are transported by drift from one place to another; in the case of viscosity, molecules are transported by momentum.

2.8.1 Diffusion

Diffusion is the spatial drift of molecules due to their kinetic motion. The process is called a "random walk" and is analogous to a person taking successive steps, with each step being unrelated to the preceding step (Figure 2.4). A given molecule will eventually drift away from its initial position. As a purely statistical effect, there will be a net movement of molecules from a region where they are in a higher concentration to a region where they are in a lower concentration (Figure 2.5). The mass transfer process is described by Fick's law:

$$J = -D\frac{dC}{dx} \tag{2.29}$$

where J is mass flux (the mass that is transported per unit area across a plane perpendicular to the concentration gradient in unit time, mg/m^2/sec), D is the molecular diffusion coefficient (m^2/sec), and $\frac{dC}{dx}$ is the local concentration gradient (mg/m^4).

The diffusion coefficient is given by

$$D = \frac{1}{2}\bar{c}\lambda \tag{2.30}$$

where $\bar{c}$ is the average molecular velocity and λ is the mean free path. For air molecules at 25°C, the average molecular velocity is 466 m/sec and the mean free path is 7.06×10^{-8} m. The diffusion coefficient calculated from Equation 2.30 is 1.6×10^{-5} m^2/sec.

2.8.2 Viscosity

The coefficient of viscosity μ of a gas is defined as a measure of the friction that is present when adjacent layers of the gas are moving with different velocities. If a fluid is moving between stationary parallel plates [Figure 2.6(a)], then the gas

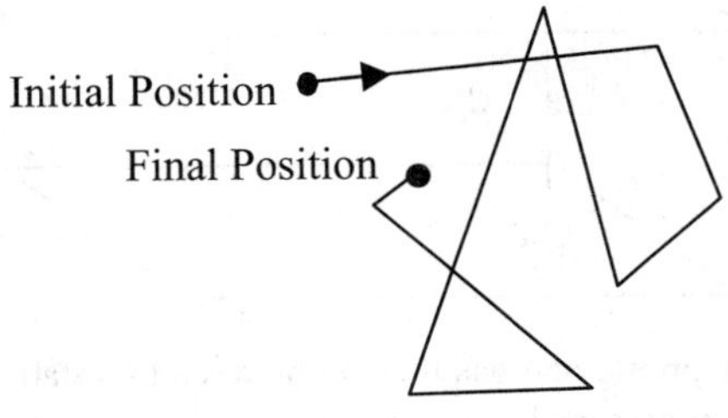

FIGURE 2.4 Random walk.

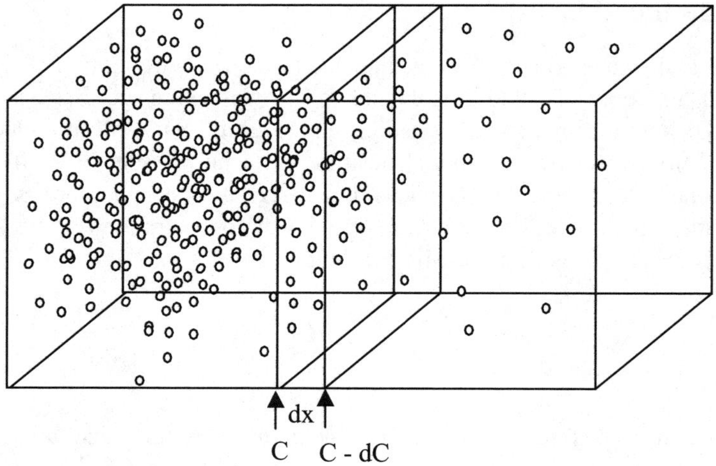

FIGURE 2.5 Molecules of a gas diffusing from a region of high concentration to a region of low concentration. The mass flux in this situation is from the left to the right in the box.

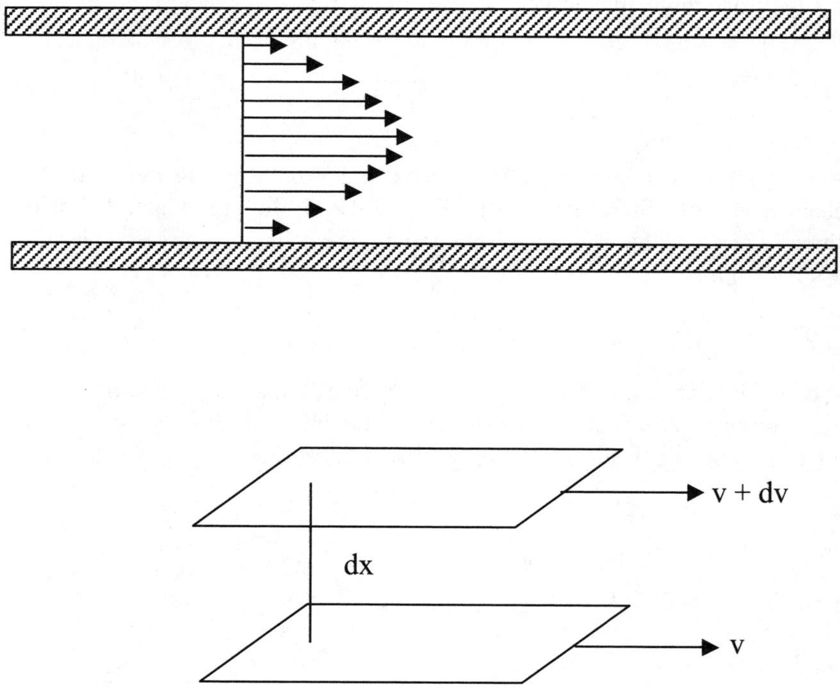

FIGURE 2.6 (a)Velocity profile of a gas flowing between two stationary parallel plates. The length of each arrow is proportional to the magnitude of the velocity at that point; (b) two layers of gas separated by a distance *dx* moving at velocities that differ by *dv*.

immediately adjacent to the walls is stationary and the gas farther away moves with increasingly higher velocity. If we now consider two gas layers separated by a distance dx, their velocities will differ by dv [Figure 2.6(b)]. If the area of each layer is A, then the frictional force F between the layers is given by *Newton's law of viscosity*:

$$F = \mu A \frac{dv}{dx} \tag{2.31}$$

On a molecular level, molecules that are in adjacent layers move randomly between the layers, transporting momentum between the layers. The coefficient of viscosity μ is given by

$$\mu = \frac{1}{2} n' m \bar{c} \lambda \tag{2.32}$$

where as before, n' is the number of molecules per unit volume, m is the mass of one molecule, $\bar{c}$ is the average molecular velocity, and λ is the mean free path. From Equation 2.26, Equation 2.28, and Equation 2.32, we see that, although gas viscosity depends on $T^{1/2}$, it is independent of any change in pressure or density at a constant temperature. The explanation is that whereas the frequency of molecules moving back and forth between adjacent layers of the gas increases proportionally with pressure, the mean free path, or effective distance between the layers, decreases proportionally with pressure, and the two effects cancel each other out.

For air at 25°C and 760 mmHg, the molecular number concentration n' is 2.46 $\times$ 10^{25} molecules/m^3, the average molecular velocity is 466 m/sec, and the mean free path is 7.06 $\times$ 10^{-8} m. Therefore, the coefficient of viscosity calculated from Equation 2.32 is 19.45 $\times$ 10^{-6} N sec/m^2.

3 Basic Concepts of Fluid Flow

3.1 INTRODUCTION

Chapter 2, with its description of gas layers moving over each other, sets the stage for developing a macroscopic picture of fluid motion. Instead of accounting for the motion of individual molecules, we simplify the problem by considering the average effects of molecules in a given volume, i.e., by considering a volume element or parcel of air whose dimensions are much larger than the intermolecular spacing. The fluid is then regarded as a continuum, i.e., as a hypothetically continuous substance. The determination of the properties of the fluid as a function of position and time is the objective of many fluid mechanics problems. Properties of the fluid include quantities such as velocity, pressure, density, and temperature.

It is sometimes useful to construct lines in the flow field to indicate the speed and direction of the flow. This is called a *flow pattern*, and the lines are called *streamlines*. Geometrically, streamlines are curves drawn such that the velocity vector at every point on the streamline is tangential to the streamline. Figure 3.1 shows an example of a flow field of relevance to air sampling — when air is being drawn from the surroundings into a tube.

Several features of the flow in Figure 3.1 are worth mentioning. Far upstream of the sampling tube, the velocity is constant, and the velocity vectors are parallel to each other. Near the sampling tube, the streamlines converge and then enter the tube. Whenever the flow moves around an object, part of the flow goes to one side and part to the other side. The streamline that forms the boundary between these two flows is called the *dividing* or *limiting streamline*. In Figure 3.1, the dashed curve shows the dividing streamline. At the point where this streamline meets the body of the sampler, the velocity is zero. This is called the *stagnation point*. The tube samples all the air flowing within the limiting streamlines (or, more precisely for a three-dimensional case, the *limiting stream surface*).

For real fluids, the velocity of fluid must fall to zero at a solid boundary because frictional forces arising due to the viscosity of the fluid retard the fluid motion (Figure 3.2). Fluid elements farther away from the solid wall move with increasingly higher velocities, until at a certain distance the fluid does not feel the presence of the solid obstacle and moves with its *freestream* velocity. This region close to the surface of the solid wall where the fluid velocity increases from 0 to 99% of its freestream value is called the *boundary layer*. Viscous forces are significant in this region, and therefore the fluid exerts a drag on the solid object.

An important kinematic property of the flow is the volumetric rate of flow Q passing through an imaginary surface S in the flow field (Figure 3.3). If the velocity

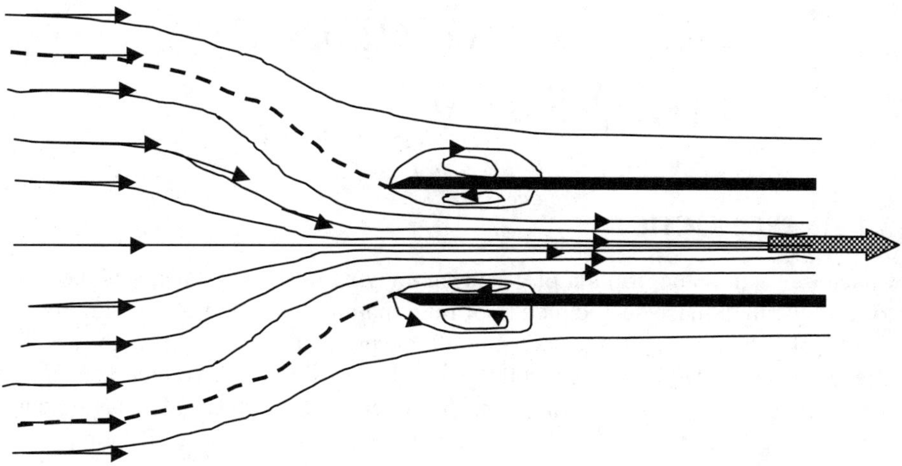

FIGURE 3.1 Flow field when air is being drawn into a thin-walled tube. The curves represent the streamlines of flow and the arrows represent the local velocity vectors. The dashed curves are the dividing streamlines.

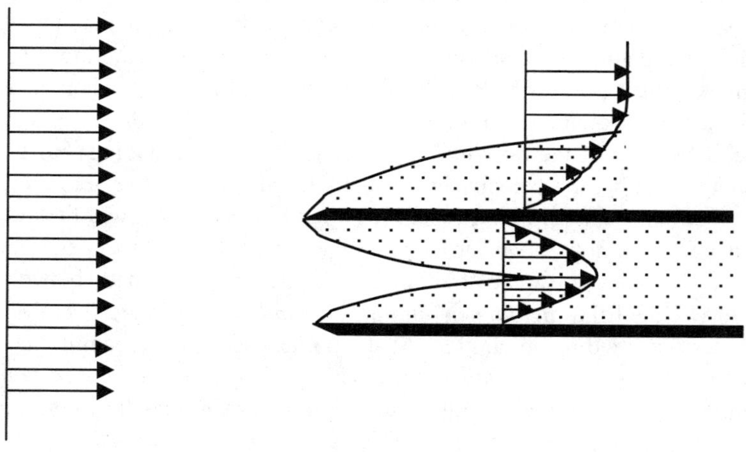

FIGURE 3.2 Development of boundary layers inside and outside a thin-walled sampling tube. The lengths of the arrows are proportional to the magnitude of the velocity. Far upstream of the tube, the flow is uniform. Outside the tube, the velocity increases from zero to the freestream velocity. Inside the tube, the velocity increases from zero at the wall to the sampling velocity, leading to a parabolic velocity profile.

vector $\vec{V}$ varies with position in the flow field, then we must integrate over each elemental surface dA. In the general case, $\vec{V}$ may pass through dA at some angle θ from the perpendicular. If V_n is the component of $\vec{V}$ perpendicular to dA, then the volume of fluid passing through the surface dA in time dt is

$$d\forall = V_n \, dA \, dt \tag{3.1}$$

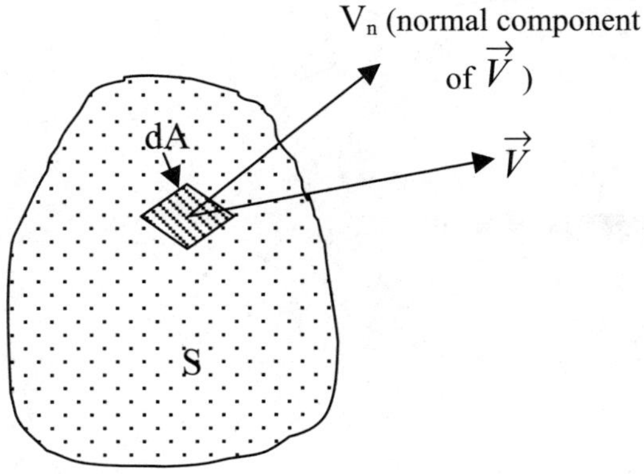

FIGURE 3.3 Fluid flow with local velocity $\vec{V}$ through a surface S in the flow field.

The integral of $\frac{d\forall}{dt}$ is the total volumetric flow rate Q through the surface S.

$$Q = \int_S V_n \, dA \tag{3.2}$$

The volume flow is often used to define an average velocity, V_{avg}, passing through the surface.

$$V_{avg} = \frac{Q}{A} = \frac{\int_S V_n \, dA}{\int_S dA} \tag{3.3}$$

3.2 EQUATION OF CONTINUITY

An important concept is the continuity principle, which is essentially the law of conservation of mass as it applies to fluids. If we consider a volume $\forall$ with surface area S through which the fluid is flowing outward with velocity $\vec{V}$, then the equation of continuity is given by

$$\int_S \rho V_n \, dA = -\frac{d}{dt} \int_\forall \rho \, d\forall \tag{3.4}$$

where V_n is the component of $\vec{V}$ perpendicular to dA. The equation states that the net rate of outflow of mass from a volume of space (called the control volume in texts on fluid mechanics) is equal to the rate of decrease of mass within the volume. Let us consider the simple case when a fluid is moving through a duct with changing cross-sectional areas, as shown in Figure 3.4.

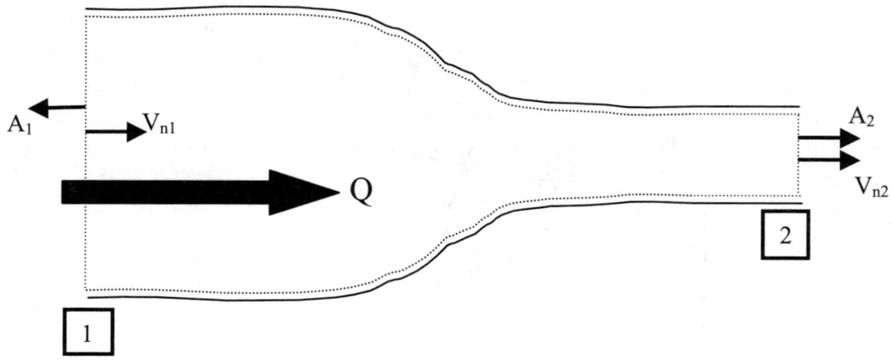

FIGURE 3.4 Fluid flow through a duct with changing cross-sectional areas.

Because there is no net decrease of mass within the control volume (the boundaries of which are shown by dashed lines), we can use Equation 3.4 to obtain a relationship between the velocities at the two sections of the conduit:

$$-\rho_1 A_1 V_{n1} + \rho_2 A_2 V_{n2} = 0$$

or

$$\rho_1 A_1 V_{n1} = \rho_2 A_2 V_{n2} \tag{3.5}$$

where the subscripts 1 and 2 refer to the two sections of the conduit with cross-sectional areas A_1 and A_2, where the velocities are V_{n1} and V_{n2}, and fluid densities are ρ_1 and ρ_2, respectively.

In the case of a constant density flow, the above equation reduces to

$$A_1 V_{n1} = A_2 V_{n2} \tag{3.6}$$

which can also be written as $Q_1 = Q_2$. Equation 3.6 is commonly used in industrial hygiene calculations, where the flow is considered incompressible.

3.3 BERNOULLI'S EQUATION

This equation describes the relationship between pressure, velocity, and elevation for frictionless flow, and is attributed to Daniel Bernoulli, who lived in the 18th century. If we consider any two points 1 and 2 in a flow field, then for steady, frictionless, incompressible flow we have

$$p_1 v_1 - p_2 v_2 = \frac{1}{2}\left(m_2 V_2^2 - m_1 V_1^2\right) + g\left(m_2 z_2 - m_1 z_1\right) \tag{3.7}$$

where p_1, v_1, V_1, and z_1 are the pressure, volume, velocity, and elevation of the fluid at point 1, respectively, and p_2, v_2, V_2, and z_2 are the corresponding quantities at point 2. The term on the left-hand side of Equation 3.7 is the energy added (or work done) to the fluid by pressure forces, and the two terms on the right-hand side are the change in kinetic energy and the change in potential energy of the fluid, respectively. Because mass is conserved, $m_1 = m_2$, and therefore, dividing both sides of Equation 3.7 by mass, we obtain

$$\frac{p_1}{\rho} + \frac{1}{2} V_1^2 + g z_1 = \frac{p_2}{\rho} + \frac{1}{2} V_2^2 + g z_2 = \text{constant} \tag{3.8}$$

Equation 3.7 is true only for a frictionless fluid, i.e., when there is no heat or work transfer in the fluid. All the terms in Equation 3.8 are energies per unit mass. Thus, it is a statement of the conservation of energy of a fluid.

In many instances in which the change in elevation is negligible, Equation 3.8 can be rewritten as

$$p_1 + \frac{1}{2} \rho V_1^2 = p_2 + \frac{1}{2} \rho V_2^2 \tag{3.9}$$

Now the two terms on either side of the equation are in dimensions of pressure. The first term is called static pressure, and the second term is called velocity pressure. The sum of these two pressures is called the total pressure.

Equation 3.9 holds true, not just for the entire flow field, but for each individual streamline. For the dividing streamline shown in Figure 3.1, the velocity becomes zero at the surface of the body. Here, the static pressure reaches its maximum value. Such a location is called a stagnation point.

3.4 CONSERVATION OF MOMENTUM

Consider an elementary packet of air that is infinitesimally small and the forces acting on it. Three kinds of forces act on the fluid packet:

1. Gravity and buoyant forces act on the entire fluid element and are called body forces. Whereas gravity acts downwards, the buoyant force acts upwards.
2. Pressure forces act perpendicularly to the surfaces of the fluid element from all sides and arise from static pressure variations in the fluid.
3. For a viscous fluid, the surface stress forces are more complex. Normal stress forces act perpendicularly to the surfaces of the fluid element, similar to pressure. Shear stresses arising from the viscosity of the fluid have a direction parallel to the surface on which they act.

The sum of all these forces on each fluid element is equal to the product of its mass and acceleration. Thus, there will be three equations of motion — one each for the force components along the three Cartesian axes. Along with the equation of continuity, there are four equations and four unknowns — pressure and the velocity components along each of the Cartesian axes. These are the so-called *Navier–Stokes equations* of fluid motion. Solving these differential equations for different conditions and flow geometries yields the position and velocity of fluid elements as a function of time. For instance, the streamlines mentioned at the beginning of this chapter arise as solutions to the Navier–Stokes equations. Whereas in the past, the solution of these equations could only rarely be accomplished, advances in computational power and the development of sophisticated numerical techniques have made this task somewhat easier.

3.5 SIMILITUDE AND REYNOLDS NUMBER

Fluid mechanics has historically been very dependent on empirical work because of the difficulties in obtaining exact analytical solutions to the Navier–Stokes equations. The approach has typically been to construct geometrically similar scale models of the actual flow conditions to study the flow. The question naturally arises as to the conditions under which flows of different fluids around geometrically similar bodies may be considered to behave similarly, i.e., the flows in the two situations will have geometrically similar streamlines. One of the key insights of fluid dynamics is that in similar flow fields at all geometrically similar points, the forces acting on an element of fluid must bear a fixed ratio at every point in time.

For an incompressible fluid, if we neglect gravity, the only forces present are frictional and inertial forces. Inertial forces arise from the product of the mass and the acceleration of fluid elements, and viscous forces due to shearing arise from the viscosity of the medium. For similarity, these two forces must have a constant ratio at all times, and therefore

$$\frac{\text{Inertial Force}}{\text{Viscous Force}} = \frac{\rho_{air}\dfrac{V^2}{D}}{\mu\dfrac{V}{D^2}} = \frac{\rho_{air}\, V\, D}{\mu} = Re \tag{3.10}$$

Here, V(m/sec) is the relative velocity between the fluid and the body, D(m) is the characteristic scale dimension of the body, ρ_{air} is the density of the fluid (air, in this instance), μ is the viscosity of the fluid, and the ratio Re is referred to as the *Reynolds number.*

For airflow in a duct, D becomes the duct diameter and V, the average air velocity in the duct. If we consider the motion of a single aerosol particle in an airstream, then D refers to the diameter of the particle and V, the relative velocity between the particle and the air.

Equation 3.10 shows that Re is the ratio of inertial forces that act on the main body of the flow and viscous forces at the flow boundaries with the body. For situations with small *Re*, viscous effects influence the flow field more than inertial forces. This type of flow is referred to as *laminar flow* and occurs when *Re* is less than 2000. Conversely, for situations with large *Re*, inertial effects influence the flow field more than viscous forces. This type of flow is referred to as turbulent flow and occurs when *Re* is greater than 2000.

4 Uncertainties in Physical Measurements

4.1 WHAT IS A MEASUREMENT?

Making measurements of physical quantities, such as temperature, flow rate, and pollutant concentration, is so commonplace an activity in occupational exposure assessment that we seldom think about the complexity of the process. A simple definition of *measurement* is "that it is the process of assigning specific numerical value to a particular characteristic of the physical world." A measurement system is a tool used for this quantification of the physical variable. The two main measurement tasks are (1) to construct a suitable "ruler" or reference scale and then (2) to compare the unknown quantity being measured with the divisions on the scale. Thus, we can describe a rectangular table by measuring its width and length using a tape measure and stating that the table is 2 m wide and 4 m long, and has an area of 8 m^2.

However, there is more to a measurement than this. A more appropriate statement might be the following: the table is modeled as a rectangle having two parameters, width and length; the best parameter estimates are 2 m for the width and 4 m for the length. This is a better description because it separates the physical object (the table) from the parameters of the mathematical model of the table. First, the actual table is not a perfectly plane object with perfectly parallel sides and sharp corners. Our plane rectangular model is, however, a useful approximation of the physical object. Second, we have no way of knowing the true value of these parameters. So, we make repeated measurements of the width and length parameters and then estimate the most likely values of these parameters, perhaps by averaging them. The repeated measurements will be different each time because of fluctuations in environmental conditions, such as temperature and relative humidity, and low-level vibrations of the table. The tape measure has a limited resolution and so a certain amount of subjectivity creeps into each reading of the tape measure.

We thus come to a more sophisticated definition of a measurement as an estimate of a parameter in a quantitative model that represents some aspect of reality. It is important to distinguish between the actual or true value of a physical quantity at some point in time (that we intuitively feel must exist) and our best estimate (or measurement) of it based on repeated trials using a quantitative model. Thus, a measurement is a random variable with a mean value, a variance, and confidence intervals.

4.2 COMPONENTS OF A MEASUREMENT SYSTEM

Figure 4.1 shows the three basic elements of any system designed to obtain physical measurements:

1. The sensor and transducer unit
2. The signal conditioning unit
3. The output unit

The *sensor* unit uses some natural phenomenon to sense the parameter being estimated. The *transducer* unit converts this sensed information into another form that is more amenable to measure, e.g., a voltage or a displacement. The *signal conditioning* unit modifies the transducer signal to a magnitude that is easily measured and removes extraneous noise. The *output* stage provides a numerical value of the measurement.

An ordinary rotameter (a device used for measuring airflow rates) consists of a solid float that moves in a tapered vertical tube (see Figure 4.2). Air enters the tube at the bottom and exits at the top, pushing the float upward. The float comes to equilibrium at a position where its weight is balanced by the force due to the velocity pressure of the gas flowing through the annular space. The force balance can be expressed as an equation (described in Chapter 5), which is the mathematical model that underpins measurements made by a rotameter.

The float is thus the sensor. It moves up the vertical tube, and so the flow rate information (e.g., in liters per minute) is converted into a linear displacement of the float. The tapered column acts as the transducer. The changing diameter of the column determines the linear extent to which the float travels in the column and thus conditions the signal. The output stage is the marked scale on the column that reads out the distance moved by the float (e.g., in inches or millimeters).

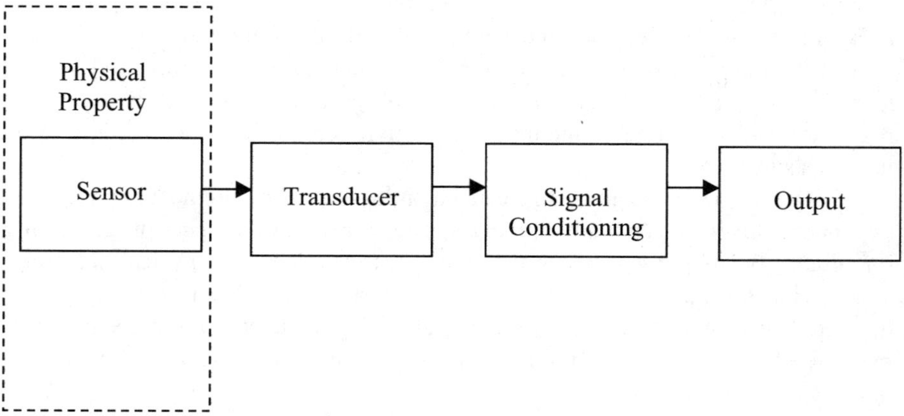

FIGURE 4.1 Components of a measurement system.

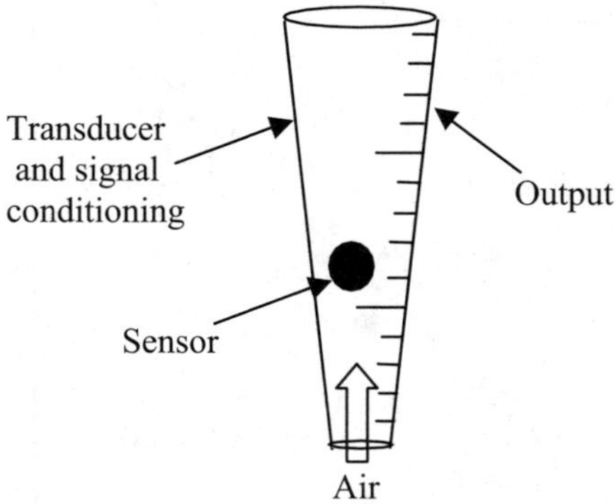

FIGURE 4.2 Components of a rotameter equivalent to sensor, transducer, and output stages.

4.3 CALIBRATION

The relationship between the input information (as acquired by the sensor) and the output information is established by a process called *calibration.* During calibration, a known value of input is applied to a measurement system and the output is observed. The known value is referred to as the *standard.*

In the case of the rotameter, a calibration procedure determines the relationship between the flow rate (the input information) and the distance moved by the float (the output information). By applying several known values of flow rate to the rotameter and observing the corresponding distances moved by the float, a direct *calibration curve* can be developed for the rotameter. The input (the known value of flow rate) is plotted along the abscissa (the x-axis), and the output (measured distance that the float travels) is plotted along the ordinate (the y-axis). Such a curve then serves to interpret the indicated output in terms of the real variable of interest (in this case, the flow rate). Once the calibration curve equation has been established, it can be used in later measurements to determine the unknown input value based on the measured output value (e.g., to determine the flow rate based on the measured value of the float position of the rotameter). An example of a calibration curve is shown in Figure 4.3, in which the measured data points describe the input–output relationship for the measurement system.

The calibration curve is obtained by applying known inputs from the minimum to the maximum values for which the measurement system can be used. These minimum and maximum values define the *input span* of the measurement system, $x_{max}–x_{min}$. The corresponding output range is from y_{min} to y_{max}, which defines the full-scale output range or *output span*, $y_{max}–y_{min}$. Measurements beyond this range are not advisable because the calibration behavior is unknown in these regions.

4.4 RANDOM AND SYSTEMATIC ERRORS

Uncertainties in the measurement system that can be revealed by repeating the measurements are called *random errors*; those that cannot be revealed by repetition

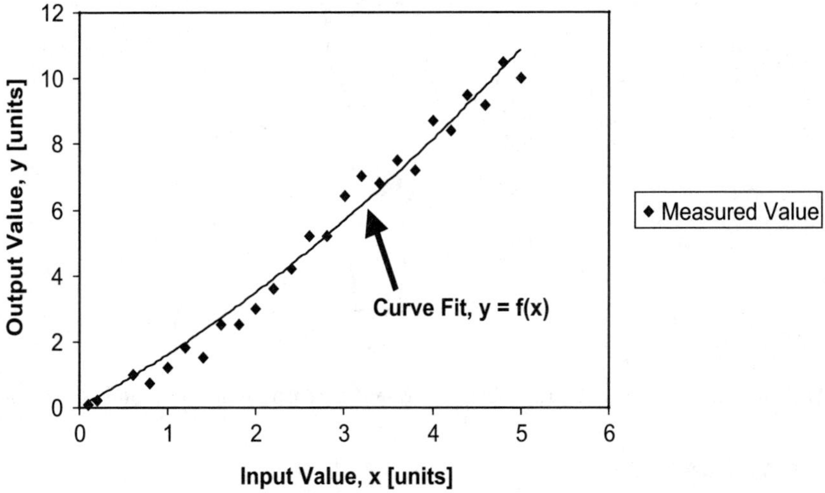

FIGURE 4.3 A calibration curve for a measurement system.

are called *systematic errors*. For instance, if a rotameter is used repeatedly to measure the same flow rate, then the measured data will be scattered around some average value. The spread in the measured values can be analyzed statistically to provide an estimate of random error. However, it is possible that the scale on the rotameter has become distorted, in which case no amount of repetition will reveal this source of error. Or the flow rate measurements are being made at a pressure other than standard pressure. This type of error is systematic. (For example, if the scale has stretched, the flow rate will be underestimated; if the scale has shrunk, it will be overestimated.) The only way to detect systematic errors is during calibration, when the measured value is compared with some standard known value.

The random variability during repeated trials of a measurement is called the *precision* of the measurement system. The difference between the average of these trials and the true value is known as the *measurement bias*. Let us consider a case where a measurement system is used to measure a variable whose value is kept constant and known exactly, as during a calibration. Ten independent measurements are made and the results are shown in Figure 4.4. The observed scatter in the data is related to the system precision. The difference between the average of the ten measurements and the true value is the bias.

However, during any measurement other than a calibration, the bias cannot be known because the true value is unknown. In Figure 4.4, if the true value were not known, we could still determine random variability and thus the precision. The following sections will describe how one can estimate random variability, along with a well-defined method for reducing it. However, systematic errors are hard to detect or quantify. An experienced industrial hygienist has to learn to anticipate possible sources of systematic bias. This process might involve, for instance, strictly following standard operating procedures for various types of measurements, regular calibration of all equipment, and reducing the effects of interference by some pollutants while sampling for other pollutants.

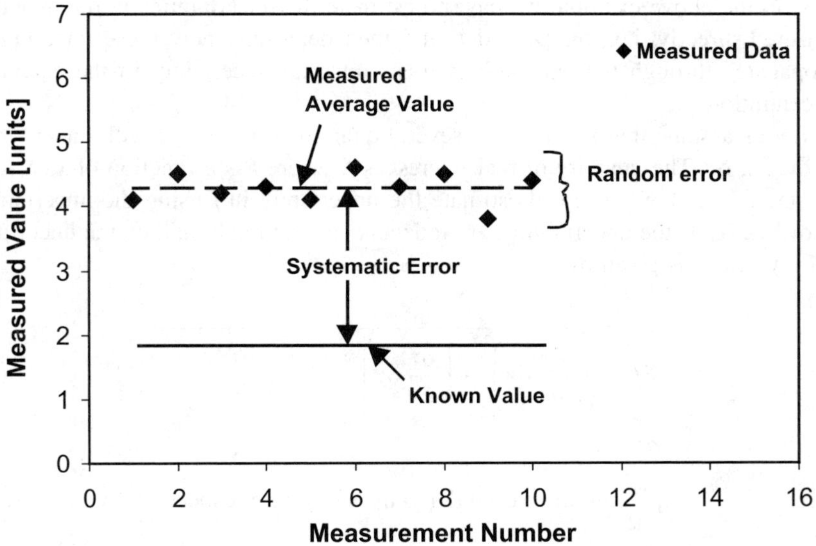

FIGURE 4.4 Precision and bias in a set of measurements during a calibration.

If we made repeated measurement of the flow rate of air through an air sampling instrument and obtained the following flow rates (say, in liters per minute) -28.3, 28.2, 28.4, and 28.3- then we could make a reasonably safe assumption that the best estimate of the flow rate is the average value, 28.3 l/min. Another safe assumption is that the correct flow rate is between the lowest value, 28.2, and the highest value, 28.4.

If we know the precision of the measurement, then the best way to report the result of a measurement is to give the best estimate of the quantity and the range within which we are confident that the quantity lies. Thus, if we are measuring some variable x, then the measured value of $x = x_{\text{best estimate}} \pm \delta x$.

This implies that our best estimate of the quantity of interest is $x_{\text{best estimate}}$ and that we are reasonably confident that the quantity lies between $x_{\text{best estimate}} - \delta x$ and $x_{\text{best estimate}} + \delta x$. The number δx is the uncertainty, or the error or margin of error. In later sections in this chapter, we will discuss the meaning of this uncertainty in greater detail.

4.5 PROPAGATION OF UNCERTAINTIES

Most quantities of interest in industrial hygiene cannot be determined in a single measurement, but are found in several steps. We measure several quantities that can be measured directly, and then the quantity of interest is calculated using these measurements. For example, when we want to find the concentration in a workplace, we measure the mass of the contaminant that is collected on some medium m and the volume of air that we have sampled V, and calculate the concentration $C = m/V$. The volume of air itself may also be determined from two other measurements: the flow rate of air Q and the sampling time t, as $V = Q \times t$. When a measurement requires several steps, then the estimation of uncertainty also involves several steps.

Thus, in the above example we have to estimate the uncertainties in the quantities measured directly, i.e., *m*, *Q*, and *t*, and then determine how these uncertainties "propagate" through the calculations to produce an uncertainty in the calculated concentration.

Let us assume that we measure several quantities, *x*, *y*, …, *z* with uncertainties δx, δy, …, δz. The quantity of real interest is *f*, where *f* is a function of *x*, *y*, …, *z*, i.e., $f(x, y, \ldots, z)$. We need to estimate the uncertainty in *f* using the uncertainties δx, δy, …, δz. If the uncertainties are independent and random, then the uncertainty in $f(x, y, \ldots, z)$ is given by

$$\delta f = \sqrt{\left(\frac{\delta f}{\delta x}\delta x\right)^2 + \left(\frac{\delta f}{\delta y}\delta y\right)^2 + \ldots + \left(\frac{\delta f}{\delta z}\delta z\right)^2} \tag{4.1}$$

where $\frac{\delta f}{\delta x}, \frac{\delta f}{\delta y}, \ldots, \frac{\delta f}{\delta z}$ are the partial derivatives of *f* with respect to *x*, *y*, …, *z*, which means that $\frac{\delta f}{\delta x}$ is the derivative of *f* with respect to *x*, assuming that *y*, …, *z* are constants, and so on for the other partial derivatives.

Let us apply this to a situation where we draw air through a filter for a certain amount of time at a given flow rate, weigh the mass of dust collected on the filter, and calculate the dust concentration in the air. As before, the concentration is obtained as $C = \frac{m}{Q \times t}$. The three partial derivatives are $\frac{\delta C}{\delta m} = \frac{1}{Q \times t}, \frac{\delta C}{\delta Q} = -\frac{m}{t}\frac{1}{Q^2}$, and $\frac{\delta C}{\delta t} = -\frac{m}{Q}\frac{1}{t^2}$, respectively. The uncertainty in the concentration is calculated as $\delta C = \sqrt{\left(\frac{\delta C}{\delta m}\delta m\right)^2 + \left(\frac{\delta C}{\delta Q}\delta Q\right)^2 + \left(\frac{\delta C}{\delta t}\delta t\right)^2}$. The fractional uncertainty in C is therefore $\frac{\delta C}{C}$, which, after some algebraic manipulation, is expressed as

$$\frac{\delta C}{C} = \sqrt{\left(\frac{\delta m}{m}\right)^2 + \left(\frac{\delta Q}{Q}\right)^2 + \left(\frac{\delta t}{t}\right)^2} \tag{4.2}$$

If we measured the mass to be 24 ± 2.3 mg, the flow rate to be 2 ± 0.1 l/min, and the sampling time to be 480 ± 5 min, then the calculated best estimate of the concentration is $C = \frac{24}{2.0 \times 10^{-3} \times 480} = 25 \mathrm{mg/m^3}$. The fractional uncertainties in the measurement of mass, flow rate, and time are 9.5, 5, and 1.04%, respectively. The fractional uncertainty in estimate of C is $\frac{\delta C}{C} = \sqrt{\left(\frac{2.3}{24}\right)^2 + \left(\frac{0.1}{2.0}\right)^2 + \left(\frac{5}{480}\right)^2} =$ 10.8%. Hence, $\delta C = 0.0108 \times 25 = 2.7$ mg/m³. Thus, we would report the result of our measurements as 25 ± 2.7 mg/m³.

4.6 QUANTIFYING UNCERTAINTY

Let us assume that we want to measure some physical variable x (e.g., a flow rate or a steady pollutant concentration in a room), and we have identified all sources of systematic error and reduced them to an insignificant level. We make N repeated measurements of the variable x and obtain the values $x_1, x_2, \ldots, x_N$. What is the best estimate of the variable x, given the measurements? The answer is that, for such measurements, the best estimate of x is usually the *arithmetic average* of the N observations.

$$\bar{x} = \frac{x_1 + x_2 + \ldots + x_N}{N} = \frac{\sum x_i}{N} \tag{4.3}$$

Suppose we make ten measurements of some gas concentration in a chamber that is at steady state (i.e., the concentration is not changing with time). We might obtain the values (in ppm) 21, 20, 23, 22, 22, 18, 20, 19, 20, and 21. The average concentration is obtained as $\bar{x} = \frac{21 + 20 + 23 + \ldots + 21}{10} = 20.6$. The average variability in the population is given by the *standard deviation*, σ_x, where

$$\sigma_x = \sqrt{\frac{1}{N}\sum_{i=1}^{N}\left(x_i - \bar{x}\right)^2} \tag{4.4}$$

Thus, the standard deviation of the population is the root-mean-square deviation of the individual values from the arithmetic mean. However, we rarely can sample all the members in a population. Typically, a subset of the population is sampled and, if we are convinced that the sample is representative of the entire population, then we can say that the standard deviation of the sample is an estimate of the population standard deviation. The sample standard deviation is given by

$$s_x = \sqrt{\frac{1}{N-1}\sum_{i=1}^{N}\left(x_i - \bar{x}\right)^2} \tag{4.5}$$

The standard deviation calculated using Equation 4.5 is a bit larger than the one calculated using Equation 4.4 and corrects for a tendency of Equation 4.4 to underestimate the uncertainty.

For the same numbers for which we calculated the mean, the sample standard deviation is

$$s = \sqrt{\frac{(21-20.6)^2+(20-20.6)^2+(23-20.6)^2+...+(21-20.6)^2}{10-1}} = 1.505$$

4.7 HISTOGRAMS

The mean and the standard deviation are commonly-used descriptors of a population, with the former describing the central tendency and the latter describing the dispersion in the population. However, they do not provide information on how the uncertainty is distributed around the mean. A better way to describe a population would provide information on the distribution of the values in a population.

Another way to calculate the mean of the numbers in the example above is

$$\bar{x} = \frac{18+19+(3\times 20)+(2\times 21)+(2\times 22)+23}{10} = 20.6$$

or, in general,

$$\bar{x} = \frac{\sum_k x_k\, n_k}{N} \tag{4.6}$$

Unlike Equation 4.3, where we sum over all the measurements, in Equation 4.6, we sum over all different values obtained, multiplying each value by the number of times it occurred. Further, because $\frac{n_k}{N}$ is the fraction of times that each value occurred, we can express the above as

$$\bar{x} = \sum_k x_k\, F_k \tag{4.7}$$

where $F_k = \frac{n_k}{N}$. The fractions F_k specify the *distribution* of the values in our sample. In the preceding example, we can say that the value 20 was observed in 3 out of 10 of our measurements, the value 21 was observed in 2 out of 10 of our measurements, and so on. Such a distribution can be graphically displayed as a *bar histogram,* as shown in Figure 4.5.

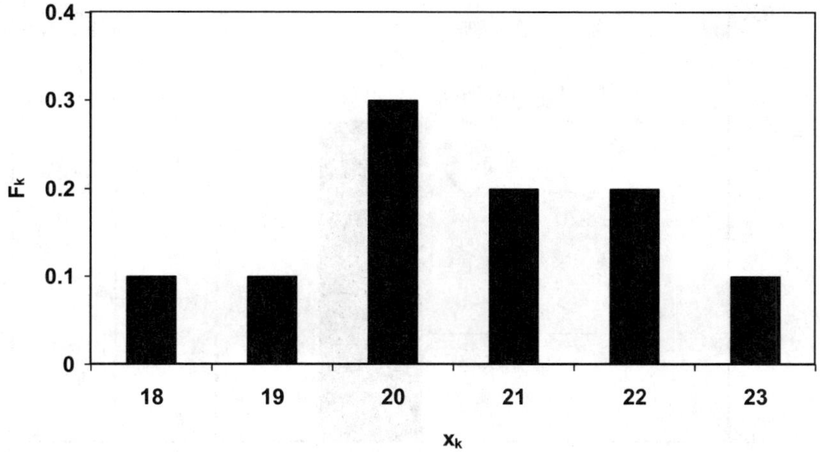

FIGURE 4.5 Histogram of ten measurements of a steady state concentration. The y-axis shows the fraction of times F_k that each value x_k was obtained.

TABLE 4.1
The Ten Measurements Grouped in Four Intervals

Interval	**18–20**	**20–21**	**21–22**	**22–23**
Measurements in interval	2	3	2	3

This kind of bar histogram is appropriate when the values x_k are uniformly spaced with integer values. Most physical measurements have a continuous range of values, and instead of the values used in the previous example, we are more likely to obtain ten values such as 21.4, 20.2, 22.9, 22.4, 22.1, 18.4, 20.1, 19.3, 20.2, and 21.3. A bar histogram of these values would consist of ten separate bars of equal height and would not be very informative. In this situation, it is more useful to divide these values into a number of intervals or bins. For example, we can count the number of measurements between 18 and 19, between 19 and 20, and so on. The measurements grouped by intervals or bins are shown in Table 4.1.

The grouped data can be plotted as a *bin histogram* shown in Figure 4.6. Here, the fraction of measurements in each interval is equal to the area of the rectangle above the interval. The height f_k is chosen such that the area $f_k\ \Delta_k$ is equal to the fraction of measurements in the kth interval. Thus, the total area under all the intervals is equal to unity, *i.e.*,

$$\sum_k f_k\ \Delta_k = 1 \tag{4.8}$$

When the total number of measurements is small, then the bin size must be chosen with care: too wide a bin width, and we might end up with just one bin in which all measurements fall; too narrow a bin width, and the histogram will contain

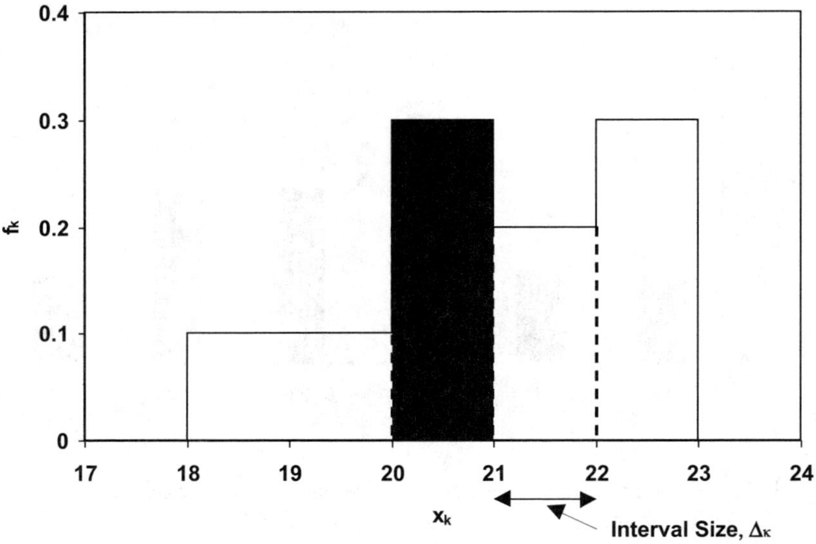

FIGURE 4.6 Bin histogram showing the fraction of ten measurements that lie in the intervals 18 to 19, 19 to 20, and so on. The area of the rectangle above each interval is the fraction of measurements in that interval. Thus, the area of the shaded rectangle is 0.3, so 30% of all measurements lie between 20 and 21.

a number of intervals with just one measurement (and therefore the same height). As the number of observations increases, it is possible to choose increasingly narrower interval sizes.

4.8 CONTINUOUS DISTRIBUTIONS

As the number of observations approaches infinity and the bin width approaches zero, the bin histogram becomes a smooth, continuous curve. This is defined by a function $f(x)$ that takes the place of the factor f_k in the bin histogram. For an infinitely large number of observations, the fraction of observations in any small interval between x and $x + dx$ is $f(x)dx$, and this equals the shaded area in Figure 4.7.

Similarly, for an infinitely large number of measurements, the fraction of observations between $x = a$ and $x = b$ is the shaded area, and is equal to the definite integral of $f(x)$, i.e.,

$$\int_a^b f(x)dx = \text{fraction of observations between } a \text{ and } b \tag{4.9}$$

In other words, $f(x)dx$ is the *probability* that a single measurement of x will lie between x and $x + dx$. $f(x)$ is called the *probability density function*. Likewise, the

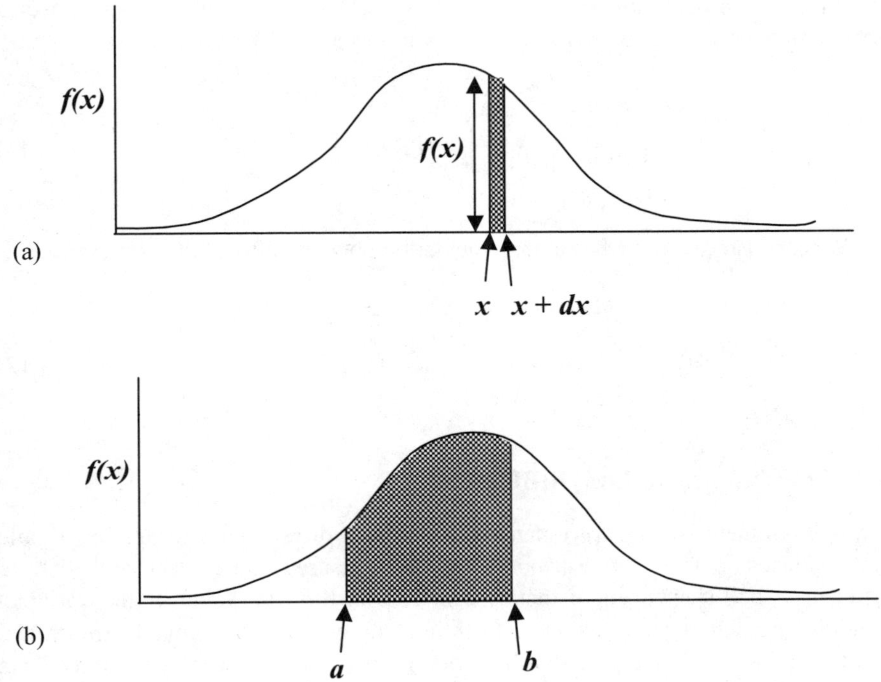

FIGURE 4.7 A continuous distribution $f(x)$. (a) The fraction of observations that are between x and $x + dx$ is the shaded area $f(x)dx$; (b) the fraction of observations between $x = a$ and $x = b$ is the shaded area.

definite integral $\int_a^b f(x)dx$ yields the probability that a single measurement lies between a and b. Similar to Equation 4.8, $f(x)$ is defined such that

$$\int_{-\infty}^{\infty} f(x)dx = 1 \tag{4.10}$$

i.e., the probability that a measurement is between $-\infty$ and $+\infty$ is one. In most situations in real life, the measurements do not range between $-\infty$ and $+\infty$, but, rather, between finite values. However, because we would not *a priori* know what these limits are, it is convenient for theoretical rigor to use the limits of $\pm\infty$.

If the measurement is very precise, then all the observations will cluster around the true value. For the limiting case when there are infinitely many measurements, the probability density function has a narrow spread. If the measurement is very imprecise, then the observations will be widely spread, and for the limiting case the probability density function will be broad.

Using the probability density function, we can calculate the mean $\bar{x}$ expected after infinite observations in a manner akin to Equation 4.7 as

$$\bar{x} = \int_{-\infty}^{\infty} x\, f(x)\, dx \tag{4.11}$$

We can also calculate the standard deviation obtained after many observations as

$$\sigma_x = \sqrt{\int_{-\infty}^{\infty} \left(x - \bar{x}\right)^2 f(x)\, dx} \tag{4.12}$$

4.9 THE NORMAL DISTRIBUTION

If a measurement is subject to many small sources of random error and negligible systematic error, then the distribution of the measured values is described by a symmetric, bell-shaped curve that is centered on the true value of the variable. Random errors are equally likely to result in readings above or below the true value. If we have only random errors, then after many measurements the number of readings above and below the true value will be the same, and our distribution of results will be centered around the true value. The sampling and analytical variability in industrial hygiene measurements follow this symmetric bell-shaped curve.

The true value is, of course, a philosophical construct because it cannot be measured exactly by any means, and it is unclear whether such a thing even exists. However, we shall assume that every physical quantity has a true value. For the sake of convenience, we shall define the true value of a physical variable as the value we approach as more and more measurements are made with increasing care.

If the true value of a measured quantity x is denoted by μ, and the measurements of x are subject to many small random errors but negligible systematic errors, then the distribution of the measurements will be a symmetric, bell-shaped curve centered on the true value μ. The mathematical function that describes this curve is called the *normal distribution* or the *Gaussian distribution.* Two parameters describe the normal distribution — its center value or mean (μ) and its standard deviation (σ).

$$G_{\mu,\sigma}(x) = \frac{1}{\sigma\sqrt{2\pi}} \exp\left(-\frac{(x-\mu)^2}{2\sigma^2}\right) \tag{4.13}$$

We know that the definite integral given by Equation 4.9 represents the probability that a given measurement lies between a and b. Using the normal function $G_{\mu,\sigma}(x)$, we can calculate the probability that a measurement lies within Z standard deviations (i.e., $Z\sigma$) of the true center value μ as

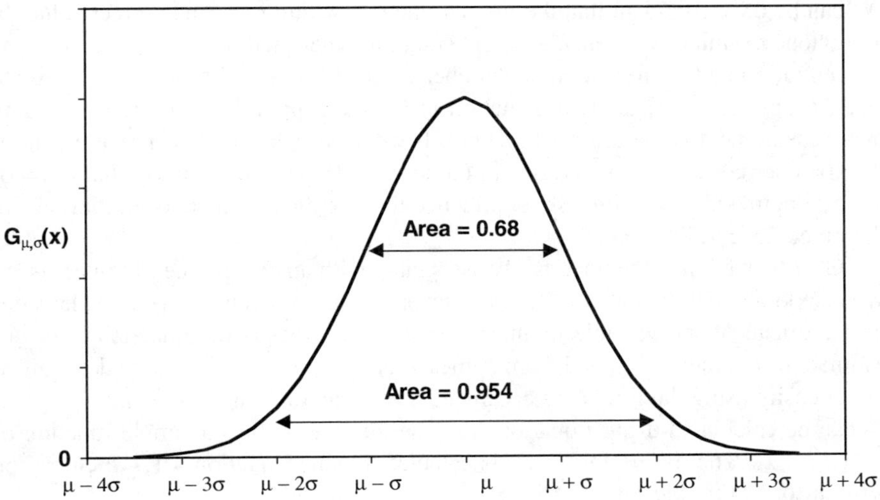

Z	0.5	1.0	1.5	1.645	1.96	2.0	2.5	3.0	3.5	4.0
Prob.(%)	38	68	87	90	95	95.4	98.8	99.7	99.95	99.99

FIGURE 4.8 The normal or Gaussian distribution, with a mean *m* and standard deviation *s*. The area under the curve between $m \pm Zs$ is shown in the table and is the probability of a measurement within *Z* standard deviations of the mean.

$$\text{Prob }(\textit{measurement is within} \pm Z\sigma \textit{ from } \mu) = \int_{\mu-Z\sigma}^{\mu+Z\sigma} G_{\mu,\sigma}(x)dx$$

$$= \frac{1}{\sigma\sqrt{2\pi}} \int_{\mu-Z\sigma}^{\mu+Z\sigma} \exp(-(x-\mu)^2/2\sigma^2)dx \tag{4.14}$$

This integral can be easily calculated using tables found in most books on elementary statistics and is equal to the area under the curve between the two limits of integration. The concept is shown graphically in Figure 4.8, which also shows a tabulation of some of the integrals as a function of *Z*.

This discussion provides us with an important interpretation of the standard deviation. If we make a single measurement, the probability is 68% that our result will be within one standard deviation of the correct value. It is, therefore, what we mean by uncertainty in the context of physical measurements. If we make one measurement of *x*, the uncertainty associated with this measurement can be taken to be

$$\delta x = \sigma_x \tag{4.15}$$

We can be 68% confident that the measurement is within δx of the correct value. In a previous example, we considered the situation where ten measurements of a gas concentration had been made in a chamber at steady state and found the average to be 20.6 ppm and the standard deviation to be 1.505 ppm. The uncertainty in any one measurement is therefore 1.505 ppm. If we now make another measurement of the chamber concentration and obtain the answer 23 ppm, we can say that $\delta C = \sigma_x = 1.505$ ppm and state with 68% confidence that the measured concentration lies in the range 23 ± 1.505 ppm.

Clearly, we know the uncertainty associated with any single measurement is σ_x. We also know that the mean, $\bar{x}$, of the several measurements we have made is our best estimate of the variable of interest. However, what is the uncertainty in our estimate of the mean obtained from N measurements, $\sigma_{\bar{x}}$? This can be determined rather easily using the following argument. The mean of N measurements $x_1, x_2, \ldots, x_N$ can be calculated using Equation 4.3. The mean $\bar{x}$ is thus a simple function of $x_1, x_2, \ldots, x_N$. The uncertainty in $\bar{x}$ is calculated using Equation 4.1, which can be written for N variables as:

$$\sigma_{\bar{x}} = \sqrt{\left(\frac{\delta x}{\delta x_1}\sigma_{x1}\right)^2 + \left(\frac{\delta x}{\delta x_2}\sigma_{x2}\right)^2 + \ldots + \left(\frac{\delta x}{\delta x_N}\sigma_{xN}\right)^2} \quad (4.16)$$

Because $x_1, x_2, \ldots, x_N$ are measurements of the same quantity, their uncertainties are all equal to σ_x,

$$\sigma_{x1} = \sigma_{x2} = \ldots \sigma_{xN} = \sigma_x \quad (4.17)$$

From Equation 4.3, we see that all the partial derivatives are equal.

$$\frac{\delta x}{\delta x_1} = \frac{\delta x}{\delta x_2} = \ldots = \frac{\delta x}{\delta x_N} = \frac{1}{N} \quad (4.18)$$

Thus, Equation 4.16 becomes

$$\sigma_{\bar{x}} = \sqrt{\left(\frac{1}{N}\sigma_x\right)^2 + \left(\frac{1}{N}\sigma_x\right)^2 + \ldots + \left(\frac{1}{N}\sigma_x\right)^2} = \frac{\sigma_x}{\sqrt{N}} \quad (4.19)$$

Let us pause and consider the significance of this result. The standard deviation σ_x represents the average uncertainty in individual measurements. Each new measurement we make will have the same uncertainty. However, the standard deviation of the mean $\frac{\sigma_x}{\sqrt{N}}$ will slowly decrease with increasing number of measurements. This makes intuitive sense, because the more measurements we make before calculating the mean, the more reliable our answer will be. Thus, we can improve the precision of our experiment by increasing *N*.

4.10 COEFFICIENT OF VARIATION

Typically, the errors in measurements of concentration due to sampling and analytical procedures are proportional to the concentration being measured. Therefore, it makes sense to express the errors as fractions or percentages of the measured concentration. Thus, the fractional error is constant and independent of the concentration being measured. This fractional error is called the *coefficient of variation* (*CV*) and is expressed as the ratio of the standard deviation to the mean, i.e.,

$$CV = \frac{\sigma}{\mu} \tag{4.20}$$

It is also called the *relative standard deviation.*

From the discussion on propagation of errors, we can also say that if the measurement procedure consists of two steps — the sampling step and the analytical step in the laboratory — then the total coefficient of variation CV_T is given by

$$CV_T = \left[CV_S^2 + CV_A^2\right]^{1/2} = \frac{\sigma_T}{\mu} \tag{4.21}$$

where CV_S is the coefficient of variation of the sampling step, and CV_A is the coefficient of variation of the analytical step.

4.11 MEASUREMENT METHOD ACCURACY

The International Standards Organization (ISO) has defined accuracy as the "closeness of the agreement between the result of a measurement and a true value of the measurand" (ISO, 1993). Thus, both systematic error (bias) and random error need to be accounted for. Let us assume that the true concentration is *C*, the bias of a measurement method is *B*, and the relative standard deviation of the measurement method is CV_T. If the mean concentration observed using the method is *c*, then the bias *B* is given by

$$B = \frac{(c - C)}{C} \tag{4.22}$$

The accuracy criterion used by the National Institute for Occupational Safety and Health (NIOSH) is called the *symmetric-range accuracy* (NIOSH, 1994; Kennedy et al., 1995). This accuracy, A_α, is the fractional range, symmetric about the true concentration, within which α (e.g., 95%) of the measurements are expected to fall. In the context of a Gaussian distribution of errors, the overall measurement uncertainty can be defined as

$$\sigma_{\text{overall}} = \left(B^2 + CV_T^2\right)^{1/2} \tag{4.23}$$

The accuracy is therefore given by

$$A_{95\%} = 1.96\,\sigma_{\text{overall}} = 1.96\left(B^2 + CV_T^2\right)^{1/2} \tag{4.24}$$

Thus, we see that the accuracy is an increasing function of both the bias and the relative standard deviation.

4.12 LIMIT OF DETECTION

The *limit of detection* (LOD) for a particular measurement method is the value of the measurement (e.g., of concentration or mass of an analyte) that is used as a cutoff point for asserting the presence of the analyte. Let the imprecision in the measurement method be given by σ, independent of the concentration. Let the false positive rate in asserting the presence of the analyte be α. Thus, only a fraction α of the measurements exceed the LOD, if the true mass sampled is zero. In other words, when a given measurement exceeds the LOD, this indicates the true presence of mass, with a false positive rate of α. Let Φ be the cumulative normal function with zero mean and a standard deviation of one. Then along the lines of Equation 4.14,

$$\Phi(X) = \int_{-\infty}^{X} G_{0,1}(x)\,\mathrm{d}x \tag{4.25}$$

Thus, we can say that $\Phi(1.645) = 0.95$, and the area under the curve from ∞ to 1.645 is 0.95. (Note that this is different from the information in Figure 4.8, in which two-sided intervals are being described, i.e., the area between 1.96 to +1.96 is 0.95). We can, likewise, define the inverse of the cumulative normal distribution Φ^{-1}, such that

$$\Phi^{-1}(1-\alpha) = Z_{1-\alpha} \tag{4.26}$$

For the above example, $\Phi^{-1}(0.95) = 1.96$. Given a false positive rate of α, the LOD is defined as

$$LOD = \Phi^{-1}(1-\alpha) \times \sigma \tag{4.27}$$

Generally, σ is not known exactly, but is estimated as s with υ degrees of freedom. This is done using the chi-square variable $\chi^2 = \upsilon \frac{s^2}{\sigma^2}$, which follows a chi-square probability distribution. This distribution is appropriate because variance estimates (s^2) are typically asymmetric and dependent on sample size. Thus, at a confidence level of γ (e.g., 95%), the single-sided confidence limit on σ is

$$\sigma_\gamma = s\sqrt{\upsilon / \chi^2_{1-\gamma,\upsilon}} \tag{4.28}$$

where $\chi^2_{1-\gamma}$ is the $1 - \gamma$ quantile value found in standard statistics tables and is defined as the value for which $prob\left(\chi^2 < \chi^2_{1-\gamma}\right) = 1 - \gamma$ (Bartley, 2001). Thus, the γ confidence limit on LOD is given by

$$LOD_\gamma = \Phi^{-1}(1-\alpha) \times \sqrt{\upsilon / \chi^2_{1-\gamma,\upsilon}} \times s \tag{4.29}$$

Traditionally, the LOD has been defined as

$$LOD = 3 \times s \tag{4.30}$$

This implies that the false positive rate has been set at ~0.001 (or ~0.1%). Thus, in order to determine the limit of detection, we need an estimate of the imprecision in the measurement method. Because it is assumed that the imprecision σ is independent of the concentration, it can be estimated from the standard deviation of the blank measurements, s. For example, if we were determining dust concentrations by weighing the mass collected on filters, a blank measurement would correspond to a blank filter being weighed pre- and posthandling. The standard deviation of the weight gains of the blank filters would be used in Equation 4.30.

4.13 LIMIT OF QUANTITATION

Limit of Quantitation (LOQ) for a specific measurement method is the limiting value for quantifying a measurement (such as a mass or a concentration) with confidence. It is the cutoff value for asserting that the relative imprecision is tighter than a specified value. It is defined as (ASTM, 2000):

$$LOQ = \frac{\sigma}{CV_{max}} \tag{4.31}$$

where CV_{max} is the maximum relative error acceptable in a quantification. For example, if σ were known to be 10 ppm, and CV_{max} is 10%, then the LOQ is 100 ppm.

As before, because we know only the estimate s of the standard deviation, the true standard deviation is determined using Equation 4.28 (Bartlely, 2001).

$$LOQ_{\gamma} = \frac{\sqrt{\upsilon / \chi^2_{1-\gamma,\upsilon}} \times s}{CV_{max}} \tag{4.32}$$

The LOQ is defined traditionally as

$$LOQ = 10 \times s \tag{4.33}$$

From Equation 4.32 and Equation 4.33, we can see that at a concentration equal to the LOQ, the relative error in the measurement is given by

$$CV_{max} = \frac{\sqrt{\upsilon / \chi^2_{1-\gamma,\upsilon}}}{10} \tag{4.34}$$

In other words, when a given measurement exceeds the LOQ (=10 × s), we can say with 95% confidence that the maximum relative error is given by Equation 4.34.

5 Measurement of Air Volumes and Flow Rates

5.1 INTRODUCTION

When quantifying the level of a pollutant in an environment, it is customary to express it in terms of the amount of some property of the pollutant per unit volume of the air in which it is dispersed. This is called the concentration of the contaminant. The relevant property for a gaseous contaminant is typically its mass or volume, whereas for an aerosol, additional properties, such as the number of particles or the surface area of the particles, can be expressed as a concentration. The units of concentration can therefore be mass/volume (e.g., $\mu g/m^3$), volume/volume (e.g., ppm), number/volume (e.g., particles per cubic centimeter, ppcc), or surface area/volume (e.g., $\mu m^2/m^3$).

5.2 ELEMENTS OF AN AIR SAMPLING SYSTEM

It is clear from our definition of concentration that we need to be able to collect a sample of air containing the pollutant and measure two properties accurately — the amount of the pollutant and the amount of air. Figure 5.1 shows the essential elements of an air sampling system. Air is drawn through the sampling train and forced to go through a *sensing zone* or *collection medium* that captures the pollutant and measures the relevant property. This can be a filter that collects airborne dust, which can be further analyzed by gravimetry or chemical means. The energy to force the air sample through the collection medium is provided by a *pump*. There is also a calibrated flow measurement device that can quantify the amount of air sampled. This type of sampling is referred to as *active sampling* because an external energy source (the pump) does the work needed to draw air through the device. *Passive sampling* devices, in contrast, depend on the random movement of air molecules to collect the contaminant.

In the rest of this chapter, we will discuss the last two elements in the sampling system, i.e., pumps and flow measurement and calibration devices.

5.3 PUMPS AND AIR MOVERS

Most pumps used for air sampling are the so-called volume displacement (or positive displacement) pumps. As the name suggests, these pumps move air by displacing it with another volume of air. Diaphragm pumps, piston pumps, and rotary vane pumps operate using this principle.

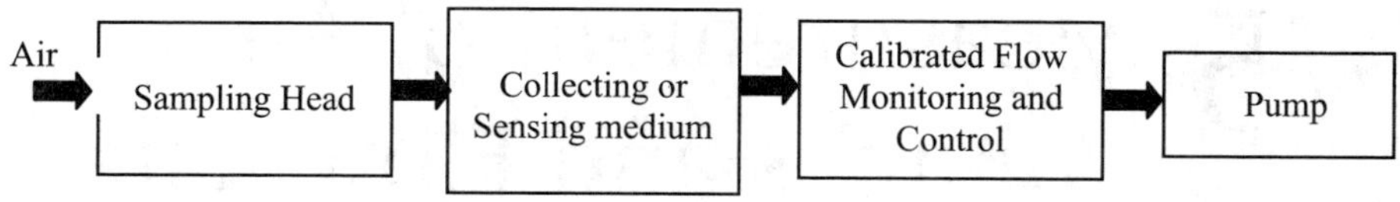

FIGURE 5.1 Schematic diagram showing elements of an air sampling system.

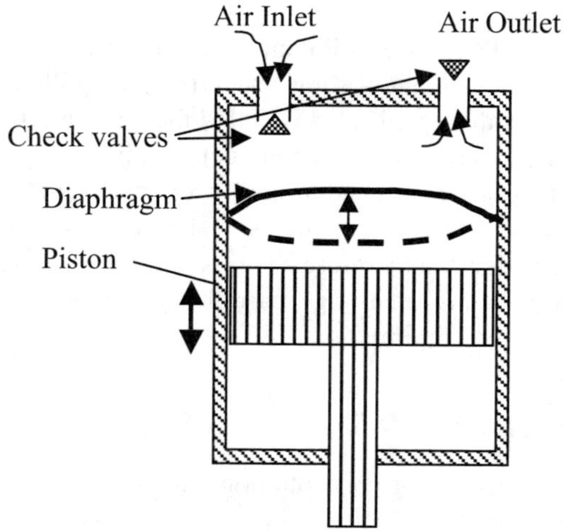

FIGURE 5.2 Diaphragm pump.

A *diaphragm pump* contains a flexible diaphragm that forms a sealed connection between the pump chamber and the plunger or crankcase. As the motor turns the crankcase or the piston, the diaphragm moves back and forth. This, in turn, causes a vacuum and pressurization of the pump chamber, which occur alternately, and is exploited by using a series of one-way check valves to draw in and expel air from the chamber. These pumps are typically lightweight, produce little noise, and can produce only relatively low flow rates. They do not need oil lubricants, which may generate contaminants during operation. They are thus ideal for personal sampling applications that need portability and flow rates of 1 to 5000 cc/min. In Figure 5.2, as the piston moves downward, a partial vacuum is created in the space between the piston and the diaphragm causing the diaphragm to flex downward. This causes air to rush in to the space above the diaphragm in the pump chamber through the inlet check valve. During this time, the outlet check valve is closed. Likewise, when the piston moves upward, the diaphragm flexes upward, and the air is pushed out of the pump chamber through the outlet valve while the inlet valve is closed.

A *piston pump* operates on the same principle as a diaphragm pump, except that a piston can displace a greater volume of air per stroke than a diaphragm. In Figure 5.3, air is drawn into the pump chamber when the piston moves downward and is pushed out when the piston moves upward. The functioning of the check valves is similar to those in the case of diaphragm pumps. Flow rates for such pumps range from a few cubic centimeters per minute for personal sampling pumps to several

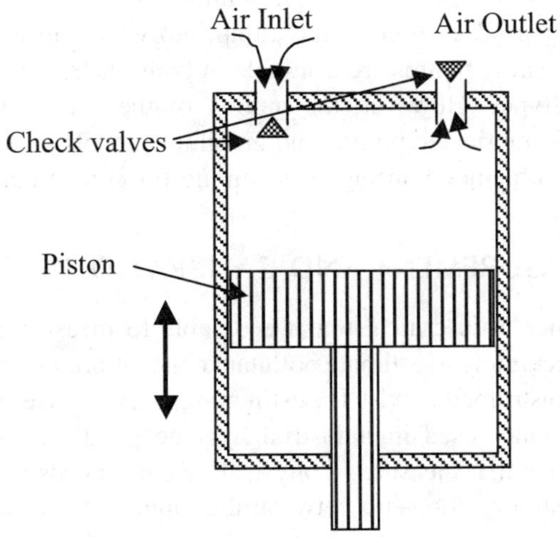

FIGURE 5.3 Piston pump.

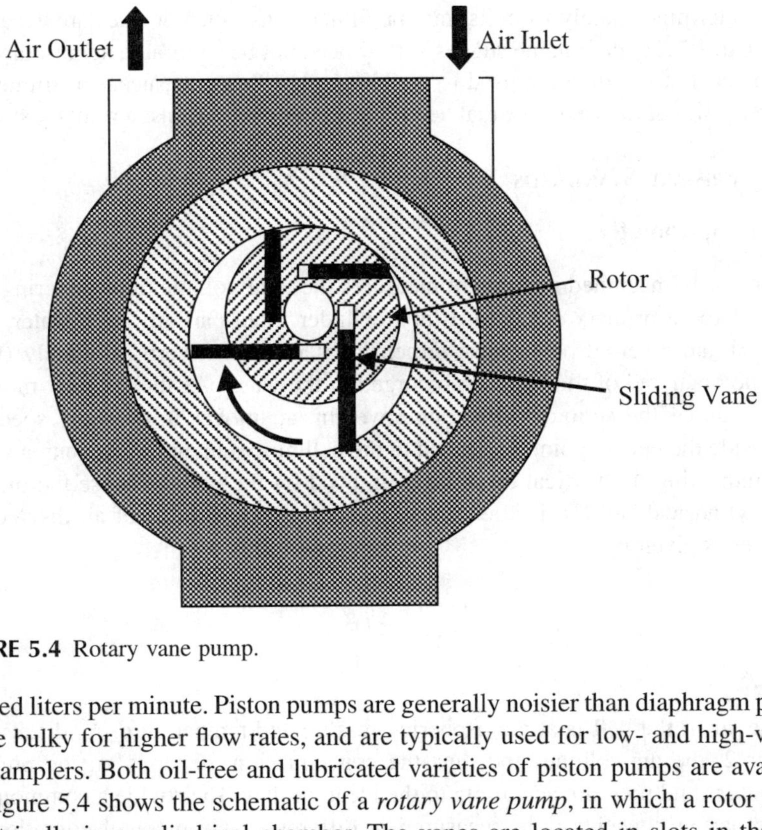

FIGURE 5.4 Rotary vane pump.

hundred liters per minute. Piston pumps are generally noisier than diaphragm pumps, can be bulky for higher flow rates, and are typically used for low- and high-volume area samplers. Both oil-free and lubricated varieties of piston pumps are available.

Figure 5.4 shows the schematic of a *rotary vane pump*, in which a rotor rotates eccentrically in a cylindrical chamber. The vanes are located in slots in the rotor and are pushed against the housing using springs. They slide in and out of the slots during the eccentric motion of the rotor, which moves the air along. The rotation of the rotor creates a partial vacuum in the pump into which air enters and is moved along by the rotor. These pumps are available in both oil-free (with graphite vanes) and oil-lubricated types. However, the motion of the sliding vanes in slots can generate oil mists in lubricated pumps and graphite aerosols in oil-free pumps, both of which may be problematic during air sampling for contaminants.

5.4 FLOW MEASUREMENT AND CALIBRATION

As mentioned earlier, it is critical that we be able to measure the volume of the sampled air very accurately to estimate pollutant concentrations accurately. Although a wide variety of instruments exist for estimating airflows, we will discuss only a few that are commonly used in industrial hygiene practice. As we discussed in Chapter 4, any device that measures a physical quantity needs to be calibrated, i.e., we need to establish a relationship between the input to the device and its output. Volume and flow rate measuring devices can be classified as primary or secondary standards depending on the extent to which they need to be calibrated.

A *primary standard* is a device in which the volume of air passing through it can be determined solely from its internal dimensions. Such devices are accurate to better than 1%. As their name suggests, they need not be calibrated against any other instrument; indeed, they are used to calibrate other flow measuring instruments. A *secondary standard* is a device that needs to be calibrated against a primary standard.

5.4.1 PRIMARY STANDARDS

5.4.1.1 Spirometer

This precisely machined instrument measures the total volume of air entering it and is considered a primary standard. It is a cylinder filled partially with water, inside which sits an inverted bell whose dimensions are known very accurately (Figure 5.5). The open end of the bell is submerged in the water. As the cylinder moves up or down under the action of the counterweight, air moves in or out, respectively, from inside the bell. A pointer attached to the bell moves up or down along a vertical scale, indicating the vertical distance (h) moved by the bell. Because the diameter of the cylindrical bell (D) is known very accurately, the volume of air displaced by the water is given by:

$$V = \frac{\pi D^2 h}{4} \tag{5.1}$$

The air in the bell is at atmospheric pressure and temperature. As discussed in Chapter 2, the air volume, and thus the concentration, depends on the prevalent temperature and pressure according to the ideal gas law. To provide a common basis for comparing concentrations measured at different environmental conditions, all volumes need to be converted to standard conditions, which are defined as 25°C (298 K) and 1 atm (760 mmHg).

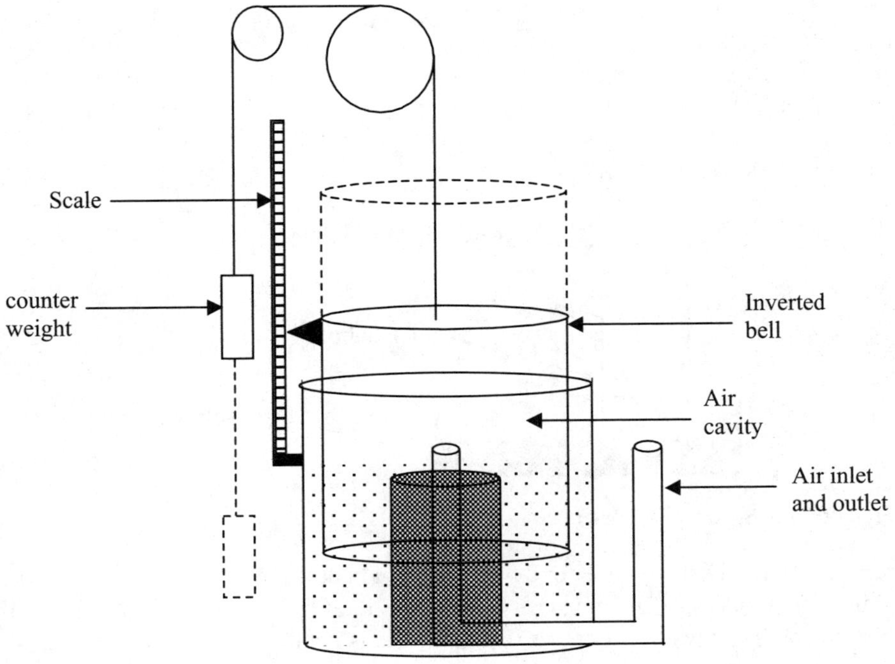

FIGURE 5.5 Spirometer.

$$V_{std} = V_{actual} \times \frac{P_{actual}}{P_{std}} \times \frac{T_{std}}{T_{actual}} \tag{5.2}$$

5.4.1.2 Soap Bubble Meter

This primary standard is used for measuring relatively small flow rates from 0.001 to 10 l/min. A soap bubble is introduced into a graduated cylinder by dipping the bottom of the cylinder into a soap solution (see Figure 5.6). The top of the cylinder is attached to a pump so that the soap bubble moves upward along with the airflow. The time it takes for the bubble to traverse a known distance is determined using a stopwatch. The volumetric flow rate is determined by:

$$Q = \frac{\pi\left(D^2/4\right)h}{t} \tag{5.3}$$

where D is the diameter of the cylinder and h is the distance moved by the soap bubble in time t.

These instruments are highly accurate. Electronic versions of the soap bubble meter are commonly used as primary flow rate standards in industrial hygiene. These electronic versions employ light beams at each end of the graduated cylinder, which, when intercepted by the soap bubble, send signals to a microprocessor, which in

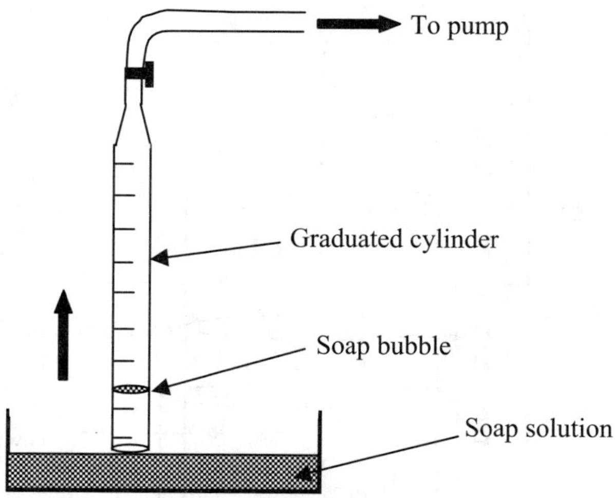

FIGURE 5.6 Soap bubble meter.

turn calculates the travel time for the bubble. The bubble moves through the cylinder almost frictionlessly, and thus very low flow rates can be measured using this instrument. The pressure drop across the bubble is negligible, and therefore the air is at ambient pressure and temperature. As in the case of spirometers, the measured flow rate needs to be corrected to standard conditions of pressure and temperature using Equation 5.2.

5.4.2 Secondary Standards

5.4.2.1 Wet Test Meter

A wet test meter consists of a cylinder that is partitioned into several rotating radial chambers that are partially filled with water (Figure 5.7). As the gas enters a chamber, the buoyant force makes the chamber rise, causing water in that chamber to be displaced into the next chamber, and so on to other chambers. This displacement process causes angular rotation of the system of chambers, which is proportional to the volume of the gas passing through, and is registered on an array of metering dials.

The volume of gas passing through in each rotation depends on the level of the water in the cylinder, and therefore the water level must be maintained at a constant level using a sight gauge. In addition, the water level in the instrument should be as close to horizontal as possible. Because the gas will dissolve in the water in the instrument, it is important to run the gas through the instrument for several hours to saturate the water in the instrument with the gas and thus prevent any additional absorption of the gas during measurement. Care should be taken to ensure that the gas passing through the water does not create a corrosive solution that may damage the internal parts of the instrument. Finally, because the wet test meter is a secondary standard, it needs to be calibrated against a primary standard such as a spirometer or a soap bubble meter.

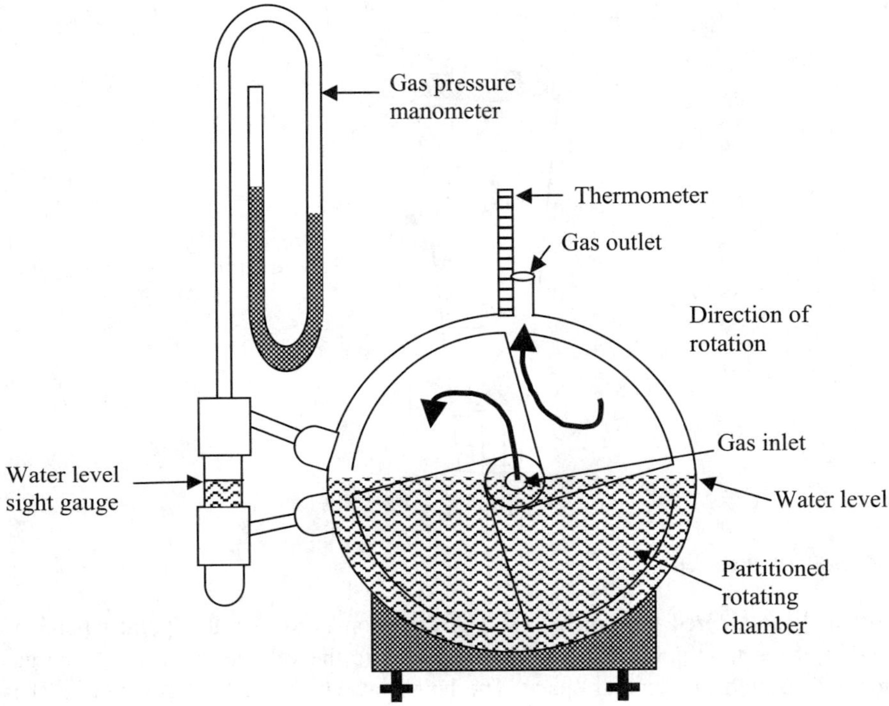

FIGURE 5.7 Wet test meter.

When the gas passes through water, it will become saturated with water vapor. This will cause an erroneously higher reading for the measured volume. To correct for this, we need to subtract the saturated water vapor pressure at that temperature from the pressure of the gas inside the wet test meter. In addition, we need to make the usual corrections to convert the measured volume to standard conditions. Thus Equation 5.2 is changed to:

$$V_{std} = V_{actual} \times \frac{\left(P_{actual} - P_{vap}\right)}{P_{std}} \times \frac{T_{std}}{T_{actual}} \tag{5.4}$$

Wet test meters can typically be used to measure flow rates from ~0.1 l/min to ~100 l/min. Very low flow rates are difficult to measure due to the inertia of the internal parts, and measurement of very high flow rates is not possible due to high pressure drops across the device.

5.4.2.2 Rotameter

A rotameter consists of a tapered vertical tube made of glass or plastic with a spherical float that can move up or down in the tapered tube (Figure 5.8). As gas flows in from the bottom to the top, the float rises due to the velocity pressure of the gas. As the float rises, the cross-sectional area of the annular space between the

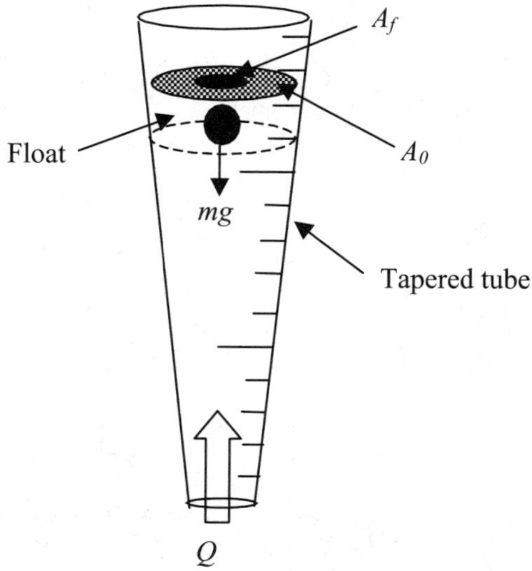

FIGURE 5.8 Rotameter.

float and the tapered tube increases. The float comes to rest at a point where the weight of the float is balanced by the force due to the velocity pressure of the gas flowing through the annular space. The height at which the float comes to rest is directly proportional to the flow rate.

The flow rate is given by:

$$Q = k A_0 \left(\frac{2m\,g}{\rho A_f} \right)^{1/2} \tag{5.5}$$

where A_0 is the area of the annular space, A_f is the cross-sectional area of the spherical float, m is the mass of the float, Q is the flow rate, ρ is the density of the gas, and k is a constant of proportionality.

Equation 5.5 clearly shows why a rotameter cannot be a primary standard. The constant of proportionality k needs to be determined by calibration against a primary flow rate standard such as a soap bubble meter. Rotameters usually come with a manufacturer-provided calibration curve that specifies the relationship between the flow rate and the height at which the float comes to rest. Hence, while using a rotameter, we read the position of the float and use the calibration curve to obtain the so-called *indicated flow rate*. Typically, these manufacturer calibrations are performed at standard conditions, i.e., 20°C and 760 mm Hg. Therefore, if the rotameter is used in the field under different conditions of pressure and temperature, the indicated reading of the instrument has to be corrected to the field conditions. However, the correction is not done according to Equation 5.2. The reason for this is that according to ideal gas law, $\rho \propto \frac{P}{T}$, and Equation 5.5 shows that $Q \propto \left(\frac{T}{P}\right)^{1/2}$-. Hence,

$$Q_{actual} = Q_{indicated} \left(\frac{T_{field\ condition}}{T_{standard}} \frac{P_{standard}}{P_{field\ condition}} \right)^{1/2} \quad (5.6)$$

where $Q_{indicated}$ is the rotameter reading in the field at standard conditions, Q_{actual} is the actual flow rate, $T_{field\ condition}$ is the temperature in the field during sampling, $P_{field\ condition}$ is the pressure at the rotameter inlet in the field during sampling, $T_{standard}$ is 293 K (20°C), and $P_{standard}$ is 760 mm Hg.

Rotameters are among the most commonly used instruments for flow rate measurements. Commercially available rotameters come in a variety of tube diameters and float configurations that correspond to flow rates from a few cm³/min to around 100 m³/min. They are factory-calibrated against a primary standard and can have accuracies of better than 1%.

5.4.2.3 Orifice Meter

This device is essentially a thin plate with a sharp-edged circular hole in the center (the orifice) that is placed in a duct or pipe; the diameter of the hole is smaller than the diameter of the duct (Figure 5.9). The flow rate through it is related to the pressure drop across the orifice, the area of cross section of the orifice, and the temperature and pressure at the inlet to the orifice, given by:

$$Q = K\,D^2 \left(\left(\frac{T_{inlet}}{P_{inlet}\,M} \right) \left(P_{inlet} - P_{outlet} \right) \right)^{1/2} \quad (5.7)$$

where Q is the flow rate, D is the diameter of the circular orifice, T_{inlet} and P_{inlet} are the temperature and pressure at the inlet, $(P_{inlet} - P_{outlet})$ is the pressure drop across the orifice, M is the molecular weight of the gas, and K is the coefficient of airflow. Equation 5.7 is valid for an orifice meter when $(P_{inlet} - P_{outlet})$ is small (generally 10% to 20% or less) compared to P_{inlet}.

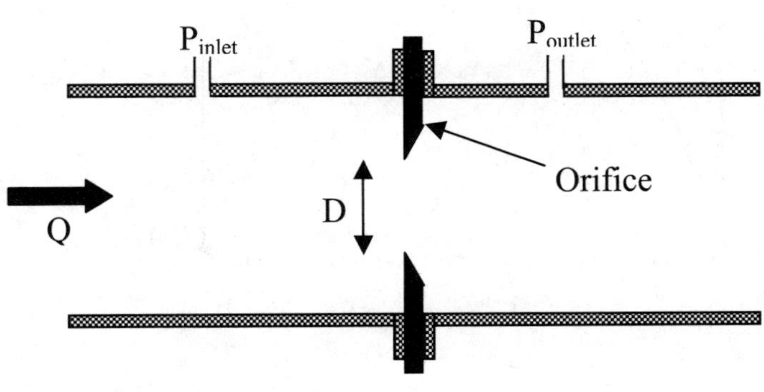

FIGURE 5.9 Orifice meter and critical orifice.

The orifice meter is generally calibrated against a primary standard to obtain a calibration curve of pressure drop vs. flow rate for a given set of operating conditions of inlet pressure and temperature. While using an orifice meter, we read the position of the pressure drop and use the calibration curve to obtain the indicated flow rate. If the device is used at some other temperature and pressure, then the indicated flow rate needs to be corrected to obtain the actual flow rate.

$$Q_{\text{actual}} = Q_{\text{indicated}} \left(\frac{T_{\text{actual}}}{T_{\text{standard}}} \frac{P_{\text{standard}}}{P_{\text{actual}}} \right)^{1/2} \tag{5.8}$$

5.4.2.4 Critical Orifice

As mentioned in the previous section, Equation 5.7 holds true only for small pressure drops across the orifice. When the pressure drop increases beyond a certain critical point, i.e., when $P_{\text{inlet}} - P_{\text{outlet}} \geq 0.47\ P_{\text{inlet}}$, the velocity of air in the constriction reaches the speed of sound (sonic velocity of 344 m/sec at STP), and the flow rate of air through the orifice reaches its maximum value for the orifice (Figure 5.10) Any further increases in pressure drop will not change the flow rate. Thus, a constant flow rate is achieved when the critical pressure drop is reached, and the orifice meter is then called a critical orifice.

Critical orifices are used in many instruments that need to sample air at a constant flow rate. They have an accuracy of better than 1% when properly calibrated. Calibration is performed against a primary standard at standard conditions, and flow

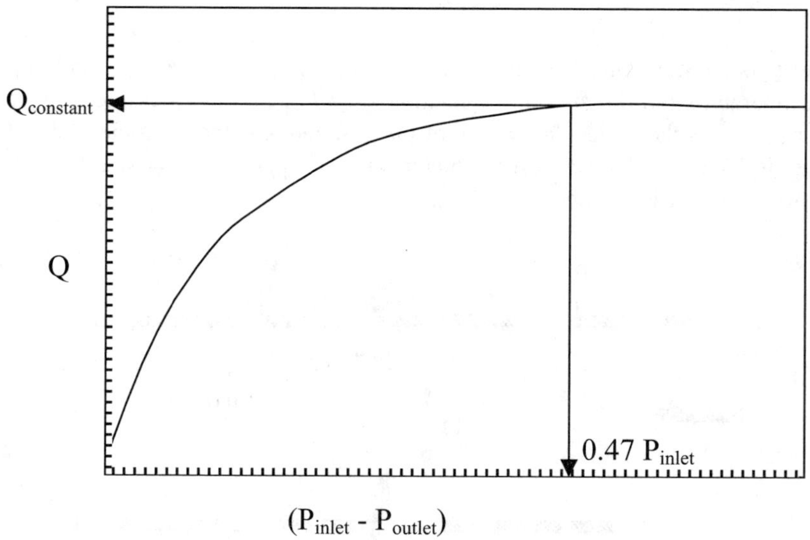

FIGURE 5.10 Schematic graphs showing the variation of flow rate with pressure drop and the critical point when a constant flow rate is achieved through the orifice.

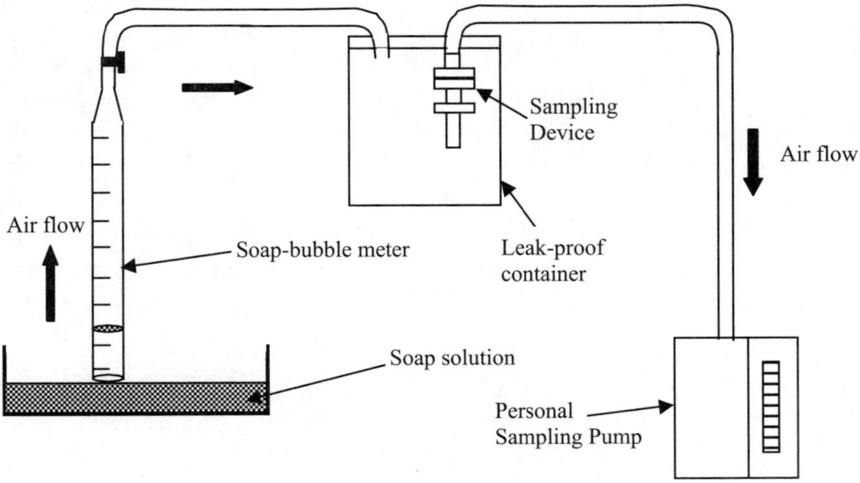

FIGURE 5.11 Set-up for calibration of a personal air sampling device attached to a pump.

measurements at other conditions need to be corrected to give the actual flow rate using Equation 5.8.

5.4.3 Calibration of Sampling Systems

Figure 5.1 shows the schematic of an air sampling train, in which the flow measuring unit is downstream of the sampling head and the sample collecting medium (e.g., a filter). There is typically a pressure drop across these two elements so that the flow measuring unit (e.g., a rotameter) observes the flow rate at a pressure different from the ambient pressure. Under these conditions, the calibration curve provided by the manufacturer is not applicable. We need to either calibrate the rotameter for the sampling conditions or correct the calibration curve for the sampling conditions of temperature and pressure. Figure 5.11 shows a calibration procedure in which the sampling device is connected to a sampling pump that has a built-in rotameter and is being calibrated against a soap bubble meter. The sampling device is placed in a leakproof container so that the airflow through the device is the same as through the primary standard. Because the soap bubble meter is operating at atmospheric pressure and temperature, it provides the true flow rate for those conditions, and the rotameter reading is calibrated against this primary standard.

6 Gas and Vapor Sampling Methods

6.1 INTRODUCTION

Sampling for gases and vapors is done to identify and quantify the amount of a pollutant in an environment. The reasons for obtaining a sample may be to assess compliance with an occupational exposure limit (OEL), to assess the health risk posed by the pollutant, to determine the efficacy of control measures for minimizing exposures, or for an epidemiological study. In this chapter, we shall discuss the various means by which gases and vapors are collected for further analysis. A gas is a substance that naturally exists in the gas phase at 760 mm Hg (101 kPa) and 20°C. A vapor is the gaseous form of a solid or liquid in equilibrium with its gas phase.

6.2 REQUIREMENTS OF A GOOD SAMPLING METHOD

A good method for gas and vapor sampling should have the following features:

- A high collection efficiency (>90%) will ensure that sampling losses are minimized. *Collection efficiency* is defined as

$$\eta = \frac{C_{\text{measured}}}{C_{\text{true}}} \tag{6.1}$$

  where C_{measured} is the concentration measured by the method, and C_{true} is the true concentration. The collection efficiency of a method can be established in the laboratory by preparing known concentrations of a gas that will be taken to be C_{true} and then measuring C_{measured} using the measurement method.
- The sampling airflow rate should be high enough to collect enough mass of the pollutant for analysis in a reasonable amount of time. The minimum volume of the air sample required should contain a mass of the pollutant greater than the *limit of detection* of the analytical method. If the expected concentration in a given environment is C (mg/m^3), the sampling flow rate is Q, and the sampling duration is t, then the minimum sample volume is given by

$$\textit{Minimum sample volume}\ (\mathrm{m}^3) = (Q \times t)_{\min} = \frac{\textit{Limit of detection}\ (\mathrm{mg})}{C\ (\mathrm{mg/m}^3)} \tag{6.2}$$

- At the same time, the sample air volume should not be so high as to overload the collection medium beyond its capacity to hold the pollutant mass. The maximum sample volume is given by

$$\textit{Maximum sample volume}\ (\mathrm{m}^3) = (Q \times t)_{\max} = \frac{\textit{Collection medium capacity}\ (\mathrm{mg})}{C\ (\mathrm{mg/m}^3)} \tag{6.3}$$

- The collected pollutant sample should stay chemically stable until analyzed. The collection medium should neither react chemically with the pollutant nor be toxic.
- The method should involve only a minimum amount of analysis in the field.

6.3 SAMPLING STRATEGIES

Sampling schemes can be divided into several categories based on the type of energy used for sampling, duration of sampling, and location of sampling.

Sampling methods can be divided into two broad categories based on whether or not a pump is required for collecting a sample. In *active sampling*, the air contaminant is aspirated through a pump on to a collection medium, i.e., an external source of energy is needed to move the air through the sampling train. In contrast, *passive sampling* uses diffusion of gas molecules to collect the pollutant.

Samples are collected over a period of time, and hence represent an average over that time interval. Of course, the time interval over which the sample is obtained may vary from a few seconds or minutes to several hours or days. A sample obtained over a very short time interval is called a *grab sample*, and typically the air contaminant is aspirated into a container. In *integrated sampling*, the contaminant is collected in a medium over a longer period of time.

Sampling can be done to determine the general background environmental conditions in a workplace or to determine the personal exposures of workers to a chemical by monitoring their breathing zone concentrations. The former is called *area sampling*, whereas the latter is called *personal sampling*.

6.3.1 GRAB SAMPLING

Grab sampling is a useful means for measuring constant concentrations or peak concentrations (when the time of the occurrence of the peak is known) and is used to measure short-term exposure limits (STELs). If the concentration varies with time, a grab sample at one instant of time will not be very informative. A common use of grab sampling is as a screening tool when it is necessary to identify all the chemicals present in a given environment. Because only a small volume of air can be drawn over a small time interval, grab samples require a very low limit of detection for the corresponding analytical method (see Equation 6.2). Thus, for sampling environments where the concentration of the pollutant is low, grab sampling may not be appropriate. The sample is usually drawn into a flask or stainless steel canister under vacuum or into a flexible plastic bag (e.g., Teflon, PVC, aluminized Mylar, and Tedlar) using a hand- or battery-operated pump. It is important that the walls of these containers do not adsorb or chemically react with the collected sample. However, adsorption to bag surfaces, diffusion through the bag walls, reactions in the containers, and leaks remain issues that need to be accounted for while using these samplers. After obtaining a sample, the container is sealed and sent to a lab for analysis.

6.3.2 Integrated Sampling

Integrated sampling is useful when the concentration in air is changing with time and there is a need to obtain an average concentration over a given time interval. The measurements obtained are time integrals of the concentration over the sampling interval. So, if the concentration in the work environment is a function of time and is denoted by $C(t)$ in units of mg/m^3, and the sampling device with a flow rate of Q m^3/min collects the pollutant over the entire sampling interval T (i.e., integrating it), then the mass of pollutant collected by it is given by

$$m = Q \int_{t=0}^{T} C(t)\,dt \tag{6.4}$$

This can be used to determine an average concentration over the time interval T as

$$C_{\text{avg}} = \frac{m}{Q \times T} = \frac{1}{T} \int_{t=0}^{T} C(t)\,dt \tag{6.5}$$

In Figure 6.1, the shaded area under the curve for $C(t)$ is the integral of $C(t)$ over the time interval T. This area is equal to the area of the rectangle whose sides are the vertical length C_{avg} and the horizontal length T. Equation 6.5 expresses this equivalence.

One advantage of integrated sampling over grab sampling is that, by increasing the sampling time, we can measure ever lower concentrations. Integrated samples are typically used to measure 8-h time weighted averages (TWAs) on which a number of occupational exposure limits are based. Although one can obtain a single sample that integrates the concentration over the entire work shift (of, say, 8 h), it might be better to obtain several consecutive samples whose individual time durations add up to the time of the entire work shift. Apart from providing (at least) a partial exposure

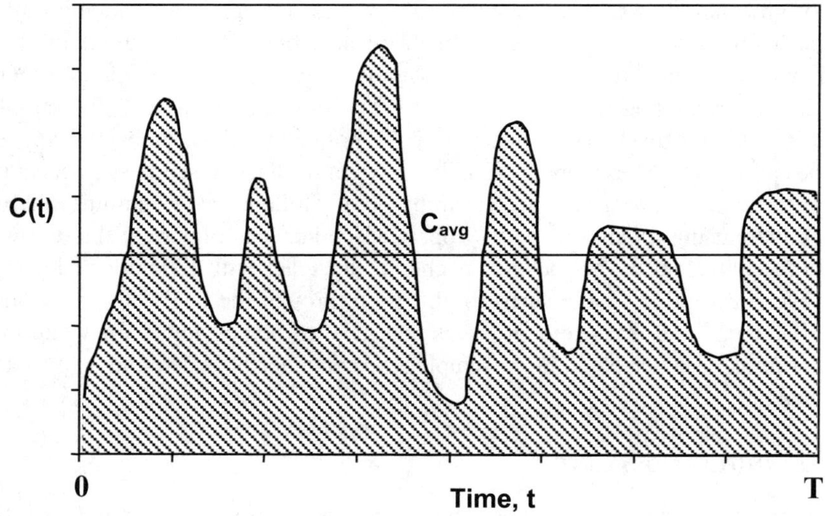

FIGURE 6.1 The concentration profile $C(t)$ and the average concentration C_{avg} over a time interval T.

value even if one of the samples is lost due to equipment malfunction, this strategy can also provide information on the variability of exposure within a work shift, which might be task-dependent. The individual measurements can be combined to yield the work shift average as

$$C_{TWA} = \frac{C_1T_1 + C_2T_2 + ... + C_nT_n}{T_1 + T_2 + ... + T_n} \tag{6.6}$$

where C_{TWA} is the time-weighted average over the entire work shift of duration T (which could be 8 h), C_1, C_2, … , C_n are the average concentrations over the time intervals T_1, T_2, … , T_n, and $T_1 + T_2 + … + T_n = T$.

6.3.3 Area Sampling

This is used to determine the general background concentration level experienced by most workers in an area. By its very nature, this type of sampling focuses more on plant conditions. Area samples are obtained by placing a sampler in the area of interest, e.g., in the vicinity of a pollutant source or far away from a source. Because the sampler is not worn by a worker, size and weight restrictions are not important. Thus, high–flow rate pumps can be used to collect enough mass to exceed limits of detection of analytical methods. A smaller number of instruments are needed to monitor a workplace, and there is less need to enlist the direct cooperation of workers. The drawback of area sampling is that it is often not representative of the actual personal exposures of the workers.

6.3.4 Personal Sampling

Personal sampling is used to determine the concentration level that a worker is exposed to during a full work shift or task by measuring the breathing zone concentration of the worker. The breathing zone is an envelope around the worker's head, which is considered to have the same concentration of pollutant as the air breathed in by the worker. It is defined as roughly the volume bounded on one side by the area between the shoulders and the midchest up to the top of the head, extending out to an arm's length away from the torso. The sampler is worn by the worker for the duration of the work shift and it follows the worker through his/her activities during the workday. This is considered the best way to estimate the dose of the pollutant inhaled by the worker. A number of studies have shown that area samples significantly underestimate personal exposures. Obviously, this type of sampling imposes a significant burden on the workers being monitored and requires their direct cooperation and consent. In addition, personal samplers need to be lightweight, necessitating the use of small pumps with low flow rates, with the consequent problem of meeting the limits of detection.

Phenomena such as absorption, adsorption, and diffusion are exploited to obtain integrated samples.

6.4 ABSORPTION

In absorption, a gas or vapor completely dissolves in a liquid. The solubility increases as the partial pressure of the gas or vapor present above the solution is increased. This relationship is described by *Henry's law*, which states that at constant pressure, the mole fraction of a gas dissolved in a solvent is directly proportional to the partial pressure of the gas.

$$p_g = K\,x \tag{6.7}$$

where p_g is the partial pressure of the gas, x is the mole fraction of the gas in solution, and K is the Henry's law constant for the gas in a particular solvent. By converting the units of the Henry's law constant from pressure to concentration, the above equation can also be written as

$$C_{\text{gas}} = K\,C_{\text{liq}} \tag{6.8}$$

Thus, during air sampling, the concentration of the vapor in the liquid increases until an equilibrium is established with the vapor concentration in air. Therefore, the collection efficiency of samplers based on absorption depends on the following factors:

1. The volume of air sampled and the volume of the absorbing liquid. For a given volume of liquid, there is a certain mass of contaminant that can

be absorbed beyond which additional air sampling will not increase the amount of contaminant in solution. Indeed, sampling more air after equilibrium has been established will lead to a measured concentration that is less than the true concentration in air, i.e., a reduced collection efficiency.

2. The greater the vapor pressure of the sampled contaminant, the greater the amount of contaminant passing into the solution. However, greater vapor pressure also increases the likelihood of contaminant loss after sampling has been completed. One way to reduce sampling losses due to evaporation of the absorbed vapor is to cool the liquid and thereby lower the vapor pressure of the contaminant.
3. The greater the amount of contact between the absorbing liquid and the vapor, the greater the collection efficiency.
4. The greater the reactivity of the vapor and the absorbing liquid, the greater is the collection efficiency.

Impingers and *bubblers* (Figure 6.2) use absorption as the principle of contaminant collection. Impingers were originally used for aerosol collection, but are nowadays used for sampling reactive gases (such as halogens), vapors, and acid mists. The sampled airstream enters through an inlet tube and exits into a known volume of liquid at the bottom of a glass flask. The airstream is accelerated to velocities greater than 60 m/sec in the orifice to increase the level of agitation in the liquid. This enhances contact between the liquid and the vapor and promotes more complete absorption. Some of the well-known impingers are the Greenburg–Smith impinger (sampling flow rate of 28.3 l/min or 1 CFM), the All Glass Impinger (8.5 to 12.5 l/min), and the midget impinger (2.8 l/min).

Bubblers typically have a fritted glass at the end of the inlet tube through which the vapor exits into the liquid. The exiting air is forced out through numerous pores, which results in a large number of small bubbles being formed. The bubble formation enhances the absorption of the vapor in the liquid solution. The number of pores in the frit depends on the vapor to be sampled. Coarse frits (with fewer pores per unit area) are suitable for vapors that are easily soluble in the liquid and finer frits (with more pores per unit area) for less soluble vapors. The finer the frit, the greater is the pressure drop across the sampler, which, in turn, necessitates a more powerful sampling pump.

The above description is for *physical absorption*, in which nonreactive gases and vapors are absorbed by a liquid in which they are highly soluble, e.g., hydrogen chloride in water and methanol in water. Impingers and bubblers can also be used for *chemical absorption*, in which the gas or vapor chemically reacts with the absorbing solution to form a more stable compound that can subsequently be chemically analyzed, e.g., ammonia vapors reacting with sulfuric acid solution. Most halogens are collected using this principle, e.g., bromine is collected using Na_2CO_3 or $NaHCO_3$ buffer solution and chlorine is collected using a 1% sulfamic acid solution.

The mass of contaminant collected in the liquid is analyzed and quantified. Frequently, only a small portion of the liquid is used for analysis, and the mass of

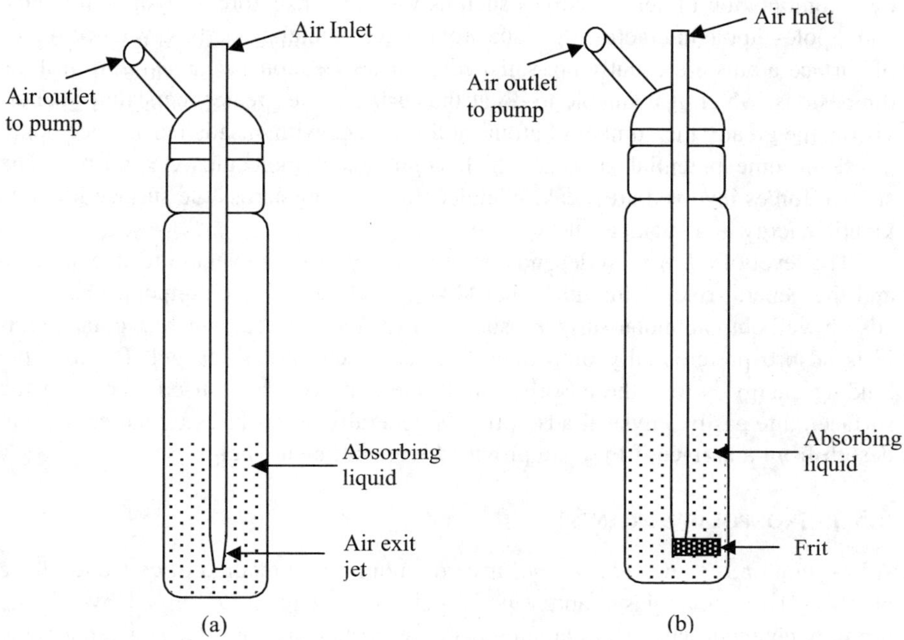

FIGURE 6.2 (a) Impinger; (b) bubbler with fritted inlet.

contaminant in that portion of the liquid is then scaled up to the total amount of liquid. Let v be the volume of liquid used for analysis in which it is determined that a mass m of the contaminant is contained. If the total volume of liquid in the impinger is V, then the total mass of contaminant collected during sampling is $\left(\frac{m}{v}\right)V$. A similar analysis is done for the blank sample, and the mass of contaminant in the blank sample is $\left(\frac{m_{\text{blank}}}{v}\right)V$. If the collection efficiency is η, the sampling flow rate is Q, and sampling is performed for a time t, then the air concentration of the contaminant is given by

$$C = \frac{\frac{V}{v}\left(m - m_{\text{blank}}\right)}{\eta \times Q \times t} \tag{6.9}$$

6.5 ADSORPTION

Adsorption refers to the movement of material from one phase of matter to the surface of another phase. For example, ammonia gas molecules move from the gaseous phase to the surface of activated charcoal. The molecules stick to the surface by a combination of surface forces such as van der Waals forces, hydrogen bonds, and dipole–dipole interaction. Surface atoms have special properties. Valence forces of surface atoms are usually not satisfied because the atom needs to bond in three dimensions, which it is unable to do at the surface. The greater the state of subdivision, the greater the number of atoms at the surface with unsatisfied valence bond. These become potential sites at which contaminant molecules can adsorb. The surface forces involved are weak. A molecule bounding across the surface loses its kinetic energy and sticks to the surface.

The level of adsorption depends on the affinity of the molecule for the surface, and the general rule of thumb is that "like adsorbs like." So, nonpolar chemicals adsorb well onto nonpolar surfaces, such as activated charcoal, whereas polar chemicals adsorb preferentially onto polar surfaces such as a silica gel. Because the binding energy is low, the adsorbed molecule can also shake itself free from the surface quite easily. Physical adsorption is generally reversible, i.e., molecules can desorb from a surface if they are provided with sufficient energy.

6.5.1 Nonpolar Sorbents

Adsorption onto *activated charcoal* is a commonly used method of collection for a number of nonpolar gases and vapors. Activated charcoal is formed by heating ordinary charcoal with steam at a temperature greater than 800°C. This renders the material porous with a network of fine tunnels extending through the body. Activated charcoal is a substance in which surface atoms are a significant fraction of the total number of atoms. The surface area on the walls of the tunnels is of the order of 100 to 1000 m^2/g. Molecules adsorb onto the surfaces by hydrogen bonding and dipole moment forces. Aliphatic hydrocarbons, alcohols, esters, aromatic hydrocarbons, and ketones are suitable for collection using charcoal media. Once these compounds are adsorbed, they can be easily desorbed using other chemicals that are preferentially adsorbed and thus displace the already adsorbed compounds. Nonpolar substances are preferentially adsorbed onto charcoal and displace more polar substances. Nonpolar substances such as aliphatic and aromatic hydrocarbons, esters, and ketones can be easily desorbed using a more nonpolar desorption solution such as carbon disulfide. More polar substances such as alcohols require other desorbers such as methanol.

Other than activated charcoal, there are a variety of media that have been used as sorbents for nonpolar compounds for very specific applications. *Porous polymers* have been tailored for high selectivity and have been used for specific gases, such as dimethyl sulfate. Tenax is widely used for sampling very low concentrations of volatile chemicals, such as those found in non-occupational indoor environments. Besides high specificity, Tenax has low affinity for water, and thus interference due to high humidity is not a problem. Porous polymers have found widespread application in gas chromatography columns, where their high selectivity and specificity is a big advantage. Some of them are quite ideal for sampling reactive molecules, while at the same time not being affected by humidity. The disadvantages include a rather low breakthrough volume and instability of the sorbent during sampling. Porous polymers also react readily with oxidizing compounds such as chlorine and

TABLE 6.1
Classes of Compounds in Decreasing Order of Polarity and Strength of Adsorption onto Polar Sorbents such as Silica Gel

Water
Alcohols
Aldehydes
Ketones
Esters
Aromatics
Alkenes
Alkanes

ozone. *Molecular carbon sieves* have a macroporous structure and retain various species according to molecular size. They are most commonly used as collection media for volatile nonpolar organic compounds at low concentrations.

6.5.2 Polar Sorbents

Silica gel is a widely used adsorber, primarily in collecting polar compounds for which activated charcoal is unsuitable. It is an amorphous form of silica obtained from the reaction of sodium silicate and sulfuric acid. More polar compounds are preferentially adsorbed onto silica gel and will displace less polar compounds. In order of decreasing polarity, Table 6.1 shows the classes of compounds that are preferentially adsorbed onto silica gel.

Thus, under high humidity conditions, water will displace other contaminants that are of greater interest. Similarly, the presence of more polar compounds in the air may interfere with the sampling and collection of less polar contaminants.

6.5.3 Breakthrough

For activated charcoal and silica gel, it is clear that, even though the amount of surface available for adsorption is enormous, it is still finite. In the presence of a large number of contaminant molecules, the adsorption sites will eventually become filled up (i.e., the collection medium becomes saturated), and no more contaminant molecules can be adsorbed. This condition is called *breakthrough*, in that the contaminants in the stream of air flowing through the adsorbent material break through to the other side (i.e., they are no longer being collected). If the concentration of the contaminant in the air exiting the collection medium is greater than 5% of the concentration in the air entering the medium, then breakthrough conditions have been reached. This definition (NIOSH, 1994) is by no means universally accepted, and others have suggested 20 to 25% as a better indicator of breakthrough. If breakthrough is reached, it implies that air was sampled for some amount of time without collecting all the contaminant mass in it. Any concentration calculated using this mass collected and this volume of air sampled will be an underestimate of the true concentration. Thus, the collected sample is no longer considered reliable and is typically discarded. *Breakthrough volume* is the volume of air sampled before breakthrough occurs, and *breakthrough time* is the time at which breakthrough occurs for a giving sampling flow rate.

$$\textit{Breakthrough Volume} = \textit{Breakthrough Time} \times \textit{Flow Rate} \tag{6.10}$$

Several factors affect the adsorption onto a surface and the occurrence of breakthrough:

1. As *temperature* increases, the contaminant molecules have sufficient energy to escape the binding attractive force of the surface, and adsorption decreases. Thus, breakthrough volume decreases with increasing temperature.
2. As the sampling *flow rate* increases, the contaminant-laden air rushes past the adsorption sites without sufficient opportunity for the molecules to stick to the adsorbent. Breakthrough volume decreases with increasing flow rate.
3. As *humidity* increases, water molecules preferentially occupy the adsorption sites and displace contaminant molecules. Thus, breakthrough volume decreases with increasing humidity. This is true not only for polar sorbents such as silica gel, but also for activated charcoal.
4. As the *concentration* of the contaminant in the sampled airstream increases, breakthrough volume decreases because a smaller volume of air will contain enough contaminant molecules to occupy the adsorption sites in the collection medium.
5. If there is a mixture of several *competing chemicals* that vie for the same adsorption sites, then the compounds that are more preferentially adsorbed displace the other chemicals from the sorbent. In some instances, two chemicals may be so similar that they have roughly the same affinity for the sorbent. In such instances, both compounds will get adsorbed in roughly equal proportions.
6. As the granules of the sorbent material become progressively finer, the surface area per gram of the sorbent material increases, and more adsorption sites become available. This increases the adsorption capacity of the sorbent, and therefore increases breakthrough volume.

Optimum sampling flow rates and sample volumes have, therefore, been determined for various compounds and media. These are available in NIOSH analytical procedure manuals.

In solid sorbent collection, a pump is used to pull air through a sorbent, such as charcoal, with a specified particle size that is sealed in a glass tube of specified dimensions. Typically, there is a front section containing 100 mg of charcoal and a rear section with 50 mg of charcoal. The two sections are separated by a urethane foam plug (see Figure 6.3). Both ends of the glass tube are sealed. Before sampling, the tips are broken and the back end of the tube is attached to a sampling pump.

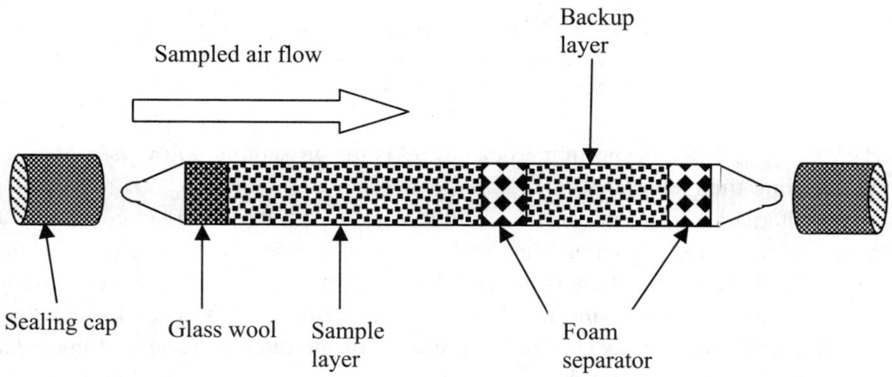

FIGURE 6.3 Activated charcoal sampling tube.

After sampling is completed, the two ends are sealed with plastic caps until desorption and chemical analysis.

6.5.4 Desorption

Compounds that have been collected on the sorbent need to be desorbed for analysis. *Desorption efficiency* or *fractional recovery* is the fraction of the total adsorbed contaminant that is removed or recovered from the adsorbent material using a desorbing compound. Although complete recovery of the analyte from the sorbent is desirable, the minimum desorption efficiency should be 75% for concentration between 10 and 200% of the exposure limit. If the desorption efficiency is less than 75%, the method is unsuitable for monitoring. As mentioned before, carbon disulfide is the preferred desorbing solvent for most nonpolar compounds adsorbed on charcoal. For polar compounds, a range of mixtures are used (alcohols mixed in various proportions with CS_2, alkanes, amines, etc.). For silica gel, common desorbents are methanol, ethanol, and diethyl ether.

Desorption efficiency varies somewhat from one batch of activated charcoal to the next. Therefore, it has to be determined each time and accounted for in calculating the sampled air concentration of the contaminant. It is determined experimentally by injecting a known amount of contaminant into a sorbent and measuring the amount that can be removed using a desorbent. Another important factor affecting desorption efficiency is the presence of water vapor. Loss of volatile contaminants during desorption is prevented by injecting the desorbent into the sorbent in a sealed container.

The air concentration of a contaminant is calculated in a manner very similar to Equation 6.9 for impingers. A volume V of the desorbent solvent is used to recover the collected contaminant. A portion of it, volume v, is used for further chemical analysis, e.g., for gas chromatography. If the mass of contaminant collected in the front section of the sorbent tube is m_{front}, the mass collected in the back section is m_{back}, and the mass of contaminant in the blank is m_{blank}, then the concentration of the contaminant in air is given by

$$C = \frac{\frac{V}{v}\left(m_{\text{front}} + m_{\text{back}} - m_{\text{blank}}\right)}{\eta_{\text{desorption}} \times Q \times t} \tag{6.11}$$

where $\eta_{\text{desorption}}$ is the desorption efficiency, Q is the air sampling flow rate, and t is the sampling time interval.

An alternative to using carbon disulfide is to desorb the adsorbed contaminant by heating the sorbent material. This is referred to as *thermal desorption*. The obvious advantage of this is that there is no need for a solvent, and thus the process can be automated easily. Also, using a solvent for desorption usually leads to less than complete desorption, especially in the presence of mixtures of polar and nonpolar contaminants. With thermal desorption, most chemicals that have boiling points in the range of 50 to 250°C can be desorbed with close to 100% efficiency. The disadvantage of thermal desorption is that it cannot be used with charcoal because the high temperatures (~300°C) needed for desorption might cause the decomposition of some contaminants. Thus, sorbents such as carbon molecular sieves or porous polymers such as Tenax need to be used.

6.5.5 Diffusive Samplers

As discussed in Chapter 2, diffusion is the mass transfer of one gas through another resulting from random motion of gas molecules in a concentration gradient. The mass transfer process is described by *Fick's law*:

$$J = -D\frac{dC}{dx} \tag{6.12}$$

where J is mass flux (the mass that is transported per unit area across a plane perpendicular to the concentration gradient in unit time, mg/m²/sec), D is the molecular diffusion coefficient (m²/sec), and $\frac{dC}{dx}$ is the local concentration gradient (mg/m⁴).

In a diffusive sampler, the random movements of gas molecules in air bring the contaminant to a solid sorbent collection medium, and the contaminant is collected by physical adsorption. Besides solid sorbents such as activated charcoal, other sorbents are used for specific applications such as sodium bisulfite solution for formaldehyde, various reagents for sulfur dioxide and nitrogen dioxide, and gold foil for inorganic mercury.

In their most common practical realization, diffusive samplers are lightweight cylindrical badges, in which the contaminant molecules pass through a membrane that minimizes the effects of convective air currents into a stagnant air layer. From this layer of air, the contaminants diffuse onto a bed of charcoal or some other adsorbent material. Figure 6.4 shows a schematic diagram of the relevant parameters affecting diffusion in the static air layer between the membrane and the charcoal bed.

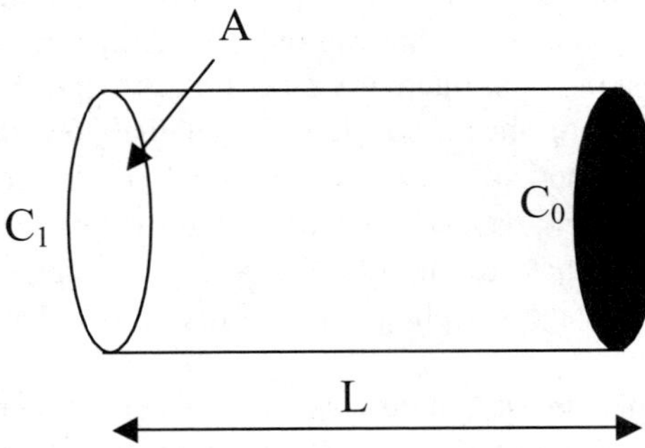

FIGURE 6.4 Schematic diagram of a diffusive sampler. C_1 is the ambient air concentration, C_0 is the concentration at the interface of the sorbent and air, A is the area of cross section of the charcoal bed (and the permeable membrane), and L is the distance between the membrane and the charcoal bed.

Equation 6.12 can be rewritten as

$$\frac{dm}{A\,dt} = D\frac{(C_1 - C_0)}{L} \tag{6.13}$$

or

$$m = \frac{DA}{L}(C_1 - C_0)t \tag{6.14}$$

where A is the area of cross section of the diffusion path (i.e., the area of the charcoal bed), L is the length of the diffusional path (i.e., the distance between the membrane and the charcoal bed), C_1 is the ambient air concentration, C_0 is the concentration at the interface of the sorbent and air, t is the sampling time, and m is the mass uptake. If the sorbent has a high affinity for the contaminant being sampled, then the air concentration at the surface of the collector is zero (i.e., $C_0 = 0$), and the air concentration is obtained as

$$C_1 = \frac{m}{t}\left(\frac{L}{DA}\right) \tag{6.15}$$

Here, the term $\frac{DA}{L}$ has units of m³/sec, m has units of mg, and t has units of seconds, and so the concentration has units of mg/m³. The units of $\frac{DA}{L}$ make it appear analogous to a sampling flow rate in an active sampling scenario. For a given gas of known diffusion coefficient and a given geometry, an "effective sampling flow rate" can be calculated. Manufacturers of diffusive samplers provide tables of such effective sampling flow rates that can be used in Equation 6.15 to calculate air concentrations. Diffusion is an inherently slow process, and the effective sampling flow rates are an order of magnitude lower than the flow rates used for active sampling using charcoal and silica gel tubes (25 to 40 cm^3/min as compared to 200 cm^3/min for most gases and vapors of occupational hygiene interest).

Many of the factors that are important in active sampling using solid sorbents are also important in passive sampling using diffusive samplers:

1. As *temperature* increases, there is an increase in random molecular motion leading to a more rapid diffusion of contaminant molecules. At the same time, adsorption decreases. Both of these factors cause more rapid saturation of the adsorption medium.
2. As *humidity* increases, water molecules preferentially occupy the adsorption sites and displace contaminant molecules, causing significant losses in sampling efficiency.
3. When there is a *mixture* of chemicals, they may compete for the same adsorption sites. Compounds that are more preferentially adsorbed displace the other chemicals from the sorbent.
4. Equation 6.15 assumes that the sorbent has a high affinity for the contaminant so that the concentration at the interface C_0 can be neglected. However, during a sampling interval, the contaminant can accumulate on the sorbent surface in significant amounts such that the true ambient concentration is underestimated.
5. The membranes on diffusive samplers are quite fragile, and even minor tears and holes in the membrane can affect the diffusion characteristics significantly. Care should also be taken not to allow water or any other liquids to touch the membrane because such contact may affect its permeability.
6. Because the effective sampling flow rate is rather low, sampling times are much longer than for sorbent tube sampling. Conversely, the mass of contaminant collected is much lower for similar sampling times.

The calculation of air concentration of contaminants is similar to Equation 6.11, and is

$$C = \frac{\frac{V}{v}\left(m - m_{\text{blank}}\right)}{\eta_{\text{desorption}} \times \left(\frac{DA}{L}\right) \times t} \tag{6.16}$$

where V is the volume of the desorbent solvent that is used to recover the collected contaminant, v is a portion of it used for further chemical analysis, $\eta_{\text{desorption}}$ is the desorption efficiency, the mass of contaminant collected in the sorbent is m, the mass of contaminant in the blank is m_{blank}, t is the sampling time interval, and $\frac{DA}{L}$ is the effective sampling flow rate.

6.6 DIFFUSIVE SAMPLERS FOR REACTIVE COMPOUNDS

Sorbent-based diffusive samplers are commonly used for many types of nonreactive and moderately reactive compounds. However, decomposition, polymerization, and irreversible adsorption are seen for very reactive compounds adsorbed on charcoal. Therefore, there have been advances in development of diffusive samplers containing reagent in solutions or reagent-coated media for sampling highly reactive compounds. One example is a combination of the principles of absorption and diffusion to sample gases in a liquid medium, i.e., a passive impinger. In a typical design (see Figure 6.5), a cassette contains a liquid that is covered with a gas-permeable membrane. The liquid solution used depends on the gas being sampled: a dilute acid is used for ammonia, a sodium carbonate solution for sulfur dioxide, and a buffered iodide solution for chlorine and chlorine dioxide. After the gas reacts with the solution, the analysis is carried out using ion chromatography.

Another approach is to coat a suitable reagent on a solid support (*chemosorption*). Figure 6.6 shows such a sampler. During sampling, a stable derivative is formed on the adsorbent. The derivative is solvent-desorbed and determined using gas chromatography (GC) or high-performance liquid chromatography (HPLC). For this method to work, the chemosorbent should be chemically stable, the reaction should be rapid and quantitative, and the desorption of the derivative should be quantitative. This approach has been effectively used for sampling reactive aldehydes such as formaldehyde, acrolein, glutaraldehyde, and acetaldehyde. For sampling formaldehyde, the reagent of choice is 2,4-dinitrophenylhydrazine (DNPH). The reaction

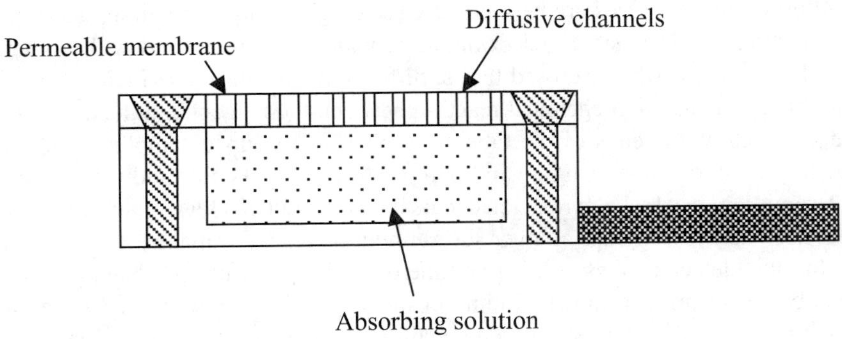

FIGURE 6.5 Diffusive sampler for liquid collection media.

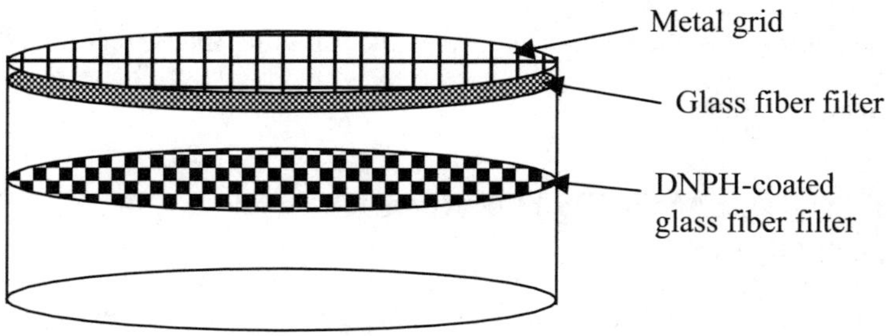

FIGURE 6.6 Diffusive sampler for reactive compounds such as formaldehyde.

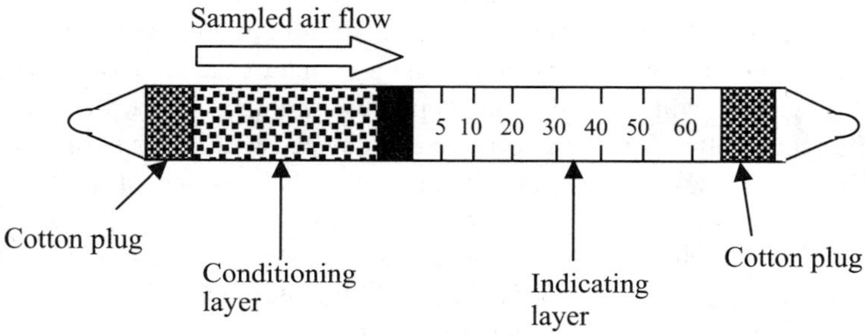

FIGURE 6.7 Length of stain colorimetric detector tube.

between formaldehyde and DNPH is rapid and quantitative. The hydrazone that is formed during the chemical reaction can be readily analyzed using HPLC.

6.7 DETECTOR TUBES

Detector tubes are used for detecting toxic gases in hazardous waste sites, measuring leaks and spills, grab sampling for screening purposes, and occasionally for personal monitoring. Such devices are hermetically sealed glass tubes containing inert granular material, such as silica gel or alumina, which is impregnated with a reagent that changes color when exposed to a specific contaminant in air (Figure 6.7). The color change is due to a chemical reaction between the reagent and the air contaminant. Typically, the ends of the tube are broken just prior to sampling, and air is drawn through the tube using a hand pump. Most detectors are used for short-term grab sampling, in which the reaction occurs over a period of a few minutes. However, detectors capable of sampling over several hours are also available.

In most detector tubes, a fixed volume of air is drawn using a hand pump that is calibrated to draw a known volume of air per stroke (Figure 6.8). As the air is drawn into the tube, the length of the stain or color change is proportional to the concentration of the air contaminant. A scale is marked on the tube to read out the length of the stain for a given number of pump strokes. The unit of the scale readout is *concentration-pump strokes,* and the scale reading is then divided by the number of pump strokes used to obtain the concentration. Thus, if it takes 10 pump strokes to reach an indicated length of stain of 1000 ppm-strokes, then the concentration in

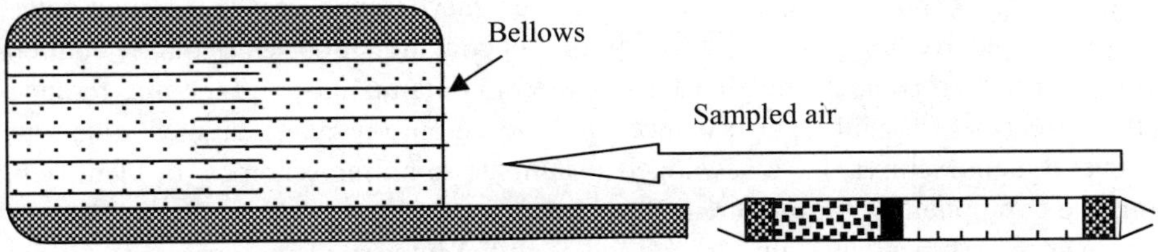

FIGURE 6.8 Hand pump (bellows type) with detector tube.

the sampled air is 100 ppm. Other scales have readouts in units of millimeters, and a conversion chart is used to convert the length of the stain into concentration. In another variation, the intensity of the color change is proportional to the air concentration. The color attained for a given number of pump strokes is compared with a reference standard tube or color chart to estimate the concentration.

Many detector tubes have a conditioning layer that helps improve the sensitivity and specificity of the instrument. The conditioning layer removes moisture and other chemicals that might interfere with the chemical reaction of interest. It might also react with the contaminant of interest that is not very reactive, to produce an intermediate compound that produces a color change more readily in the indicating layer of the detector tube. Often, an entire tube is used for preconditioning, and the gas passes through it before moving into the indicator tube.

A wide variety of detector tubes are available, and the appropriate tube should be selected on the basis of the chemical as well as the range of concentration expected in the environment. The instructions for each tube are also highly specific, and a proper sequence of events needs to be followed in order for the chemical reaction to occur correctly. Because the tubes operate by chemical reaction, temperature and humidity are important factors that affect their operation. These affect the rate of reaction, and if the tubes are used in conditions beyond those specified by the manufacturer, then appropriate corrections need to be made to the measurements. The chemical reactions are also prone to interference by other contaminants in the air, i.e., the same detector tube may react with more than one chemical, causing very similar color changes. This might cause an over- or underestimate of the true air concentration of the contaminant.

Two types of hand pumps are available for use with detector tubes — piston pumps and bellows pumps. The hand pumps that are used with the tubes are highly specific to each kind of tube, and, unfortunately, one type or even brand of pump cannot be replaced with another without errors in measurement. In addition, the flow rate may not be constant while drawing air through the pump, with higher flow rates at the beginning of the stroke and lower flow rates toward the end. This might lead to inaccurate concentration estimates. However, several brands have orifices to maintain constant flow rate. Some pumps have a mark that indicates the volume drawn when the piston is pulled up to a certain mark, as well as stroke counters. Most pumps draw a nominal volume of 100 ml per stroke, with the capability to draw partial strokes.

Detector tubes are used primarily for grab sampling for qualitative and quantitative estimation of air contaminants in occupational settings. Common uses include monitoring of spill sites, hazardous waste sites, inaccessible sites (e.g., pits); detection of explosive hazards; and detection of soil contamination with volatile contaminants. Frequently, such sites have a mixture of contaminants, and the interferences that affect detector tube performance prove to be an advantage in such situations. Several manufacturers have developed systematic sampling schemes for identifying all the components of a mixture.

Detector tubes have also been used for time-integrated measurements over a period of 4 to 8 h. Personal sampling pumps are used with the tubes to obtain a time-weighted average value over the sampling interval. Both area and personal samples can be obtained using this method.

6.8 ACCURACY OF GAS AND VAPOR SAMPLING METHODS

Several standards-setting bodies have developed criteria of acceptance for gas and vapor samplers. When a new method is developed for sampling, it needs to be tested and evaluated to ensure that the data collected provide precise and accurate results with low bias. The accuracy of different sampling methods is obtained experimentally. A key requirement in method evaluation is to have the samples collected from an environment that is as close as possible to actual sampling conditions. The concentrations of the generated atmosphere should be verified using a reference method. The precision and bias of the method should be homogeneous over the range of concentrations tested. Sampler results of analytical recovery, experiments involving measuring concentrations at 0.1, 1.0, and 2.0 times the exposure limit value, sample stability data, and other factors are used in estimating the method precision. Method bias is also estimated from these experiments. The knowledge of method precision and bias are used together to estimate method accuracy. NIOSH recommends that samplers produce results of ± 25% for 95% of the samples tested in the range of 0.1 to 2 times the occupational standard, and the bias should be less than 10%.

Most charcoal tube samplers have an accuracy of ±10 to ±15%. Diffusive samplers are not significantly different from active tube samplers and have accuracies in the range of ±10 to ±15%. Detector tubes need to meet a slightly different set of criteria for NIOSH certification. For concentrations above the permissible exposure limit (PEL), an accuracy of ±25% is required; for concentrations between 50% and 100% of the PEL, an accuracy of ±35% is required; and for lower concentrations, an accuracy of ±50% is needed. Detector tubes have much lower accuracies than charcoal tubes or diffusive monitors, and these range from ±25 to ±50%. It is recommended that the measurements be presented as a range rather than a single number.

7 Analytical Methods for Gases and Vapors: Gas Chromatography and Mass Spectroscopy

7.1 INTRODUCTION

After a gas or vapor sample has been collected on a sorbent surface, it is extracted by desorption using a solvent such as carbon disulfide. The sample is then analyzed using one of several methods to quantify the contaminant concentrations in the sample. This chapter describes two of the more common methods used for analyzing air samples obtained in occupational environments.

7.2 GAS CHROMATOGRAPHY

Few methods for chemical analysis are truly specific. Therefore, the separation of the contaminant of interest from other potential interferences is a critical first step in many analytical procedures. The most common method to separate the components of a mixture of chemicals is *chromatography*. Although the term encompasses a wide variety of techniques used for separation, all of them make use of a *stationary phase* and a *mobile phase*. In *gas chromatography*, the components of the mixture are carried through the stationary phase (solid or liquid) by the flow of a gas, which is the mobile phase. The different components migrate at different rates. The stronger the interaction between the compound in the gas phase and the stationary phase, the stronger is the retardation of its movement through the column. Thus, each component gets separated out according to its characteristic retention time. The separated substances are subsequently detected as a function of time as the gas leaves the column. In *gas–liquid chromatography*, the gas moves through glass capillary columns or packed solid material that is coated with a liquid, and the interaction between the two phases is essentially a partitioning of the contaminant between the mobile and stationary (i.e., gas and liquid) phases. In *gas–solid chromatography*, the gas moves through a packed solid material and the interaction is based on adsorption. Gas–solid chromatography has limited application due to the semipermanent retention of active and polar molecules. Most of the discussion in this chapter is focused on gas–liquid chromatography.

Figure 7.1 is a pictorial representation of how a mixture of two contaminants A and B gets resolved by chromatography. The sample (the contaminant mixture

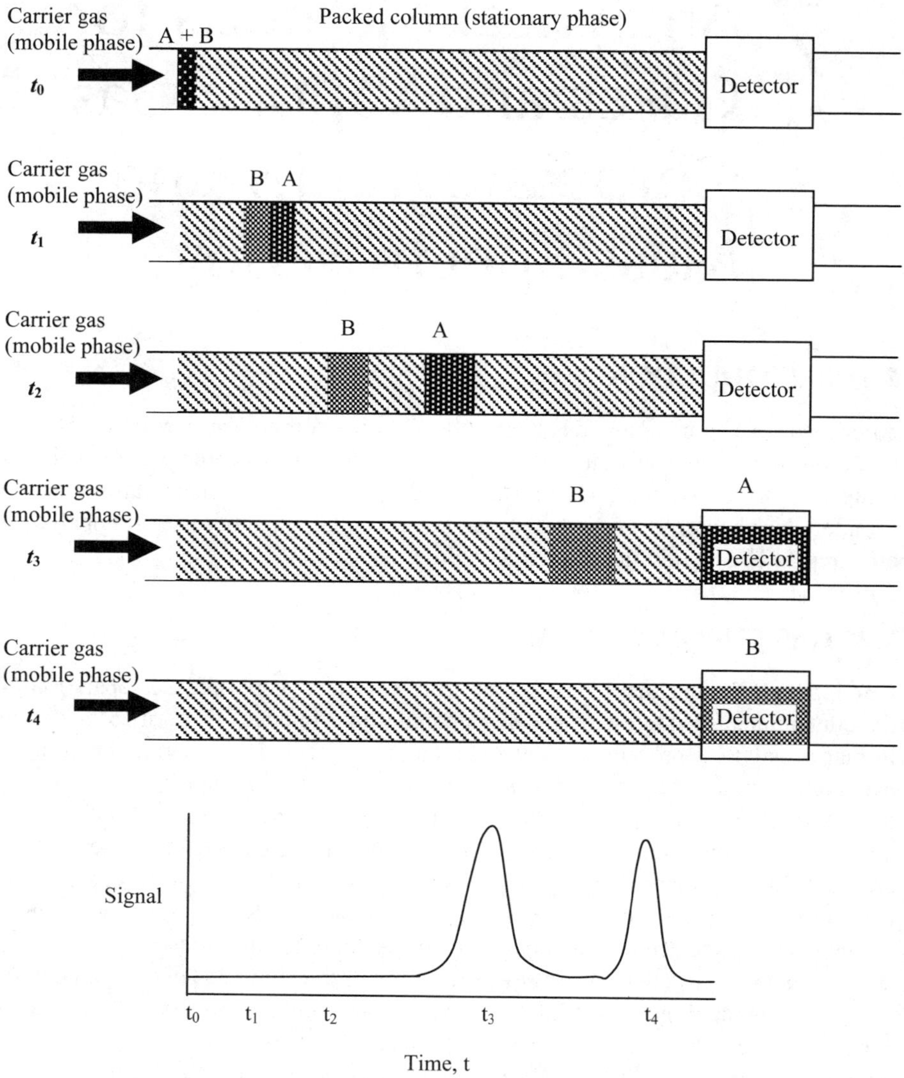

FIGURE 7.1 Pictorial representation of separation of components A and B in a mixture injected into a column of a gas chromatograph.

desorbed in a solvent) is introduced at the head of the column at time t_0. The components of the mixture distribute themselves between the mobile and stationary phases. Introduction of an additional mobile phase (carrier gas) forces the sample down the column, where further partitioning between the mobile phase and downstream portions of the stationary phase occurs (time t_1). Because the movement of the sample constituents can only occur in the mobile phase, the rate of migration of each constituent depends on the fraction of time it spends in that phase. This fraction is small for constituents with partition coefficients that favor retention in the stationary phase, and is large for constituents that favor retention in the mobile phase. Ideally, the differences in rates cause the components in a mixture to separate into bands along the length of the column (time t_2). The isolation of the separated components is achieved by passing a sufficient quantity of carrier gas through the column to force the individual components to exit out of the other end and be detected (times t_3 and t_4).

A detector that responds to the contaminants of interest is placed at the end of the column, and its signal as a function of time is obtained (bottom of Figure 7.1). This plot is called a *chromatogram*. For a given temperature and column length, each contaminant has a characteristic retention time in the column. Thus, the positions of the peaks in the chromatogram are used to identify the components of the contaminant mixture. The signal strength is proportional to the mass of each contaminant exiting the column at a given time. Therefore, the areas under the peaks are proportional to the total masses of the contaminants in the mixture injected into the gas chromatograph (GC) column. In this manner, the chromatogram identifies each contaminant and quantifies its amount.

7.2.1 Calibration Standards

A series of solutions of known concentrations is prepared and injected into the GC column. Chromatograms for the standards are obtained, and the peak heights or areas are determined as a function of the concentration for each component. These are the calibration curves for the GC, and further analysis of an unknown sample is based on these curves. Injection of the standard solutions can introduce errors in the amount of volume injected. This is especially true when the mixture is injected into a heated inlet, where evaporation from the needle tip can cause substantial variability in the volume injected. Most high-performance GCs avoid this problem by using internal standards that are not injected from the outside.

7.2.2 Resolution

This term denotes the ability of the column to completely separate the components of a mixture (see Figure 7.2). Because the components travel through the column

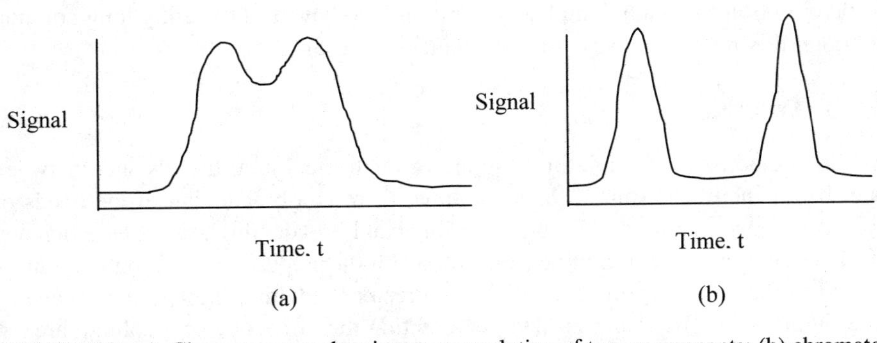

FIGURE 7.2 (a). Chromatogram showing poor resolution of two components; (b) chromatogram showing good resolution of two components.

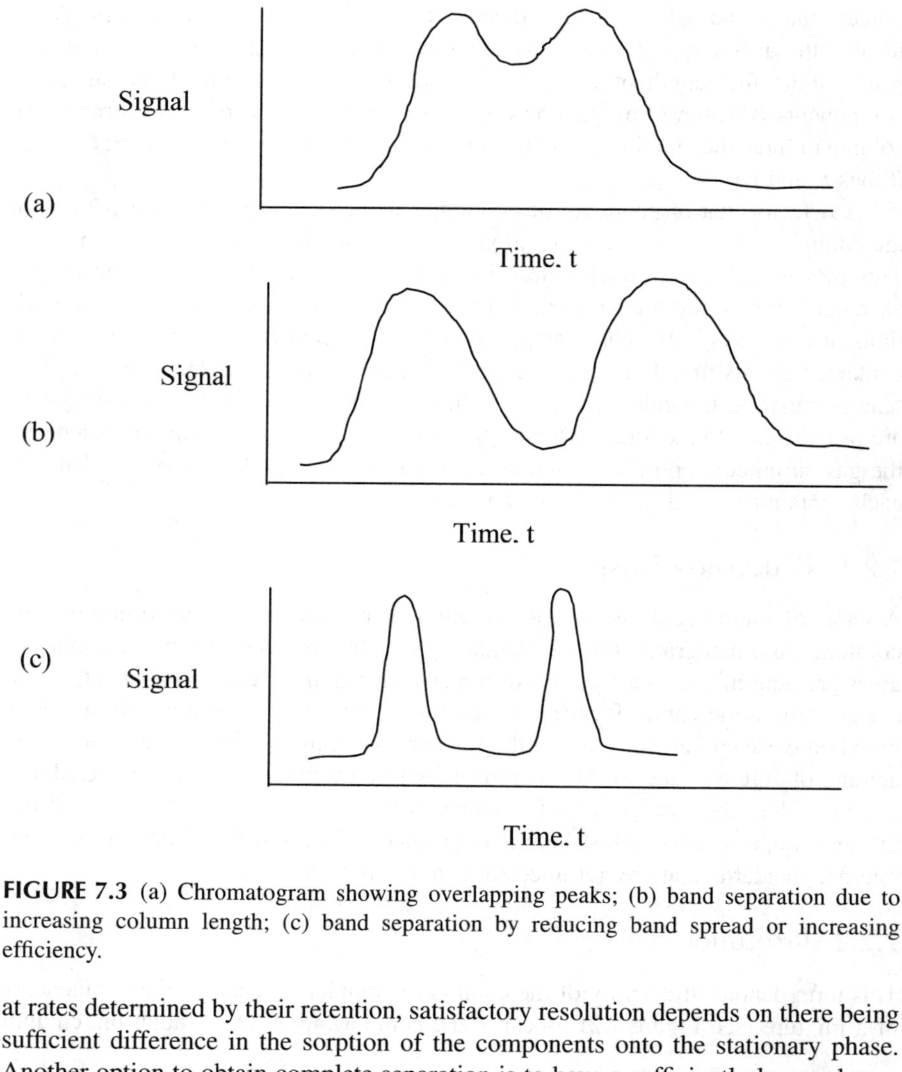

FIGURE 7.3 (a) Chromatogram showing overlapping peaks; (b) band separation due to increasing column length; (c) band separation by reducing band spread or increasing efficiency.

at rates determined by their retention, satisfactory resolution depends on there being sufficient difference in the sorption of the components onto the stationary phase. Another option to obtain complete separation is to have a sufficiently long column, although this may not always be feasible (see Figure 7.3).

7.2.3 Efficiency

As the components of a mixture migrate through a column, the distance between their bands increases. But, at the same time, there is a broadening of the bands of each component, as seen in Figure 7.1. This band broadening lowers the efficiency of the column as a separation device. The width of the peaks in a chromatogram is related to the efficiency of separation; the greater the width, the less the efficiency (see Figure 7.3). The important factors affecting the efficiency of a column are:

1. Particle sizing of the solid support material: The finer the particles, the greater the specific surface area and the smaller the width of each band.
2. Thickness of the stationary liquid phase: The smaller the thickness, the better the efficiency.
3. Uniformity of packing: More uniformity leads to better separation.
4. Carrier gas velocity: Plots of band thickness vs. velocity show a minimum at which maximum separation is achieved.

7.2.4 Components of a Gas–Liquid Chromatograph

Figure 7.4 shows the basic components of a gas–liquid chromatograph, which include a means for injecting the sample, a column for separating the components of the sample, and a detector.

The *carrier gas* needs to be chemically inert, and typically helium, hydrogen, nitrogen, or argon is used. The choice of the gas depends on the type of detector used. The flow rates are controlled by a pressure regulator and range between 25 to 200 ml/min. The flow rates are measured using a highly precise and accurate flow meter such as a soap bubble meter.

The *sample injection system* is typically heated to prevent condensation of low volatility compounds at low temperatures. The sample should be rapidly introduced as a small plug of vapor. A slow injection will cause the sample to spread out over a greater length in the column, resulting in poor separation of the components. A

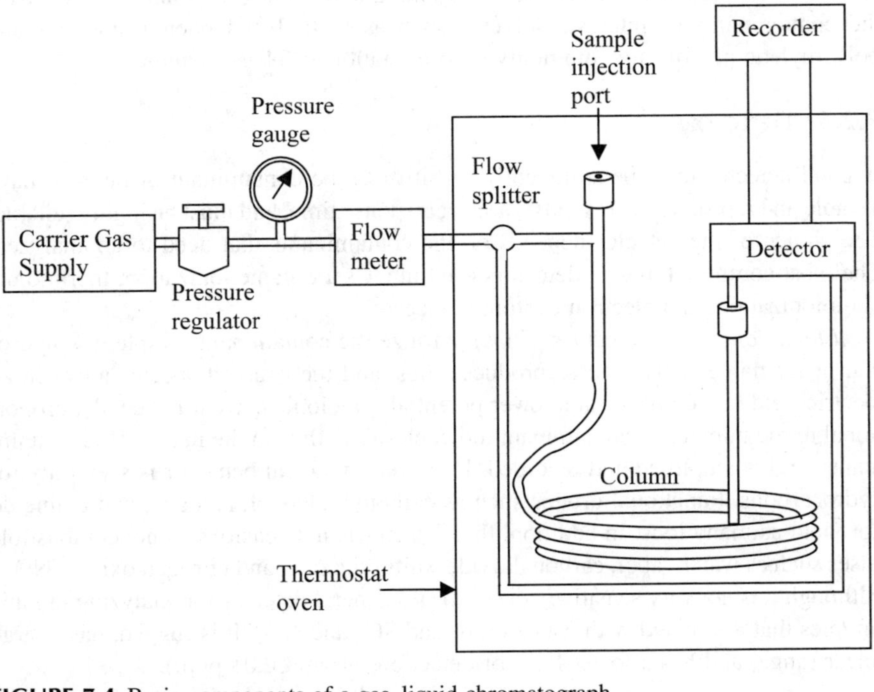

FIGURE 7.4 Basic components of a gas–liquid chromatograph.

syringe is used to inject liquid samples into a port at the head of the column. The port is heated to ~50°C above the boiling point of the least volatile component of the sample. Sample volumes range from ~0.1 µl to 25 µl. Column temperature is controlled to a high degree of precision, and is changed according to the boiling point of the sample and the degree of separation required.

The columns are made of coiled metal tubes with diameters less than 5 mm and lengths of up to 5 m. *Packed columns* contain a fine inert solid material (the support phase), which is coated with a known volume of a nonvolatile liquid (the stationary or liquid phase). The purpose of the support material is to provide a large surface area for the mobile phase, and typical surface areas are 1 to 10 m^2/g. Commonly used support materials are sand (silica), Teflon, glass beads, and diatomaceous earth (e.g., Chromosorb). As mentioned earlier, the smaller the size of the particles, the greater the efficiency of the column. This increased efficiency comes at the cost of a greater pressure drop across the column to maintain a given carrier gas flow rate. Typical particle sizes range from 150 µm to 250 µm. The narrower the size distribution of the particles, the greater the efficiency of the column. In *capillary columns*, the liquid is coated on glass or silica tubes. Capillary columns have much better ability to separate the components of a mixture than packed columns, although they can accommodate only rather small sample volumes and have a tendency to get clogged.

The *stationary phase* is a liquid that (1) has low volatility, i.e., having a boiling point that is much higher than the maximum operating temperature for the column, (2) has thermal stability, (3) is chemically inert, and (4) has sufficient selectivity for the contaminants of interest. Solvents such as methyl and phenyl silicones and polyethylene glycols are commonly used as stationary-phase liquids.

7.2.5 Detectors

A good detector must be sufficiently sensitive to the contaminant of interest, have a stable and reproducible response, a short response time, and must be highly reliable. The choice of the detector depends on the contaminants that need to be analyzed. The most common types of detectors used in GCs are flame ionization, thermionic, photoionization, and electron capture devices.

Flame ionization detectors (FIDs) pyrolize the contaminant sample in a hydrogen or air flame. This process produces ions, and the charged species move in an electric field to a collector at a lower potential. The ionic current is, ideally, proportional to the number of contaminant molecules (and thus to the mass of the contaminant), and is amplified and recorded. However, this ideal behavior is seen only for hydrocarbons. Functional groups such as carbonyl, alcohol, halogen, and amine do not yield as many ions. In addition, this detector is not sensitive to noncombustible gases such as water vapor, carbon dioxide, sulfur dioxide, and nitrogen oxides (NO_x). Although it is not very sensitive, it is used as a general detector for analyzing organic samples that are mixed with water vapor and SO_x and NO_x. It is rugged, has a large linear range, and has a lower limit of detection (around 0.01 ppm).

Thermionic detectors pass the hydrogen and the sample along with excess air through a flame tip assembly similar to that in a flame ionization detector, and then around a rubidium silicate bead that is heated to ~ 800°C. This produces a large number of ions, which are then detected as in FIDs. Thermionic detectors are used for analyzing organic compounds containing phosphorus and nitrogen. Their response to a phosphorus or nitrogen atom is roughly 10^4 to 10^6 times greater than their response to a carbon atom, and they are much more sensitive than FIDs to these compounds.

Photoionization detectors (PIDs) contain a UV light source that emits photons of sufficient energy to ionize the contaminant molecules. The ionic current moves toward a collector electrode where the current is amplified and recorded. The current is proportional to the number of contaminant molecules. PIDs are commonly used for detecting aromatic compounds. Other compounds that are easily detectable are aliphatics, halogenated hydrocarbons, and hydrogen sulfide. PIDs are also rugged devices with a large linear range and have lower limits of detection that are in the ppb range.

Electron capture detectors (ECDs) use a β-emitter such as ^{63}Ni or tritium to generate a stream of electrons. These electrons cause ionization of the carrier gas (e.g., nitrogen) and the production of more electrons, and a constant current is maintained between the electrodes. When there are electron-capturing contaminant molecules in the carrier gas stream, however, this current decreases, and the decrease in current intensity is related to the concentration of the contaminant molecules. By their nature, ECDs are highly sensitive and selective toward molecules of halogens, peroxides, and nitro groups. They are insensitive to amines, alcohols, and hydrocarbons. They have relatively low detection limits that are in the ppb range.

7.3 MASS SPECTROMETRY (MS)

In this analytical method, the molecules of the sample are bombarded with ions or electrons. This collision results in the sample molecules being fragmented into a number of smaller charged particles, each with its own characteristic mass-to-charge (*M/e*) ratio. A mass analyzer separates the charged particles on the basis of their *M/e* ratios. This pattern of fragmentation, called a *mass spectrum,* is characteristic for each molecule, and is used for identifying the parent molecule or atom. MS provides qualitative and quantitative information on both the atomic and molecular composition of organic and inorganic chemicals. Over the last several decades, it has been increasingly used as a detector for gas chromatography.

Figure 7.5 shows the basic components of a mass spectrometer. Because this method is crucially dependent on the interaction between electrons and the sample molecules, a characteristic feature of MS is the need to maintain very low pressures (10^4 to 10^5 mm Hg) in all the components. A very small quantity of the sample is injected into the source chamber. The molecules of the sample are ionized and fragmented by collision with a stream of electrons or ions. The positive ions are separated from the negative ions by a large negative potential that attracts the positive ions through a slit.

Conversely, one might use a positive potential to attract negative ions toward a slit. The ions are then accelerated to a high enough velocity and led into the mass analyzer. The mass analyzer most commonly uses a magnetic field to separate the

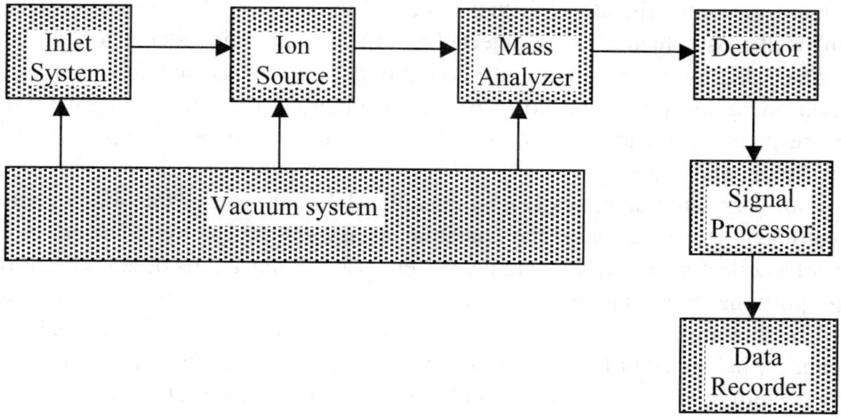

FIGURE 7.5 Basic components of a mass spectrometer.

components. When a magnetic field is applied to a charged particle, the ion is deflected from its original path and moves in a circular arc. The radius of this arc is dependent on the strength of the magnetic field and, most importantly, on the particle's *M/e* ratio. Once the particles are separated, they are directed toward a collecting electrode. The resulting ion current is amplified and recorded as a function of time.

7.3.1 Inlet Systems

Although there are several methods of introducing the sample into the ion source, the two most common methods are the *batch inlet* and the *gas chromatographic inlet*. In the batch inlet, the sample is volatilized externally and then allowed to leak into the ionization region that is under high vacuum. A small measured volume of the gas or vapor is expanded into a reservoir that is maintained at an elevated temperature to prevent condensation of the vapor. The sample is then leaked into the ionization chamber by means of a glass or metal diaphragm containing several very small pinholes.

Because the amount of sample mass needed for chromatography is roughly the same as that for MS (~1 μmole), the gas sample exiting a GC column is an ideal source for the mass spectrometer. Chromatographic inlet systems interface a GC with a mass spectrometer. A major problem arises because of the presence of the GC carrier gas, which overwhelms the vacuum pumping system of the spectrometer. The inlet system, therefore, forces the exit gases from the GC into a glass jet, which increases the momentum of the gas molecules. From the jet nozzle, the heavier contaminant molecules travel in a straight line toward the inlet of the MS ion source. The lighter carrier gas molecules (e.g., helium) are deflected from the straight path due to an applied vacuum (see Figure 7.6). The flow rates in GC columns are small enough that direct coupling of the GC and MS is feasible.

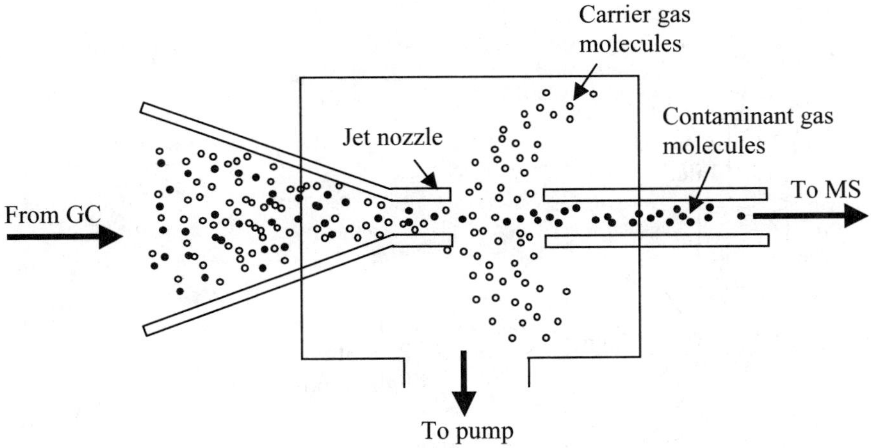

FIGURE 7.6 Interface between gas chromatograph column and mass spectrometer. [Skoog, 1985].

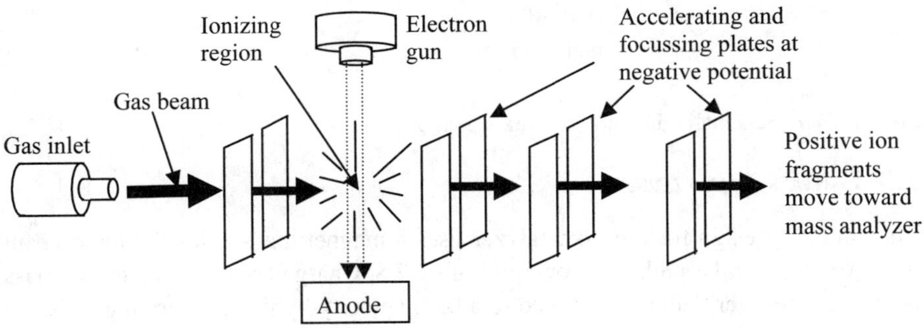

FIGURE 7.7 Schematic diagram of an electron gun ion source.

7.3.2 Ion Sources

The classic method for producing ions for bombardment of the sample is to use an electron gun. The electrons are produced by a heated tungsten wire and accelerated toward an anode by an electric potential. The electrons run into the sample molecules that are diffusing through a pinhole into the ionization chamber. The collision between the electrons and the sample molecules produces both positive and negative ions. The positive ions are accelerated to a high velocity by a series of plates that have progressively larger negative potentials.

Figure 7.7 shows a schematic diagram of an electron gun ion source. Other designs are being commonly used for generating ions, such as field ionization, chemical ionization, and fast atom bombardment sources.

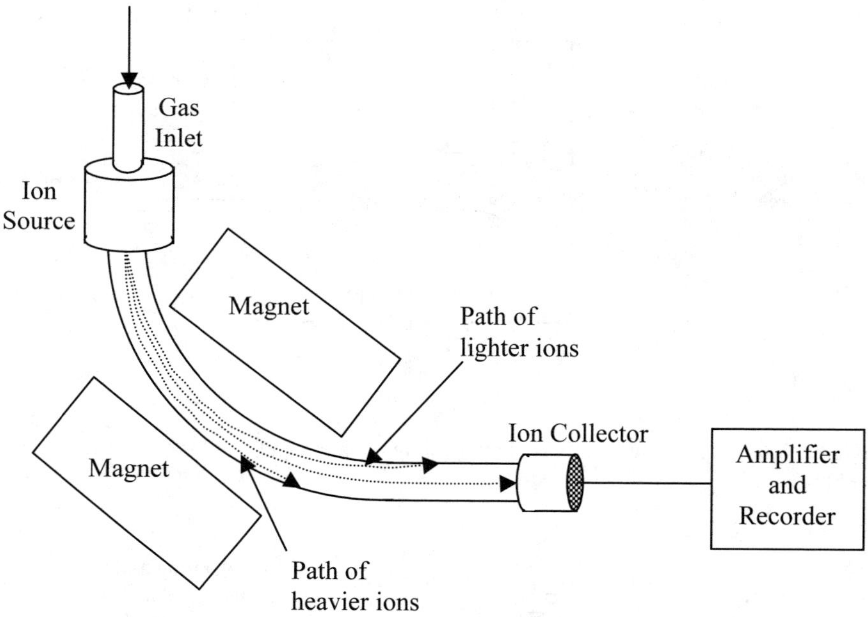

FIGURE 7.8 Schematic diagram of a mass analyzer.

7.3.3 Mass Analyzers

The simplest design for a mass analyzer uses a magnet that causes the ionic beam to move in a circular path, as shown in Figure 7.8. Charged particles enter the mass analyzer tube after being accelerated to a high velocity by the accelerating plates in the ion source. A particle of mass M and charge e, when acted upon by an electric potential V, will have an energy E and velocity v, where

$$E = eV = \frac{1}{2}Mv^2 \tag{7.1}$$

The analyzer tube is maintained at a very low pressure (~ 10^{-7} mm Hg), and has a circular arc section. The particles entering this section are acted upon by the magnetic field H, which pulls the particles inward, and by the centrifugal force acting outward. For a particle to traverse the centerline of the circular section to the ion detector, the magnetic force must equal the centrifugal force. Thus,

$$H\,e\,v = \frac{M\,v^2}{r} \tag{7.2}$$

From Equation 7.1 and Equation 7.2, we obtain

$$\frac{M}{e} = \frac{H^2 r^2}{2V} \tag{7.3}$$

From Equation 7.3, we see that *M/e* can be varied by changing either *H* or *V* (for an analyzer that has a given radius *r*). Most spectrometers vary the magnetic field strength, *H*, while keeping *V* constant to sequentially select ions with desired *M/e* ratios to move along the circular arc and reach the detector.

The above is by no means the only design used for mass separation. Older spectrometer models kept *H* and *V* constant, and the ions were directed toward a photographic plate. The positions where the ions hit the photographic plate were related to the radii of the circular paths taken by particles of different *M/e* ratios. Other designs employ double focusing, quadrupole analyzers, and time-of-flight analyzers. A discussion of these designs is outside the scope of this chapter.

7.3.4 Ion Collectors

Most modern mass spectrometers utilize an electron multiplier for detection. The positive ions from the analyzer are accelerated by a potential difference and fall on the first plate of the multiplier. The plate, made of a metal alloy, emits two electrons for every ion striking it. These electrons are accelerated to the next plate by a potential difference. After 20 to 25 stages, an amplification of 2^{20} to 2^{25} (10^7 to 10^8) is obtained.

The output from the ion collector and amplifier is sent to a recorder that produces a mass spectrum such as the one shown in Figure 7.9.

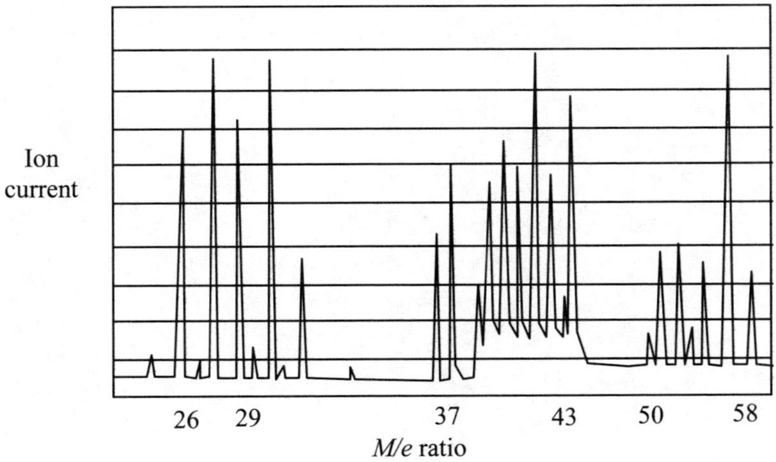

FIGURE 7.9 Mass spectrum for *n*-butane.

7.3.5 Resolution

An ideal mass analyzer should be able to differentiate between very small mass-to-charge ratios while still allowing a sufficiently large number of ions to pass through to produce a measurable ion current. However, these two criteria are often at odds with each other. For example, if the ions are classified into very narrow bins, then the number of ions per bin would be very small, leading to a small ionic current. The ability of a mass spectrometer to distinguish between *M/e* ratios is called its *resolution* and is defined as $\frac{(M/e)}{\Delta(M/e)}$, where *M/e* and $(M/e + \Delta(M/e))$ are the mass-to-charge ratios of two particles that give just-separable peaks. Two peaks are considered distinguishable if the height of the valley between them is less than 10% of the height of the peaks. The resolution needed depends upon the particular application. If we need to discriminate between particles that differ from each other by a tenth or a hundredth of a molecular mass number, then we would need a resolution of several thousand. However, particles differing from each other by one molecular mass number or more can be differentiated with a resolution of 50 to 100. For most organic samples, a resolution of 200 to 500 is more than adequate.

8 Direct Reading Instruments for Gases and Vapors

8.1 INTRODUCTION

As the name suggests, direct reading instruments provide a measurement of the gas or vapor property, usually the concentration, very quickly (within a few seconds or minutes after sampling). As such, they find use in a wide variety of applications in occupational hygiene, ranging from detecting leaks of hazardous vapors in workplaces to checking the performance of control equipment to assessing worker exposures in workplaces. Because they provide readings in near-real time, they are very useful in determining concentrations over very short time intervals and in assessing whether short-term exposure limits (STELs) are being exceeded. Thus, they can be used for personal as well as area monitoring. For the purposes of this chapter, we will classify real-time instruments into several categories: (1) instruments based on absorption or emission of electromagnetic radiation by gases and vapors, (2) instruments based on the electrochemical properties of gases and vapors, and (3) instruments based on the thermal properties of gases and vapors.

8.2 INSTRUMENTS BASED ON ABSORPTION OR EMISSION OF ELECTROMAGNETIC RADIATION

The electromagnetic spectrum can be divided into several regions, as shown in Figure 8.1. These divisions are somewhat artificial in that they are based on technological methods used for detecting specific regions of the spectrum. Fundamentally, all electromagnetic radiation travels at the same speed, c, also called the speed of light, which is 2.997×10^8 m/sec. The radiation is characterized by its wavelength, λ, or its frequency, ν, where

$$c = \nu\lambda \tag{8.1}$$

Quantum theory tells us that atoms and molecules have only a limited number of discrete energy levels. So, when radiation passes through a region of a gas (or any phase of matter), for absorption of radiation to occur, the energy of the radiation must be exactly equal to the difference between the ground state and one of the excited states of the gaseous species. These energy differences are unique for each chemical, and a study of the wavelengths of absorbed radiation provides a method

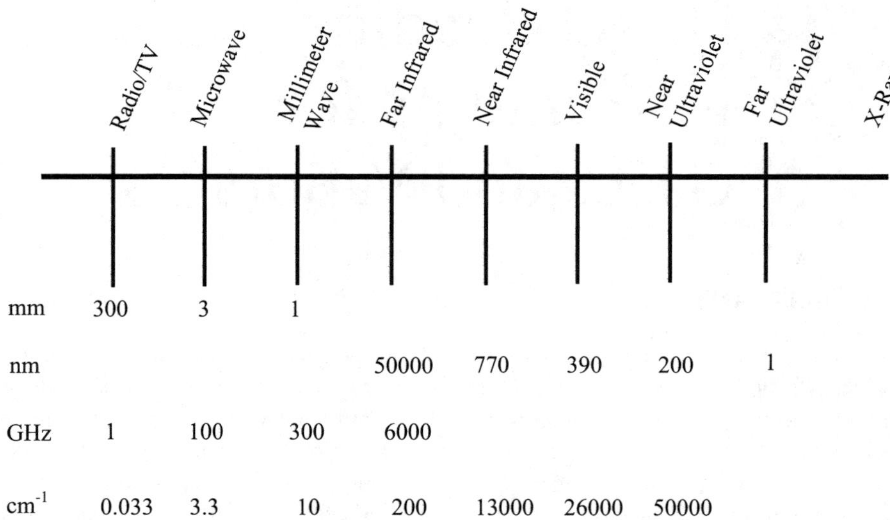

FIGURE 8.1 The electromagnetic spectrum.

of characterizing the constituents of a sample. In spectroscopy, we take advantage of the fact that molecules absorb and emit radiation at specific wavelengths. Using this information, we can determine the presence of various gases and vapors in a sample, as well as their concentrations.

The energy of radiation, E (of photons), is related to its frequency, ν, by the well-known equation

$$E = \mathrm{h}\,\nu \tag{8.2}$$

where h is Planck's constant (6.63×10^{-34} J sec).

The energy of an atom, molecule, or ion is described as

$$E = E_{\mathrm{electronic}} + E_{\mathrm{vibrational}} + E_{\mathrm{rotational}} \tag{8.3}$$

where $E_{\mathrm{electronic}}$ describes the electronic energy of the species, $E_{\mathrm{vibrational}}$ is the energy resulting from the various atomic vibrations, and $E_{\mathrm{rotational}}$ is due to the energy associated with the rotation of the molecule about its center of gravity. For each electronic energy state of the molecule, there are several possible vibrational energy states, and, for each of these, there are several rotational energy states, as shown in Figure 8.2.

As we can see from Figure 8.2, the transitions between electronic energy states require a large amount of energy (which is provided by higher frequency ultraviolet, visible, or x-ray radiation) that is used for atomic absorption spectroscopy. In comparison, the transitions between the vibrational energy states require much less energy (lower by 1 to 2 orders of magnitude), which can be provided by infrared wavelengths in infrared spectroscopy. Rotational spectra for gases are seen in the microwave region of the spectrum.

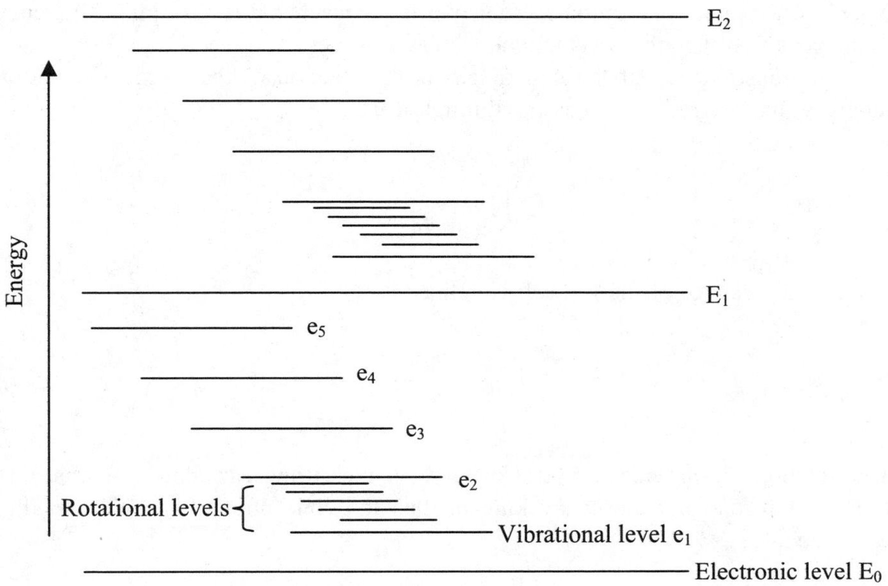

FIGURE 8.2 Energy level diagram for a hypothetical molecule.

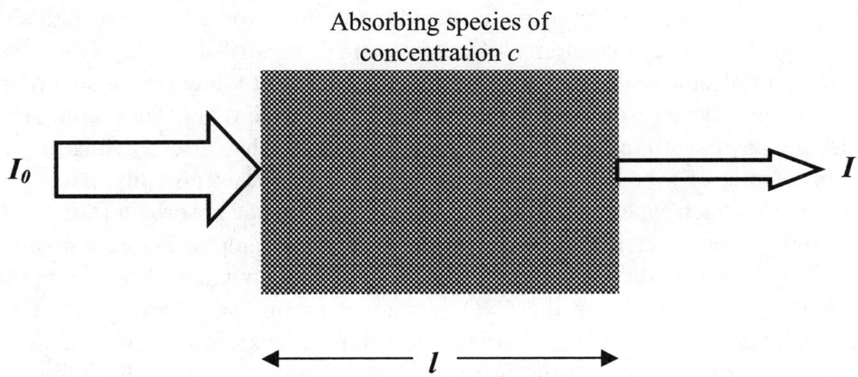

FIGURE 8.3 Attenuation of a beam of radiation by an absorbing gas.

8.2.1 Lambert–Beer Law

Figure 8.3 shows a beam of electromagnetic radiation passing through a region of space of thickness l, containing a gas whose concentration is c. The molecules of the gas absorb some of the radiation, and as a result the intensity of the beam is reduced, or attenuated, from I_0 to I. The relationship between the incident and emergent intensities is given by the Lambert–Beer law,

$$I = I_0 \exp(-\varepsilon c l) \tag{8.4}$$

where ε is the molar absorption coefficient. ε is a measure of the absorption efficiency at the peak wavelength and is unique for each species.

The transmittance of the cell of gas is the fraction of the incident radiation intensity that emerges after passing through it, i.e.,

$$T = \frac{I}{I_0} \tag{8.5}$$

The absorbance of the gas cell is defined as

$$A = \log\left(\frac{I_0}{I}\right) = \varepsilon c l \tag{8.6}$$

This relationship provides a useful method for measuring gas concentrations. If A is measured, and if l and ε are known, then the concentration c can be readily calculated.

8.2.2 Infrared Spectrophotometers

As mentioned earlier, infrared spectroscopy makes use of the transitions in the vibrational energy of atoms of molecules due to absorption of infrared radiation ($\lambda = 10^3$ to 10^6 nm). A two-atom molecule is capable only of stretching vibrations, whereas a molecule with three or more atoms can exhibit vibrations of subgroups of atoms, which may also bend and twist relative to each other. Thus, a complex molecule may absorb radiation at a number of wavelengths corresponding to each possible mode of vibration of the molecule. In practical terms, this means, for instance, that each functional group in organic compounds absorbs infrared radiation over a very specific range of wavelengths. For example, Figure 8.4 shows the infrared absorption spectrum of acetone in the vapor phase. The absorption bands due to the C–H and the C=O functional groups are clearly seen. Each chemical, therefore, has a characteristic spectrum. An unknown species can therefore be identified by comparing its absorption spectrum pattern with a library of thousands of such spectra.

The *infrared radiation source* is commonly an inert solid heated to a high temperature so that it emits radiation akin to a black body. Typically, a tightly wound spiral of nichrome wire is heated to 1100 K by passing electrical current through it. An ordinary tungsten filament lamp is another convenient source that emits infrared radiation over a broad range of wavelengths (0.78 to 2.5 μm).

A *wavelength selector* or *monochromator* is used to pick the wavelength of radiation that is transmitted through the gas sample. The wavelength selector can be *dispersive* or *nondispersive*. Dispersive devices use prisms or gratings to disperse the infrared radiation into its component wavelengths (much as a beam of visible white light is dispersed into the colors of the rainbow after passing through a glass

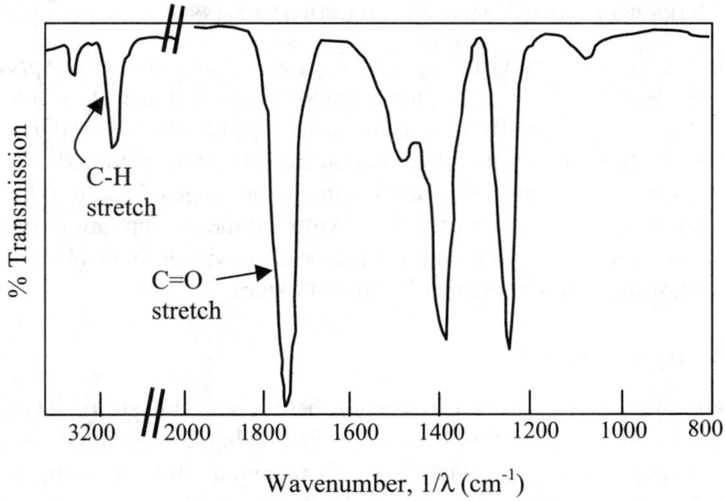

FIGURE 8.4 Infrared absorption spectrum of acetone (2-propanone).

prism). A slit is then used to select the desired region of the wavelength spectrum created by the prism, and that radiation is transmitted to the gas cell and then on to the light detector. The width of the slit is an important parameter that defines the selectivity of the instrument. Nondispersive devices use interference filters for the identification of specific contaminants, or filter wedges or wheels that provide narrow and continuously variable bands of infrared radiation. This provides for great flexibility in analyzing a wide variety of compounds using customized filters.

The radiation then passes through the *gas cell*, which may have a fixed or a variable path length. From the Lambert–Beer law, it is clear that a longer path length will enable the detection of lower concentrations of a contaminant, i.e., a longer path length leads to greater sensitivity. Some well-known infrared analyzers such as the MIRANs (miniature infrared analyzers) have path lengths that can be varied over more than an order of magnitude, and can detect concentrations as low as 1 to 5 ppm. The gas contaminant is drawn into the cell by means of a pump that samples at a constant flow rate.

The primary drawback of such instruments is that at most infrared wavelengths, several contaminants absorb radiation. Thus, analyzing mixtures of chemicals by using this technique can be problematic. If a unique wavelength is not chosen for each chemical in the mixture, then the concentration of each chemical may be overestimated. Similarly, even while analyzing single compounds, we need to assure ourselves that any potentially interfering chemicals are absent in the environment being sampled. The presence of interfering compounds could lead to a measured concentration being higher than the true concentration. Water vapor and carbon dioxide are ubiquitous and absorb over a wide range of infrared wavelengths. Thus, they need to be removed from the gas sample or minimized prior to analysis.

8.2.3 Ultraviolet and Visible Spectrophotometers

In principle, ultraviolet and visible spectroscopy are similar to infrared spectroscopy in that they depend on electromagnetic radiation absorption that is governed by Lambert–Beer's law. Typically, deuterium or hydrogen lamps are used to produce a continuous spectrum in the ultraviolet region from 160 nm to around 375 nm, and xenon lamps are used to produce wavelengths in the range of 250 to 600 nm.

Ultraviolet photometers are used for monitoring the concentrations of chlorine, mercury vapors, sulfur dioxide, and ozone, whereas visible light photometers are used for measuring concentrations of nitrogen oxides.

8.2.4 Chemiluminescence

In chemiluminescence, a chemical reaction between an analyte of interest and a reagent results in a product that is in an excited or higher electronic energy state. The molecules in the excited state then emit radiation while returning to a lower energy state (ground state). The amount of energy emitted is proportional to the number of molecules of the chemical of interest. Chemiluminescence is much more sensitive and selective than absorption spectroscopy, and typical detection limits range from the ppb range to a tenth of a ppm range. However, it is less widely used than absorption spectroscopy because of the limited number of chemical reactions that produce luminescent radiation.

The instrumentation required for measuring chemiluminescence is relatively simple, and typically consists of a reaction vessel in which the contaminant gas reacts with a reagent, and a photomultiplier that converts the photons released in the process into an amplified electrical signal. Typically, the signal from a chemiluminescence reaction rises as a function of time to a maximum as the mixing of the analyte and the reagent is complete, and then exponentially decays. The signal is integrated as a function of time and compared with a standard concentration that is treated the same way.

Chemiluminescence is commonly used for measuring atmospheric pollutants such as ozone and oxides of nitrogen with great sensitivity. For example, in the determination of nitric oxide, the reactions that occur are

$$NO + O_3 \rightarrow NO_2^* + O_2$$

$$NO_2^* \rightarrow NO_2 + h\upsilon \qquad (\lambda = 600 \text{ to } 2800 \text{ nm}) \tag{8.7}$$

Ozone is generated internally in the instrument and is mixed with the atmospheric sample in a reaction vessel, where the chemiluminescence reaction is monitored using a photomultiplier tube.

Chemiluminescence is also used for detecting ozone by reacting it with ethylene (C_2H_4). The chemiluminescence reaction produces photons whose number is directly proportional to the number of ozone molecules in the sample.

8.3 INSTRUMENTS BASED ON ELECTROCHEMICAL PROPERTIES

These techniques are based on the electrical properties of a solution of the analyte when it is made part of an electrochemical cell. They can be used to establish a relationship between analyte concentration and electrical properties such as current, potential, or conductance. When an electrical voltage V is applied across the ends of a conducting medium, the current flowing through it is I, and they are related by Ohm's law

$$V = I \times R \tag{8.8}$$

where R is the resistance of the medium to the flow of current. The change in any of these three parameters can be used to relate it to the analyte concentration.

8.3.1 Conductance Devices

The *conductance*, G, of a medium is the reciprocal of its electrical resistance R (ohms). The unit of conductance is ohms^{-1} or siemens. The conductance of an electrolytic solution depends on the number of ions in the solution, their charge, and their rate of movement under an electrical field. In instruments based on electrical conductance of solutions, a gaseous sample is drawn through an aqueous solution, which results in the formation of electrolytes that change the conductance of the electrolytic solution. The electrolyte should be so chosen that the instrument is specific to a given chemical. The gas diffuses through a membrane into an electrolyte in which are immersed a cathode and an anode. These membranes are sometimes selectively permeable to some compounds and not to others. At low electrolyte concentrations, the conductance of the solution is directly proportional to the concentration of the gas.

Conductance devices are used to measure gases, such as sulfur dioxide, in the ambient environment by passing the gas through a hydrogen peroxide solution. The reaction produces H_2SO_4, which dissociates into H^+ and SO_4^{2-} ions. The change in conductivity of the solution is proportional to the number of ions in the solution, which, in turn, is proportional to the concentration of gaseous sulfur dioxide. Other instruments are used for measuring other gases that are easily oxidized or reduced, such as ammonia or hydrogen sulfide.

8.3.2 Potentiometry

The change in electrical potential in an electrochemical cell can be used for quantifying the concentration of a chemical, and this class of methods is referred to as *potentiometry*. These devices are based on the Nernst equation, which relates the electrode potential to concentration. For example, if there is a reaction between a gaseous species A and a reagent B producing a species C, so that

$$aA + bB \rightarrow cC$$

where a, b, and c are the number of moles of A, B, and C, then the Nernst equation is given by

$$E = E_0 - \frac{RT}{nF}\log\left[\frac{[C]^c}{[A]^a[B]^b}\right] \tag{8.9}$$

where E is the cell potential, E_0 the standard potential for the cell, R the gas constant, T the absolute temperature, n the number of moles of electrons associated with the oxidation–reduction process, and F the Faraday constant (96,487 Coulombs per mole).

Like conductance devices, potentiometric devices also commonly utilize a permeable membrane to selectively allow the gas of interest into the electrochemical cell. The chemical reaction between the gas and the electrolyte changes the electrical potential of the electrode, and this change in potential is related to the concentration of the gaseous species. Potentiometric devices are commonly used for detecting gases such as oxygen, hydrogen sulfide, carbon monoxide, chlorine, and a variety of combustible gases. As Equation 8.9 makes clear, such devices are very sensitive to temperature, and thus temperature needs to be controlled very precisely.

Another variation is to use the electrical current in an electrochemical cell to quantify the gas concentration. Oxygen monitors are the most common example of this class of devices. Oxygen diffuses into the cell through a permeable membrane. The oxidation–reduction reactions that then occur lead to an electrical current between the two electrodes that is proportional to the concentration of oxygen.

The previous chapter discussed sensors based on ionization of a gas sample by various means. A variety of instruments are based on flame ionization, photoionization, and electron capture. However, these will not be discussed here again.

8.4 INSTRUMENTS BASED ON THERMAL PROPERTIES

The *heat of combustion* is the most commonly used thermal property for detection of gases and vapors. The heat of combustion is the amount of energy released when a given mass of a substance undergoes complete combustion, and it is somewhat unique for a given combustible chemical. A combustible gas or vapor is passed over a filament heated above the ignition temperature of the gas. The contaminant gets ignited, and the resultant heat of combustion changes the temperature of the filament. The change in temperature is related to the change in the electrical resistance of the filament, which can be easily measured. The change in electrical resistance is related to the gas concentration using standard known gas concentrations in a calibration procedure. Although each chemical has a unique heat of combustion, the differences between the heats of combustion of similar chemicals are much smaller than the precision of the sensors. Thus, these detectors are quite nonspecific.

A variation on the above scheme is the use of catalysts to lower the temperature of combustion. The reduced temperature results in lower power consumption and increased stability of the sensor. Heated catalytic filaments (e.g., platinum or palladium filaments) are used to ignite a gas, resulting in a change in the temperature of the filament (and hence its resistance). In some instances, the choice of the catalyst may result in somewhat better selectivity for the device.

These instruments provide measurements in terms of ppm or the lower explosive limits (LELs) of combustible gases. They are commonly used in confined space surveys, industrial safety surveys, and leak monitoring. Oxygen monitors are used to alert workers to oxygen deficiency hazards, whereas other instruments are used to detect dangerous levels of various combustible gases in work areas, as well as flue gases. Catalytic heat-of-combustion instruments are used for detection of specific gases such as methane, benzene, toluene, various hydrocarbons, and carbon monoxide.

Section III

Properties and Measurement of Aerosols

9 Basic Aerosol Properties

9.1 INTRODUCTION

An *aerosol* is a suspension of solid or liquid particles in a gas. The sizes of these suspended particles range from 0.001 μm to greater than 100 μm (1 μm = 10^{-6} m). In contrast, gas molecules have sizes ranging from 0.0002 to 0.0005 μm (or 2 to 5 Å). Thus, a wide range of airborne particles is encompassed by the above definition. Naturally occurring smoke, dust, snow, mist, and clouds, as well as particles created by human activities such as cutting and grinding a solid during mining, spraying a paint, or spraying pesticides in agricultural settings are all examples of aerosols. Aerosols play a very important role in a number of areas that affect humans. Our everyday atmospheric climate is profoundly influenced by aerosols that affect the formation of clouds. Aerosols are generated in a number of basic industries such as petroleum refineries, metallurgical operations, nonmetallic mineral product industries, production and processing of chemicals, pulp and paper industries, cotton production and processing, and power plants. The aerosols generated in such industries, although essential to the useful product being manufactured, may be harmful to the workers involved in the production. In addition, aerosols are generated in indoor environments such as residential areas, schools, and offices. Activities such as cooking, vacuuming a carpet, and smoking generate different kinds of aerosols. Indoor environments also harbor biological particles such as fungi, bacteria, dander, pollens, and viruses.

Everyday usage includes a number of words that refer to different types of aerosols. *Dusts* are solid particles that are created by the disintegration of a bulk solid and range in size from less than 1 μm to greater than 100 μm. *Fumes* and *smokes* are formed from condensation of gases and vapors which result in very small primary particles which aggregate to form secondary, larger particles. However, even the secondary particles are typically less than 1 μm in size. *Mists* refer to very small liquid droplets (~1 μm) formed by condensation or atomization, whereas *sprays* refer to larger droplets (1 to 100 μm) that are created by the mechanical disintegration of a bulk liquid. To put these sizes in context, it might be helpful to realize that the diameter of the period at the end of this sentence is roughly 300 μm. Figure 9.1 shows the size ranges of different types of common aerosols found in the ambient environment as well as in occupational settings.

The size of particles plays an important role in their inhalation by humans and deposition in various regions of the respiratory tract, where they may cause adverse health effects. Figure 9.1 also shows the size ranges of particles that can be inhaled and deposited in three broadly defined regions of the respiratory tract. In this chapter and in Chapter 10 to Chapter 14, the focus is on aerosols that are encountered in occupational environments — the types of aerosols that are generated by different processes, their properties, the physical mechanisms by which they are inhaled and deposited in the respiratory tracts of human beings, and their measurement.

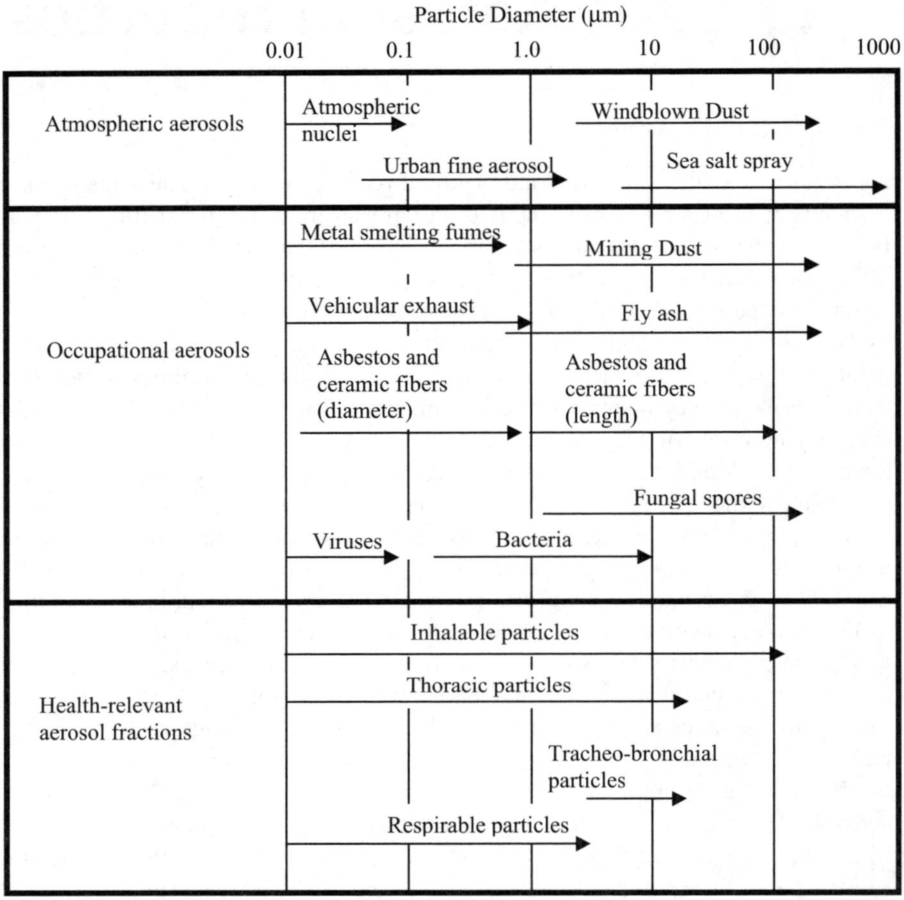

FIGURE 9.1 Types of aerosols and size ranges.

9.2 PARTICLE SHAPE AND DENSITY

As might be expected, aerosol particles come in a variety of shapes. They include well-defined geometries such as spheres (e.g., mist droplets), cylinders (e.g., fibers), and crystals, as well as irregularly shaped particles (e.g., a quartz particle). Particle shapes can be divided into several categories. *Isometric particles* have sizes that are roughly the same in all three dimensions, i.e., their length, width, and height are similar, although not equal. Most particles encountered in nature and in occupational settings are isometric. *Platelets* have two dimensions (length and width) that are much larger than the third (height). *Fibers* have one dimension (length) that is much larger than the other two (width and height), and examples include mineral fibers such as those of asbestos and ceramic. In addition, there are more complex particle shapes such as those of aggregates and agglomerates (e.g., soot particles made of smaller primary particles). For such shapes, the common ideas of geometry do not apply and one needs to invoke concepts of fractal geometry to describe their shapes.

This naturally means that a parameter such as diameter, which can aptly describe the size of one type of particle shape (e.g., a sphere), may not be appropriate for another shape (e.g., a cylinder).

Particle density is another important property that affects particle behavior. Here, particle density refers to the mass per unit volume of the material of which the particle is composed, and has units of kg/m^3.

9.3 AEROSOL GENERATION AND PROPERTIES

As mentioned above, aerosols are generated in a number of workplaces. The sizes of particles generated in a workplace depend on the types of processes underway there. For example, granite mining might involve drilling and cutting into a rock face, whereas quartz extraction processes involve additional crushing and grinding of the extracted mineral ore. Coal mining involves blasting and subsequent removal of the extracted coal. The transport of raw or intermediate industrial products, agricultural tilling, heavy construction activities, and unpaved roads act as open dust sources. These are examples of solid aerosols being generated by *mechanical* means such as cutting, breaking, fracture, abrasion, agitation, transportation, and reentrainment. Energy is supplied to a bulk material to break it into smaller pieces by overcoming the adhesive forces holding the material together. The sizes of aerosol particles and their concentration depend on the ratio of the energy being supplied and the energy of the adhesive bonds (that are specific to the material as well as ambient conditions such as humidity). Although no theoretical models for aerosol generation can encompass the wide range of such processes, empirical emission factors have been determined that estimate the amount of aerosol produced per unit activity, e.g., per unit of raw material handled. For example, the amount of nickel aerosol (oxides and sulfides) produced per ton of nickel ore processed into Bessemer matte is known because it represents a loss of nickel ore that could otherwise have been made into pure nickel. Liquid aerosols can also be generated mechanically, although in this case, the energy supplied externally is used to overcome the surface tension forces holding the bulk liquid together. Examples include atomizers for perfume bottles, nebulizers such as those in room humidifiers, and nozzle jets used for spraying paints.

Besides mechanical means, aerosols are also created by physical and chemical processes such as *nucleation*, *condensation*, and *coagulation*. These are quite common in high-temperature processes in industry, such as in coke ovens, metal ore smelters, and municipal and hazardous waste incinerators. Nucleation refers to the transfer of molecules from the gas phase to the solid or liquid phase. In heterogeneous nucleation, the molecules of a vapor condense onto extremely small preexisting nuclei to form larger particles. The conditions for such processes are created when a gas that is saturated with a vapor undergoes rapid cooling, creating supersaturation of the vapor. Thus, metal ore being smelted at high temperature produces saturated vapor in the reaction vessel, and as the vapor exits the high-temperature region, it rapidly cools and creates small aerosol particles by nucleation. Another example is the formation of primary soot particles from the tail pipe emissions of vehicles. Once these aerosol particles are formed, they can continue to increase in size by condensation (i.e., if molecules of the vapor continue to condense on the surface of the particles), or decrease in size by evaporation (i.e., if molecules leave the particle surfaces). The particles may also collide and stick to each other, creating particles that are larger. Although the mass of the aerosol is unchanged, the total number of particles will be reduced. This process is called coagulation, and it is an important mechanism when there is a high concentration of aerosol particles in a region.

Thus, once an aerosol is created either mechanically or by nucleation, its particles can change in size by mechanisms such as condensation, evaporation, and coagulation. These phenomena play an important role in the exposure to workplace aerosols that human beings face. Depending on where the workers are located with respect to the aerosol generation source and the relative importance of the various phenomena described in the preceding text at that location, they will be exposed to very different aerosol size characteristics, concentrations, and compositions.

9.4 EQUIVALENT DIAMETERS

Two particles with the same shape (e.g., spherical) and same diameter may have very different chemical and physical properties (e.g., different densities or colors) that may cause them to behave very differently in the way they move through air or interact with light. The situation becomes even more complex when we consider the myriad shapes, sizes, and chemical compositions of particles. This makes the task of characterizing them challenging.

One way to manage this complexity is to assume that the particles are spherical and have some invariant property, and describe the particle in terms of the diameter of this sphere. We can, therefore, define an *equivalent diameter* as the diameter of a sphere that has the same value of a physical property as that of the particle in question. A variety of equivalent diameters can be defined for a given particle, depending on the physical property that we are interested in. Equivalent diameters can be based on geometrical properties as well as on particle behavior when subjected to gravitational, inertial, and electrical fields, diffusional gradients, or when particles interact with electromagnetic radiation. Thus, the *volume equivalent diameter* (d_v) for a particle of arbitrary shape is the diameter of a sphere that has the same volume as the particle under consideration. The *surface area equivalent diameter* (d_A) is the diameter of a sphere that has the same surface area as the particle under consideration. The *projected surface area diameter* (d_P) is the diameter of a sphere that projects the same area in two dimensions as the particle in question. As mentioned above, particle behavior can be used to define several equivalent diameters. The *aerodynamic diameter* (d_{ae}) of a particle is the diameter of a sphere with the density of water (ρ_p = 10^3 kg/m^3), which settles down with the same velocity under the effect of gravity as the particle under consideration. Similarly, we can define an *electrical mobility equivalent diameter* (similar motion in an electric field) and an *equivalent light scattering diameter* (similar patterns of light scattering). Figure 9.2 illustrates the fact that the same particle may be described by several equivalent diameters, depending on the geometrical or physical property of interest.

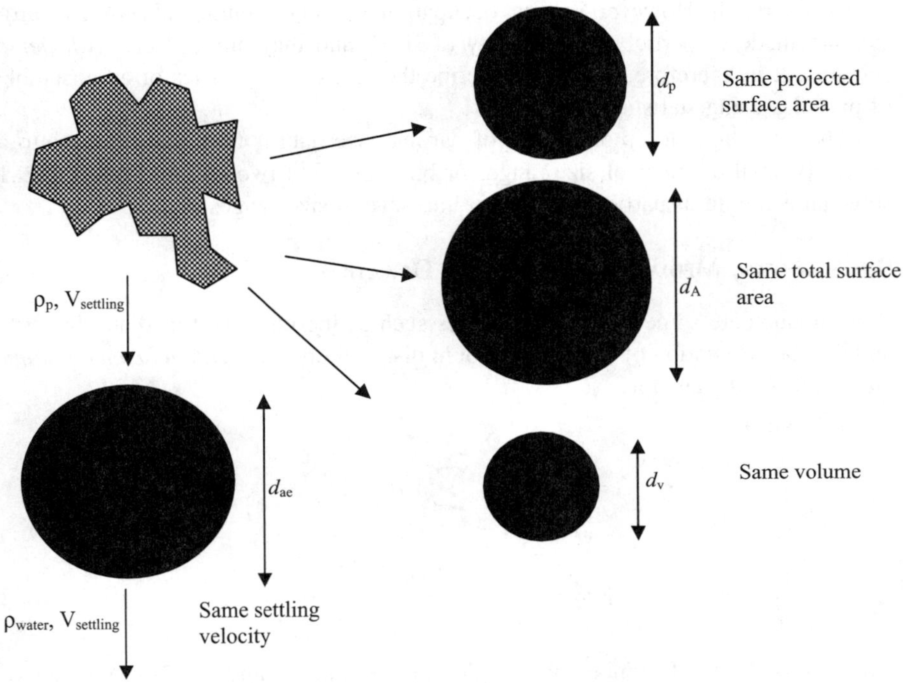

FIGURE 9.2 The same irregularly shaped particle can be described by several different equivalent diameters based on projected surface area, total surface area, volume, and gravitational settling.

9.5 AEROSOL CONCENTRATION

Several measures are used in industrial hygiene to express how much of an aerosol is in a given volume of air. The first measure, and the one most commonly used, is the mass concentration, which is expressed as the mass of aerosol particles in a given volume of air. Mass concentrations are typically expressed in units of mg/m^3 (milligrams per cubic meter) or µg/m^3 (micrograms per cubic meter). Many of the occupationally relevant aerosols have occupational exposure limits that are expressed in these units, as the adverse health effects of these aerosols depend on the mass of the aerosol to which a worker is exposed. The occupational exposure limits for different types of aerosols fall in the range of 0.01 to 10 mg/m^3. However, there are a few exceptions in which it is the number of particles in a given volume of air that is of interest. A notable example is asbestos fibers, in which occupational exposure limits are set in terms of fibers/cm^3. Particle number concentration in clean rooms used in semiconductor manufacturing is roughly 10^3/m^3.

9.6 PARTICLE SIZE DISTRIBUTIONS

It takes careful effort under highly controlled conditions to generate an aerosol composed of particles that are all of the same size. Such aerosols are called *mono-*

disperse aerosols. However, in most occupational and environmental settings, aerosols are made of particles of a variety of sizes, and they are called *polydisperse* aerosols. It is, therefore, useful to describe the size characteristics of an ensemble of particles using statistical descriptors.

The first stage of simplification of particle size data is to classify them into a relatively small number of size ranges or bins. The first two columns of Table 9.1 show an example of particles classified into several size ranges.

9.6.1 Mean, Median, and Standard Deviation

We can calculate some summary statistics such as the mean and median diameter, and standard deviation of the particle count distribution. The *arithmetic mean diameter* ($\bar{d}$) is calculated as

$$\bar{d} = \frac{\sum_{i=1}^{N} n_i d_i}{\sum_{i=1}^{N} n_i} \tag{9.1}$$

where N is the total number of particles in the sample, and n_i is the number of particles with diameter d_i. In our example, using the calculations shown in Table 9.1, $\bar{d} = \frac{1181.1}{832} = 1.42$ µm.

The *count median diameter* is the diameter that half the particles are smaller than and half the particles are larger than in size. In our example, we have 832 particles and the diameter of the 416th particle is the median diameter, which is between 0.5 and 0.8 µm.

The *count mode diameter* is the diameter that is observed most frequently in the sample. In our example, the count mode diameter is between 0.5 and 0.8 µm.

The standard deviation, σ, is calculated using the formula

$$\sigma = \sqrt{\frac{\sum_{i=1}^{N} n_i \left(d_i - \bar{d}\right)^2}{\sum_{i=1}^{N} n_i - 1}} \tag{9.2}$$

where $\bar{d}$ is the mean diameter, calculated from Equation 9.1. In our example, using the calculations shown in Table 9.1, $\sigma = \sqrt{\frac{2877.4}{832-1}} = 1.56$ µm.

TABLE 9.1
Particle Counts Classified into Several Size Ranges

Particle Size Range (μm)	Particle Count, n_i	Midpoint of Size Interval, d_i (μm)	$n_i \times d_i$	$n_i \times (d_i - \bar{d})^2$
0.1–0.5	120	0.3	36	150.4
0.5–0.8	380	0.65	247	225.1
0.8–1.4	146	1.1	160.6	14.9
1.4–2.7	96	2.05	196.8	38.2
2.7–5.6	53	4.15	219.95	395.1
5.6–8.9	22	7.25	159.5	747.9
8.9–12.6	15	10.75	161.25	1305.8
	$\sum n_i = 832$		$\sum n_i d_i = 1181.1$	$\sum n_i \left(d_i - \bar{d}\right)^2 = 2877.4$

9.6.2 Histograms

Table 9.2 contains the same data as Table 9.1. We can easily plot the data in the first two columns of Table 9.2 as in the histogram shown in Figure 9.3. However, this type of plot has an inherent flaw in that the shape of the histogram depends very much on the size ranges that we choose. For example, we could combine the ranges 1.4 to 2.7 μm and 2.7 to 5.6 μm to form a new range, 1.4 to 5.6 μm with 96 + 53 = 149 particles. The height of this interval is thus increased. To avoid this kind of a problem, we can plot the particle count per micrometer (column 4 in Table 9.2), $n_i/\Delta d$, as a histogram (Figure 9.4). The advantage of this type of histogram is that the interval heights are independent of the size interval. Additionally, because the height of each block is $n_i/\Delta d$ and the width is the interval size Δd, the area of each block of the histogram is equal to the number of particles n_i. Therefore, the total area of all the blocks of the histogram is equal to the total number of particles, i.e., Σn_i.

One drawback of Figure 9.4 is that the heights of the intervals are still dependent on the number of particles. To circumvent this problem, we can plot the fraction of particles per micrometer in each size interval instead of the number of particles. In other words, we plot $\left(\dfrac{n_i}{\sum n_i}\right)/\Delta d$ as shown in Figure 9.5. In the given figure, the area of each block is equal to the fraction of particles in that size interval. Therefore, the total area of all the blocks is equal to 1.

Next, we can draw a smooth curve through the midpoints of the tops of the rectangular blocks to obtain a particle size distribution curve. This is shown in Figure 9.6. This is an approximation to the probability density function that we first encountered in Chapter 4. In fact, the discussion in the following text is very much like the section on Continuous Distributions in Chapter 4. As the width of each block approaches zero, the histogram becomes a smooth, continuous curve. This is defined by a function $n(d)$ that takes the place of the fraction per micrometer in the bin histogram. The fraction of

TABLE 9.2
Particle Counts Classified into Several Size Ranges

Particle Size Range (μm)	Particle Count, n_i	Midpoint of Size Interval, d_i (μm)	Count/μm, $n_i/\Delta d$	Fraction/μm, $\left(\frac{n_i}{\sum n_i}\right) / \Delta d$
0.1–0.5	120	0.3	300	0.3636
0.5–0.8	380	0.65	~1267	1.5357
0.8–1.4	146	1.1	~244	0.2957
1.4–2.7	96	2.05	~74	0.0896
2.7–5.6	53	4.15	~18	0.0218
5.6–8.9	22	7.25	~7	0.0085
8.9–12.6	15	10.75	~5	0.0060
	$\sum n_i = 832$			

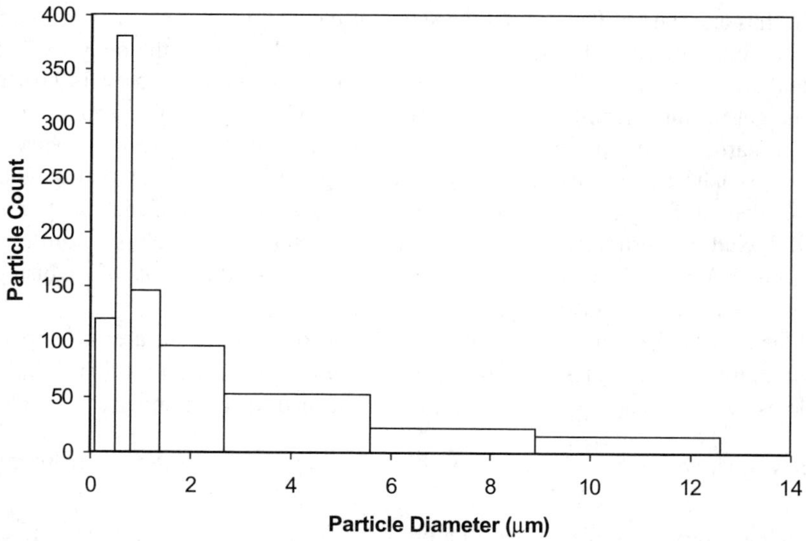

FIGURE 9.3 Histogram of particle count vs. particle size.

observations in any small interval between d and $d + \mathrm{d}d$ is $f(\mathrm{x})\ \mathrm{d}d$, and this equals the shaded area in Figure 9.7. $n(d)$ is the probability density function or the particle size distribution function. Just as the total area of all the blocks of the histogram in Figure 9.5 is equal to 1, the total area under the curve of $n(\mathrm{d})$ is equal to 1.

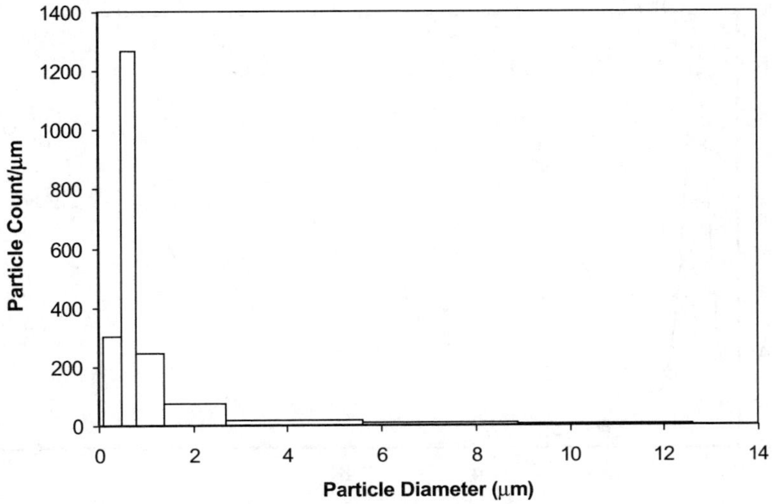

FIGURE 9.4 Histogram of count per micrometer vs. particle size.

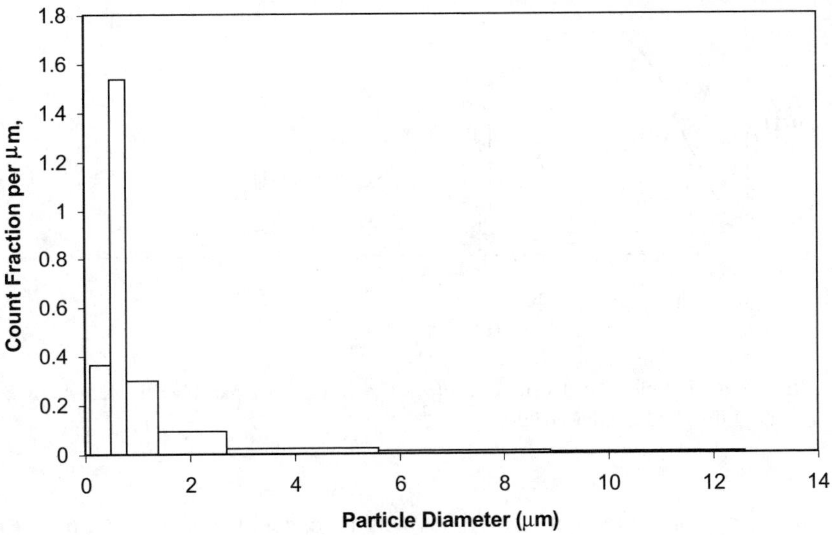

FIGURE 9.5 Histogram of count fraction per micrometer vs. particle size.

$$\int_0^\infty n(\mathrm{d})\mathrm{d}d = 1 \tag{9.3}$$

The shaded area under the curve between diameters a and b is likewise given by the definite integral of n(d), i.e.,

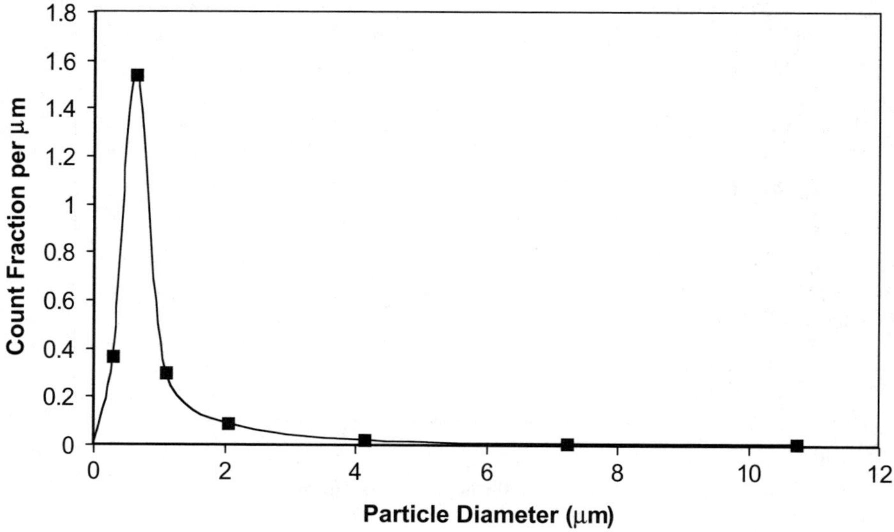

FIGURE 9.6 Particle size distribution curve.

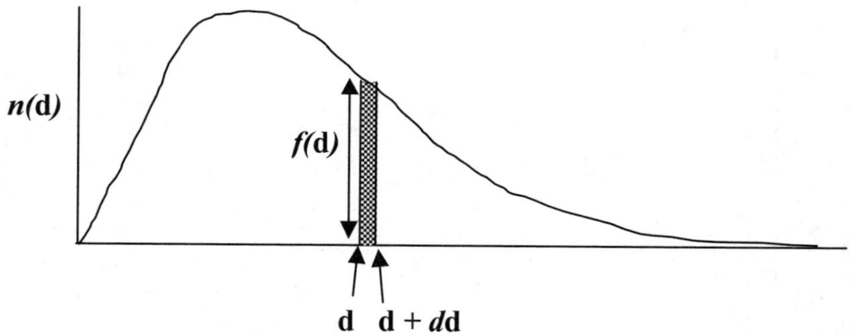

FIGURE 9.7 A particle size distribution $n(d)$. The fraction of particles that are between d and d + dd is the shaded area $n(d)$dd.

$$\int_a^b n(d)\mathrm{d}d = \text{fraction of particles with diameters between } a \text{ and } b \qquad (9.4)$$

Another way of representing particle size information is in the form of a cumulative probability distribution. A cumulative size distribution $C(a)$ is defined as the fraction of all particles with diameter less than a, i.e.,

$$C(a) = \int_0^a n(d)\mathrm{d}d = \text{fraction of particles with diameters less than } a \qquad (9.5)$$

TABLE 9.3
Obtaining a Cumulative Size Distribution from Particle Count Data

Particle Size Range (μm)	Particle Count, n_i	Fraction of Particles, $\frac{n_i}{\sum n_i}$	Cumulative Fraction Smaller than the Upper Diameter, C_i
0.1–0.5	120	120/832 = 0.144	0.144
0.5–0.8	380	380/832 = 0.457	0.601
0.8–1.4	146	146/832 = 0.176	0.777
1.4–2.7	96	96/832 = 0.115	0.892
2.7–5.6	53	53/832 = 0.064	0.956
5.6–8.9	22	22/832 = 0.026	0.982
8.9–12.6	15	15/832 = 0.018	1.000
	$\sum n_i = 832$	$\sum \frac{n_i}{\sum n_i} = 1.000$	

The data that were plotted in Figure 9.6 as a frequency distribution can be plotted as a cumulative distribution. The third column in Table 9.3 shows the fraction of the number of particles in each size range. Thus, 14.4% of the particles are in the size range 0.1 to 0.5 μm, 45.7% of the particles are between 0.5 and 0.8 μm, and so on. The fourth column shows the cumulative fraction. Figure 9.8 shows a plot of the cumulative fraction in column 4 vs. the upper size limit of each size range in Table 9.3. Thus, 14.4% of the particles are less than 0.5 μm, 60.1% of the particles are less than 0.8 μm, etc. Finally, 100% of the particles are less than 12.6 μm. A smooth curve can be drawn through these points, as shown in Figure 9.8.

Figure 9.8 is thus a plot of the areas under the curve shown in Figure 9.6 between 0 and a particular diameter plotted against particle diameter. This relationship also holds in the case of a continuous distribution, as illustrated in Equation 9.5. Because the cumulative distribution is the integral of the probability density function, we can conversely state that the probability density function (particle size distribution) is the derivative of the cumulative distribution function, i.e.,

$$n(\mathrm{d}) = \frac{\mathrm{d}C(d)}{\mathrm{d}d} \tag{9.6}$$

9.6.3 The Lognormal Size Distribution

We have discussed the properties of the normal distribution in Chapter 4, in the context of measurement errors. The symmetrical normal (or Gaussian) distribution is ideal for describing measurement uncertainties that are distributed symmetrically about a central value, and the uncertainties can take positive or negative values. However, aerosol size distributions are seldom symmetrical. Typically, they are positively skewed with a long tail to the right. This can also be noted in the example

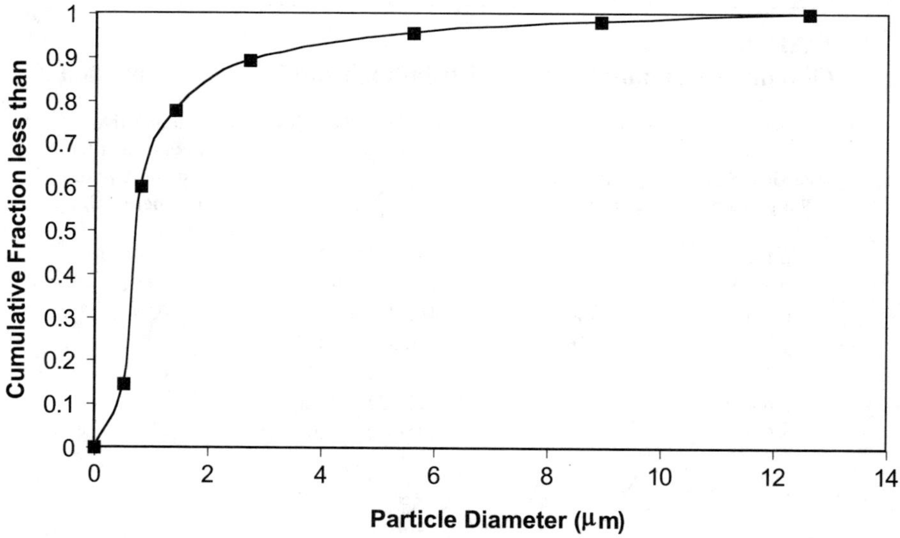

FIGURE 9.8 Cumulative distribution of data in Table 9.3.

data set shown in Table 9.1 and plotted in Figure 9.5 and Figure 9.6, in which the diameter values are distributed asymmetrically about the mean value of 1.42 μm. Additionally, unlike measurement errors, particle sizes cannot have negative values. However, whereas the frequency distributions of particle sizes have a skewed shape, the log of the particle sizes often has a symmetric distribution that can be described well using the normal distribution. In these cases, the log of the particle sizes has a normal distribution. Thus, the particle sizes are said to have a *lognormal distribution*. The lognormal distribution is good way to describe particle size distributions in workplaces as well as in ambient environments.

Just as a normal distribution is described by its mean and standard deviation, the lognormal distribution is described by the geometric mean and *geometric standard deviation* (GSD). The geometric mean diameter (d_g) can be calculated as

$$\log(d_g) = \frac{\sum_{i=1}^{N} n_i \log(d_i)}{\sum_{i=1}^{N} n_i} \tag{9.7}$$

and the GSD, σ_g, is calculated as

$$\log(\sigma_g) = \sqrt{\frac{\sum_{i=1}^{N} n_i \left(\log(d_i) - \log(d_g)\right)^2}{\sum_{i=1}^{N} n_i - 1}} = \sqrt{\frac{\sum_{i=1}^{N} n_i \left(\log\left(\frac{d_i}{d_g}\right)\right)^2}{\sum_{i=1}^{N} n_i - 1}} \tag{9.8}$$

Note that Equation 9.7 and Equation 9.8 are similar to Equation 9.1 and Equation 9.2, except that the diameter is replaced by its log transform. The data used in Table 9.1 can be used to illustrate the calculation of the geometric mean and GSD.

$$\log(d_g) = \frac{\sum n_i \log(d_i)}{\sum n_i} = \frac{-30.67}{832} = -\,0.036 \tag{9.9}$$

$$d_g = 10^{-0.036} = 0.92\ \mu\text{m} \tag{9.10}$$

$$\log(\sigma_g) = \sqrt{\frac{107.04}{831}} = 0.36 \tag{9.11}$$

$$\sigma_g = 10^{0.36} = 2.29 \tag{9.12}$$

The GSD is dimensionless because it is calculated by obtaining ratios of diameters, as shown in Equation 9.8. The above calculations were performed by using logarithms in base 10, and then taking their antilogarithms.

The lognormal distribution has a form analogous to the normal distribution described in Chapter 4.

$$L(d) = \frac{1}{d\ln(\sigma_g)\sqrt{2\pi}} \exp - \left(\frac{\left(\ln(d) - \ln(d_g)\right)^2}{2\ln^2(\sigma_g)} \right) \tag{9.13}$$

An example of a lognormal distribution is shown in Figure 9.9. A log transformation of the x-axis converts the distribution into a normal function (i.e., the Gaussian function described in Chapter 4). Thereafter, the useful properties of the normal distribution can be exploited as described in Chapter 4. For example, we can state that 68% of the particles lie between the diameters $\exp(\ln(d_g) \pm \ln(\sigma_g))$. In a normal distribution, the standard deviation is defined as the distance between the 84th and 50th percentiles (or the distance between the 50th and the 16th percentiles):

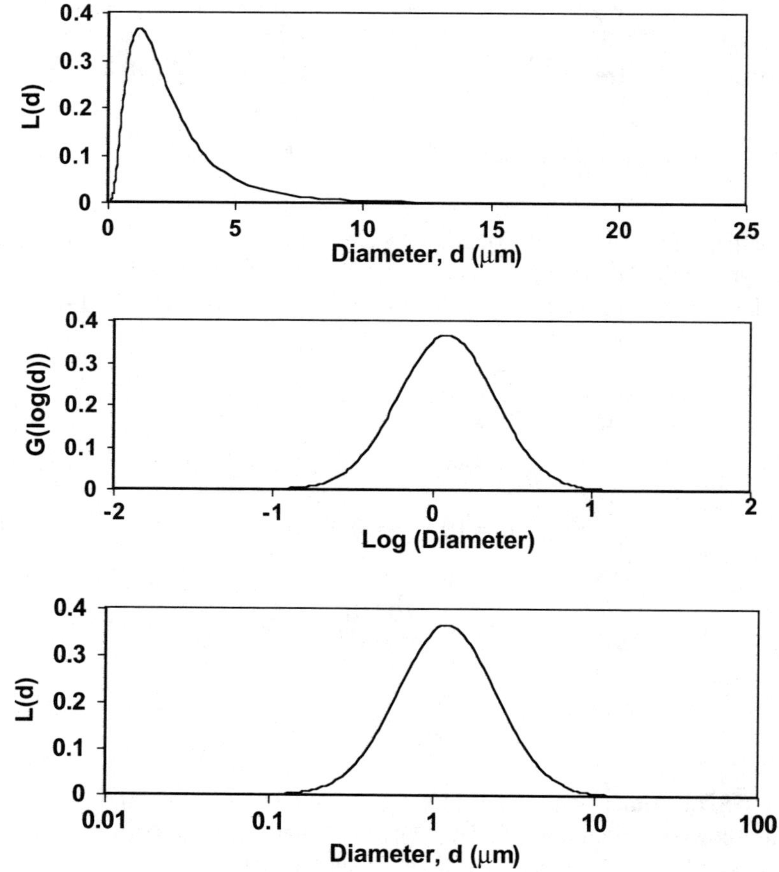

FIGURE 9.9 The top figure is a lognormal probability density function ($d_g = 2\ \mu$m; $\sigma_g = 2$) plotted against particle diameter showing the skewed nature of the distribution. The middle figure shows the same function plotted against the logarithm of the diameter, a transformation that makes the distribution symmetrical and normal. The bottom figure is the same as the middle, with the same function being plotted against particle diameter except that the x-axis is a log axis.

$$\ln(\sigma_g) = \ln(d_{84}) - \ln(d_{50}) = \ln\left(\frac{d_{84}}{d_{50}}\right) = \ln\left(\frac{d_{50}}{d_{16}}\right)$$

or

$$\sigma_g = \frac{d_{84}}{d_{50}} = \frac{d_{50}}{d_{16}} \qquad (9.14)$$

Thus, we see that a monodisperse aerosol (all particles have the same diameter) has a GSD of 1. Using the same data that we have used previously in Table 9.1 to Table 9.4, we can obtain a plot akin to Figure 9.6, except that the logarithm of

TABLE 9.4
Calculation of the Geometric Mean and Geometric Standard Deviation

Particle Count, n_i	Midpoint of Size Interval, d_i (μm)	$\log(d_i)$	$n_i \times \log(d_i)$	$n_i \times (\log(d_i)-\log(d_g))^2$
120	0.3	–0.52	–62.7	28.45
380	0.65	–0.19	–71.1	8.67
146	1.1	0.04	6.04	0.87
96	2.05	0.31	29.93	11.61
53	4.15	0.62	32.76	22.67
22	7.25	0.86	18.93	17.68
15	10.75	1.03	15.47	17.09
	$\sum n_i = 832$		$\sum n_i \log(d_i) = -30.67$	$\sum n_i \left(\log(d_i) - \log(d_g)\right)^2 = 107.04$

TABLE 9.5
Calculations for Plotting Fraction per Log Diameter against Log Diameter

Particle Size Range, (μm) d_1 d_2	Particle Count, n_i	Midpoint of Size Interval, d_i (μm)	$\log(d_i)$	$\Delta\log(d) = \log(d_2) - \log(d_1)$	$\left(\frac{n_i}{\sum n_i}\right) \Big/ \Delta \log d$
0.1–0.5	120	0.3	–0.52	0.70	0.21
0.5–0.8	380	0.65	–0.19	0.20	2.24
0.8–1.4	146	1.1	0.04	0.24	0.72
1.4–2.7	96	2.05	0.31	0.29	0.40
2.7–5.6	53	4.15	0.62	0.32	0.20
5.6–8.9	22	7.25	0.86	0.20	0.13
8.9–12.6	15	10.75	1.03	0.15	0.12
	$\sum n_i = 832$				

particle diameter is plotted along the x-axis, and the count fraction per log diameter is plotted on the y-axis. The calculations are shown in Table 9.5, and the curve is plotted in Figure 9.10. All the particles in a particular size range are assumed to have a diameter equal to the midpoint of the size interval, as shown in the third column. The fractional count for each size range is divided by the difference of the logarithms of the upper and lower size limits of the size range.

A comparison of Figure 9.6 and Figure 9.10 shows that the log transformation has made the distribution more symmetrical and much closer to a normal distribution.

We can also use the above data to obtain the volume distribution of the aerosol. If all the particles in the aerosol have the same density, then the volume distribution

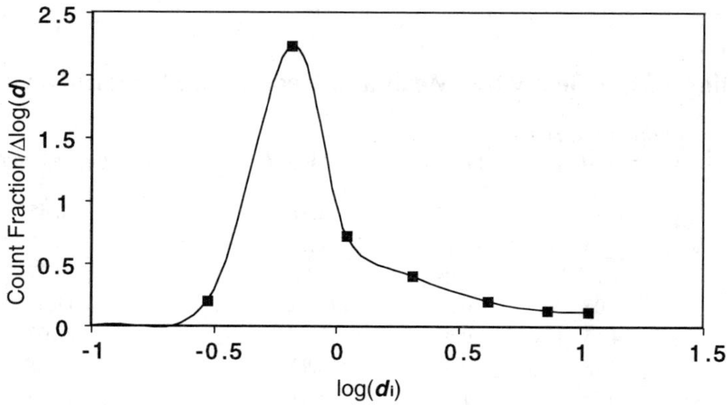

FIGURE 9.10 Plot of data from Table 9.5.

TABLE 9.6
Calculations for Obtaining the Mass (or Volume) Distribution of the Aerosol Whose Count Distribution is Provided

Particle Count, n_i	Midpoint of Size Interval, d_i, (μm)	$m_i = n_i\ \rho_p \frac{\pi}{6} d_i^3$ (μg)	log(d_i)	Δlog(d)	$\left(\frac{m_i}{\sum m_i}\right) \Big/ \Delta \log d$
120	0.3	1.70 E–6	–0.52	0.70	1.45 E–4
380	0.65	5.46 E–5	–0.19	0.20	0.016
146	1.1	1.02 E–4	0.04	0.24	0.025
96	2.05	4.33 E–4	0.31	0.29	0.091
53	4.15	1.98 E–3	0.62	0.32	0.374
22	7.25	4.39 E–3	0.86	0.20	1.305
15	10.75	9.76 E–3	1.03	0.15	3.865
$\sum n_i = 832$		$\sum m_i = 1.67$ E–2			

is equal to the mass distribution as well. The calculations are shown in Table 9.6, in which the particle density is assumed to be 1000 kg/m^3 or 10^{-6} μg/μm^3. All the particles in a particular size range are assumed to have a diameter equal to the midpoint of the size interval, as shown in the second column. The mass corresponding to each particle size is equal to the product of the number of particles of that size and the mass of each particle, as shown in the third column of Table 9.6. In turn, the mass of each particle is the product of particle density and the volume of each particle. The mass fraction per log diameter calculation is similar to that for the count fraction per log diameter. Figure 9.11 shows a plot of the mass distribution calculated in Table 9.6.

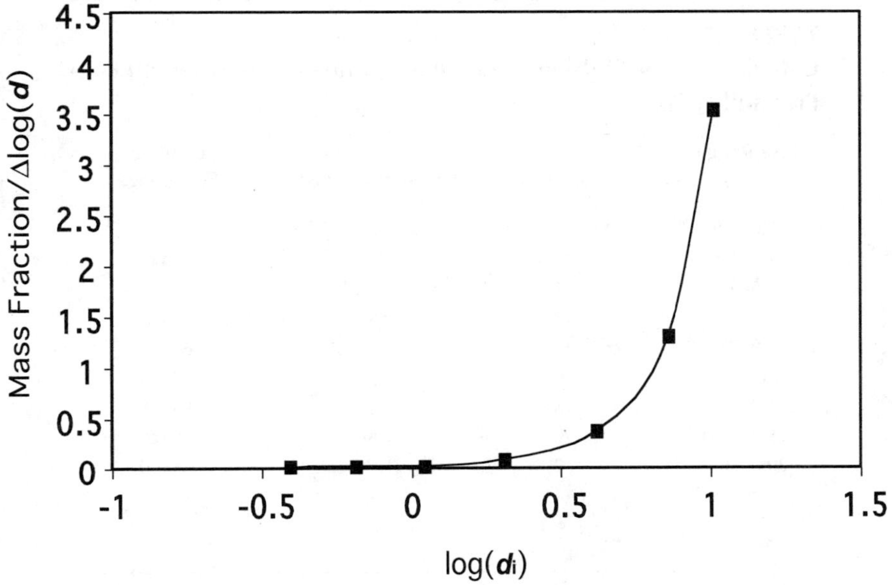

FIGURE 9.11 Plot of mass distribution calculated in Table 9.6.

From Figure 9.10 and Figure 9.11, we can infer that, whereas the particle numbers are mostly in the smaller size ranges, most of the particle masses are in the larger size ranges, even though there are fewer of the larger particles. The reason for this is straightforward. The mass of a particle is proportional to the cube of its diameter. So, the mass of a single 10 μm particle is equal to the mass of 1000 particles with a diameter of 1 μm. Therefore, larger particles have a disproportionate impact on the total mass of an aerosol.

9.7 LOG-PROBABILITY PLOTS

Using the above data, we can also construct a cumulative mass distribution similar to the cumulative number distribution plotted in Figure 9.8. For lognormal distributions, however, a great simplicity in analysis is achieved by plotting such data on *log-probability graphs*. The cumulative data are plotted with the cumulative percentage of particles (number, mass, or any other metric) less than the largest size in each size interval on the x-axis and the upper size limit of the size interval on the y-axis. The x-axis uses a probability scale such that it is compressed near the 50% point and expanded near the tails, and the y-axis uses a log scale. Log-probability graphs have the convenient property that the cumulative plot of a lognormal distribution will result in a straight line. Table 9.7 shows mass data collected in several size ranges. The third column calculates the cumulative mass less than the upper limit of the corresponding size interval, and the fourth column calculates the cumulative percentages.

TABLE 9.7
Calculations for Plotting a Cumulative Mass Distribution on Log-Probability Axes

Size Range, (μm)	Mass, m_i (μg)	Cumulative mass	Cumulative Percentage
0.0–1.0	4	4	3.31
1.0–1.5	5	9	7.44
1.5–3.0	21	30	24.79
3.0-5.0	18	48	39.67
5.0–7.0	30	78	64.46
7.0–11.0	7	85	70.25
11.0–15.0	18	103	85.12
15.0–20.0	6	109	90.08
20.0–30.0	12	121	100.00

$\sum m_i = 121$

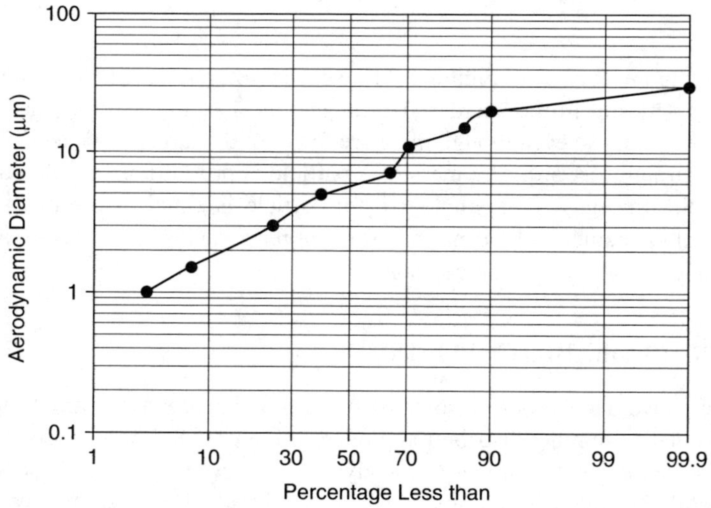

FIGURE 9.12 Log-probability plot of the data shown in Table 9.7.

The data are plotted on a log-probability graph in Figure 9.12. We can fit a straight line to the data. In Figure 9.12, we have merely connected the data points; however, we could have fit a straight line through all the data points, excluding the last one. If a straight line fit is reasonable, we can assume that the size distribution is lognormal. The mass median diameter (MMD) can be obtained by reading off the 50th percentile diameter for the fitted line, and the GSD can be

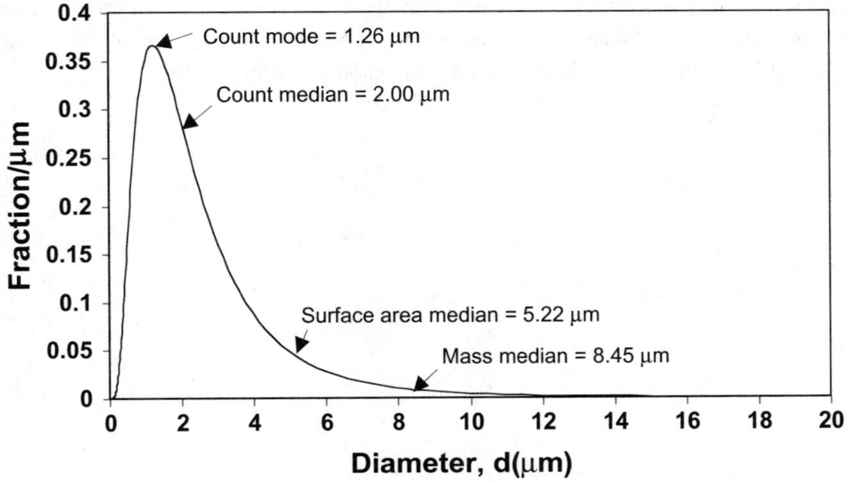

FIGURE 9.13 Lognormal number distribution with count median diameter of 2 μm and geometric standard deviation of 2.0, showing the surface area median and mass median diameters.

obtained using Equation 9.14. For the data plotted in Figure 9.12, the MMD is approximately 7.0 μm, and the GSD is ~d_{84}/d_{50} = 15/7 = 2.14.

The last data point for 30 μm does not fall on the straight line, and therefore the straight line fitted through the other points appears to curve near the top. Typically, the last data point is not plotted. This is because particles larger than 30 μm are unable to enter the instrument that generated this data set. Thus, the instrument is sampling only part of the aerosol size distribution.

9.8 THE HATCH–CHOATE RELATIONSHIPS

Most aerosols found in occupational settings are lognormally distributed, with GSDs between 1.5 and 3.5. Table 9.5 and Table 9.6 show how one can calculate the mass distribution for an aerosol given its count distribution. However, this tedious process can be simplified by exploiting the lognormality of the size distribution. The Hatch–Choate equations describe a simple relationship that can be used to convert a mass distribution into a number distribution or surface area distribution (or vice versa).

$$MMD = CMD \exp\left(3 \ln^2 \sigma_g\right) \tag{9.15}$$

$$SMD = CMD \exp\left(2 \ln^2 \sigma_g\right) \tag{9.16}$$

where MMD is the mass median diameter, CMD is the count median diameter, SMD is the surface area median diameter, and σ_g is the GSD. The GSD remains unchanged during these conversions, which means that the number, mass, and surface area distributions have the same σ_g. Figure 9.13 shows a hypothetical lognormal number distribution that also shows the locations of the count median, count mode, surface area median, and the mass median diameters. The derivation of the above relationships can be found in standard aerosol texts such as Hinds (1999).

10 Particle Motion in a Viscous Medium

10.1 INTRODUCTION

In this chapter, we will consider the motion of aerosol particles through a medium that is composed of gas molecules, which offer resistance to the movement of the particles. The driving force of the motion is usually some external force such as gravity, and this is opposed by the resistance of the medium. The motion may be steady and rectilinear (i.e., in a straight line), or accelerated and along a curved path.

10.2 DRAG FORCE ON A PARTICLE

Using some simple arguments and assumptions, Newton developed an expression for the drag force on an object (such as an aerosol particle) moving through air. Consider a particle moving through a medium composed of molecules such that the particle is much larger than the molecular dimensions, as in Figure 10.1.

The particle moves through a medium at a velocity v, and its diameter is d. The mass rate at which the total number of molecules hit the sphere is $\dot{m} = \rho_g \frac{\pi}{4} d^2 v$, i.e., it is equal to the mass of air in a cylinder of diameter d and length v. Due to the fact that momentum is conserved, the sphere moving with a velocity v will impart a velocity of Kv, on average, to each molecule it collides with, where K is a constant of proportionality. Therefore, the gas molecules will experience a net force that is equal to the rate of change of their momentum, $K\rho_g \frac{\pi}{4} d^2 v^2$. The spherical particle experiences an equal and opposite force that is called the *drag force* on the particle:

$$F_D = K\rho_g \frac{\pi}{4} d^2 v^2 \tag{10.1}$$

It is more customary to express the above equation as

$$F_D = C_D \rho_g \frac{\pi}{8} d^2 v^2 \tag{10.2}$$

Equation 10.2 is Newton's expression for drag on an object due to air resistance, in which the constant C_D is the coefficient of drag. The above derivation implicitly

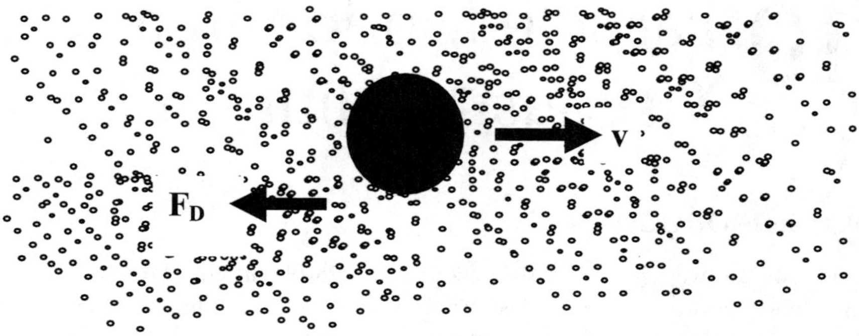

FIGURE 10.1 A sphere of diameter *d* moving with velocity *v* through a medium comprising many small molecules.

assumes that resistance arises only on the projected surface area of the particle, and that the coefficient of drag is constant. However, this is true only for large values of *particle Reynolds numbers* ($Re_p > 1000$) when, in fact, C_D has a constant value. For large values of particle Reynolds numbers, resistance is thought to arise due to frictional resistance on the surface of the particle and pressure drag due to compression of the medium. In this scenario, the drag is associated with the projected surface area of the particle. However, for smaller values of particle Reynolds numbers, viscous drag predominates, and this force acts on the entire surface of the body. The drag force is correspondingly higher.

For laminar flow ($Re_p < 1$),

$$C_D = \frac{24}{Re_p} \tag{10.3}$$

and for $1 < Re_p < 1000$,

$$C_D = \frac{24}{Re_p}\left[1 + 0.15\,Re_p^{\,0.687}\right] \tag{10.4}$$

For $Re_p > 1000$,

$$C_D = 0.44 \tag{10.5}$$

10.3 STOKES' LAW

When the flow is laminar ($Re_p < 1$), Stokes' law provides an expression for the drag force experienced by a sphere moving through a viscous medium. This expression is a solution of the Navier–Stokes equations for fluid motion around a sphere when several simplifying assumptions are made. The assumptions are that the fluid medium is an incompressible and viscous continuum, and that the inertial forces are negligible compared with the viscous forces. Using these assumptions, the drag force on the spherical particle is obtained as

$$F_D = -3\pi\mu d v \tag{10.6}$$

where μ is the viscosity of the medium ($\mu \approx 18 \times 10^{-6}$ N s m^{-2} at 20°C in SI units), d the diameter of the particle, and v the relative velocity between the particle and the medium. The negative sign indicates that the drag force acts in a direction opposite to the particle's motion. Equation 10.6 is referred to as Stokes' law. We also notice that a comparison of Equation 10.2 and Equation 10.6 for $Re_p < 1$ yields $C_D = \dfrac{24}{Re_p}$, a result already presented in Equation 10.3.

10.4 MODIFICATIONS TO STOKES' LAW

Although Stokes' law is broadly applicable to a range of aerosol motion, it is not applicable when the assumptions underlying its derivation do not hold. The first assumption is that the medium is made up of a large number of molecules that are much smaller than the aerosol particles. In such a case, the particle "sees" the medium as a continuum and cannot distinguish between individual collisions with the molecules. However, when the size of the particle becomes small enough that it approaches the mean free path of the gas, one can think of the particles as "slipping" between the molecules, so that it does not collide with as many molecules. The reduced number of collisions leads to a smaller drag force on the particle. This necessitates the use of a correction factor known as the *Cunningham slip correction factor,* C_c, which modifies Stokes' law:

$$F_D = -\frac{3\pi\mu d v}{C_c} \tag{10.7}$$

where

$$C_c = 1 + \left(\frac{2.52\lambda}{d}\right) \tag{10.8}$$

when 0.1 μm < d < 1.0 μm, and

$$C_c = 1 + \left(\frac{\lambda}{d}\right)\left\{2.514 + 0.8\exp\left(\frac{-0.55\,d}{\lambda}\right)\right\} \tag{10.9}$$

when 0.01 μm < d < 0.1 μm.

As discussed in Chapter 2, the mean free path for air molecules at 25°C is 0.07 μm. The preceding discussion makes it clear that the slip correction factor needs to be applied when we are dealing with fine aerosols less than 1 μm in size, such as those resulting from combustion processes.

The second assumption underlying Stokes' equation is that the flow is laminar, i.e., $Re_p < 1$. For $Re_p > 1$, the coefficient of drag, C_D, is given by Equation 10.4, and Stokes' law needs to be modified accordingly for *non-Stokesian flow.* The drag force is therefore expressed as

$$F_D = -\left(\frac{C_D\, Re_p}{24}\right) 3\pi\mu\, d\, v \tag{10.10}$$

where the first term contains the modification for non-Stokesian flow.

The third assumption underlying Stokes' law is that the aerosol particles are spherical. However, nonspherical particles are encountered in a wide variety of occupational and nonoccupational settings. For such nonspherical particles, a *dynamic shape correction factor,* ϕ, is applied to Stokes' law

$$F_D = -\,3\pi\mu\, d_V\, v\phi \tag{10.11}$$

where d_V is the equivalent volume diameter of the particle. The dynamic shape factor has a value of 1.00 for perfect spheres. Nonspherical particles have larger values, e.g., isometric particles such as quartz (1.36) and coal dust (1.05 to 1.11), platelet-like particles such as talc (1.88), and cylindrical particles such as fibers (1.35, which is an orientation-averaged value for L/d = 5).

Thus, Stokes' law can be modified for (1) particle slip, (2) non-Stokesian flow, and (3) nonspherical shape, using Equation 10.8 to Equation 10.11. These can be combined into one equation as

$$F_D = -\left(\frac{C_D\, Re_p}{24}\right)\left(\frac{3\pi\mu\, d\, v}{C_C}\right)\phi \tag{10.12}$$

10.5 EQUATION OF MOTION FOR AN AEROSOL PARTICLE

In a general sense, the motion of an aerosol particle can be mathematically described by setting the net force acting on it equal to its rate of change of momentum.

$$m\frac{d\vec{v}}{dt} = \sum_i \vec{F}i \tag{10.13}$$

The above is a vector equation that needs to be solved for each of the coordinate directions along which the force and velocity can be resolved. The external forces may be due to gravity or electric or magnetic fields, besides the drag force due to the medium that is described by Stokes' law with the relevant modifications.

10.6 PARTICLE MOTION UNDER GRAVITY

A common example is that of a particle falling through air under the influence of gravity. The forces acting on the particle are gravity (acting downward), the drag force (acting upward), and the buoyant force (acting upward). The buoyant force is the upward force exerted on the particle by the volume of air displaced by the particle and is equal to the weight of the displaced air. Because the density of air is much less than the density of the particle, the buoyant force is typically very small compared with the other two forces, and is therefore neglected.

Figure 10.2 shows the forces acting on a spherical particle. For this case, Equation 10.13 can be expressed as

$$m\frac{dv_y}{dt} = -3\pi\mu d v_y + mg = -3\pi\mu d v_y + \frac{\pi d^3}{6}\rho_p g \tag{10.14}$$

where v_y is the velocity of the particle in the vertical direction, m is the mass of the particle, ρ_p is the density of the particle, and g is the acceleration due to gravity (9.81 m/sec^2). We have chosen the downward direction to be positive. Equation 10.14 can be rearranged as

$$\frac{dv_y}{dt} + \frac{v_y}{\tau} - g = 0 \tag{10.15}$$

where

$$\tau = \frac{\rho_p d^2}{18\mu} \tag{10.16}$$

We also assume that the particle starts off with an initial velocity equal to zero. Equation 10.15 is a first-order differential equation whose solution (for the specified initial condition) is given by

$$v_y = \tau g\left[1 - e^{-\frac{t}{\tau}}\right] \tag{10.17}$$

Figure 10.3 shows how the vertical particle velocity changes with time. The particle starts off with a zero velocity that initially increases rapidly with time. During this time, the force of gravity is much more than the drag force retarding its motion. However, as the particle velocity increases, the drag force increases proportionately. This decreases the rate of change of velocity (i.e., its acceleration) until

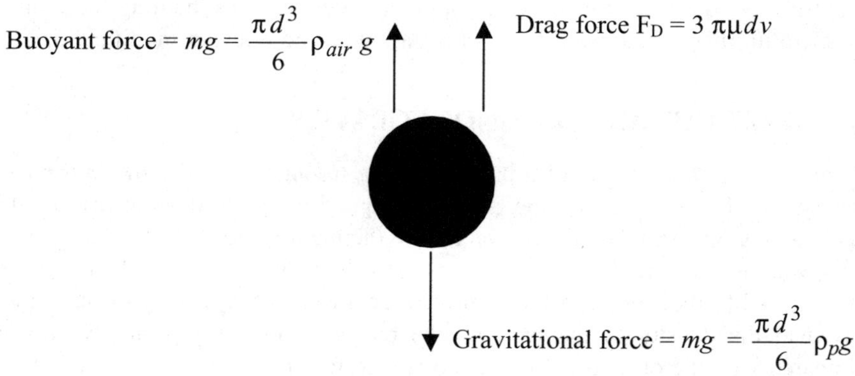

FIGURE 10.2 Forces acting on a spherical particle moving under the influence of gravity.

finally the drag force equals the gravity force, and the particle stops accelerating. After this point, the particle continues to move at a constant velocity that is called the *terminal settling velocity.*

The quantity τ defined by Equation 10.16 has dimensions of time and is called the *particle relaxation time*. We see that if we set $t = \tau$ in Equation 10.17, then $v_y = 0.63V_{TS}$. Thus, it is the time needed for a particle to reach 63% of its final steady state velocity after it has started moving under the influence of a new force (in this case, gravity). In more general terms, it is the characteristic time related to how long a particle takes to come into equilibrium (or "relax") with a new set of forces acting on it, i.e., how long it takes to reach a constant velocity.

The terminal settling velocity is attained asymptotically at $t = \infty$ and is given by

$$V_{TS} = \tau g = \frac{\rho_p d^2}{18\mu} g \tag{10.18}$$

However, after $t = 3\tau$, the particle attains 95% of its final velocity, i.e., $v_y = 0.95\,V_{TS}$, and stays nearly constant after that. Thus, 3τ can be taken as a good measure of the time taken to reach terminal settling velocity. For most particle sizes encountered in industrial hygiene settings, terminal settling velocity is reached very quickly. For example, the values of 3τ for particles with aerodynamic diameters of 0.1 μm, 1.0 μm, and 10 μm are 2.7×10^{-7} sec, 11×10^{-6} sec, and 940×10^{-6} sec, respectively.

It should be recognized that Equation 10.18 was obtained by assuming that the drag force is given by Stokes' law without any modifications. If we need to account for non-Stokesian flow, particle slip, and particle shape effects, the corresponding expression for terminal settling velocity becomes

$$V_{TS} = \tau g = \left(\frac{24 C_c}{C_D \, \mathrm{Re}_p \, \phi} \right) \tag{10.19}$$

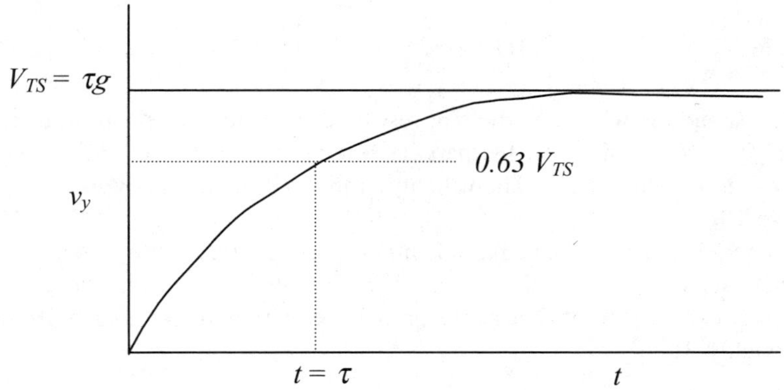

FIGURE 10.3 Velocity of a particle falling vertically through air under the influence of gravity as a function of time.

It can be seen from Equation 10.19 that several of the quantities are dependent on each other. For example, Re_p can be calculated only after knowing the particle settling velocity. However, the value of Re_p is necessary to know whether to apply the correction for non-Stokesian flow or not. Similarly, C_D and Re_p are related to each other. Therefore, the calculation of terminal settling velocity needs an iterative procedure. A reasonable approach is to first see if the particle size is less than 1 μm. If it is, then we need to apply the slip correction formula given by Equation 10.8 or Equation 10.9. Particles of size greater than 1 μm do not require slip correction. The next step is to calculate V_{TS} using Equation 10.18 and use this value of settling velocity to calculate the particle Reynolds' number Re_p. If $Re_p < 1$, then no further calculations are needed. If $Re_p > 1$, then V_{TS} is calculated using Equation 10.19 and the calculated value of Re_p. Then, this new value of V_{TS} is used to calculate a new value of Re_p, which in turn is used to calculate a newer value of V_{TS}. This iterative procedure is repeated until the calculated value of V_{TS} does not change too much from one iteration to the next.

If, in solving the differential equation in Equation 10.15, we had different initial conditions, e.g., if the initial velocity had a nonzero value of V_i, then the solution would become

$$v_y = V_i e^{\frac{-t}{\tau}} + \tau g \left[1 - e^{-\frac{t}{\tau}}\right] \tag{10.20}$$

Thus, the effect of the initial velocity undergoes a rapid exponential decay, and the particle ultimately reaches the same terminal settling velocity of τg.

10.7 FURTHER GENERALIZATIONS

Equation 10.20 can be generalized so that it is expressed only in terms of initial and final velocities, V_i and V_f, and can refer to motion in some arbitrary direction.

$$v(t) = V_i e^{\frac{-t}{\tau}} + V_f \left[1 - e^{-\frac{t}{\tau}}\right] \quad (10.21)$$

One example is when a particle at rest is released into a stream of air moving with velocity U. In this case, the particle velocity will increase until it reaches a velocity U in roughly 3τ sec. The velocity profile will look exactly like that shown in Figure 10.3.

Another example is when a particle moving along with air at a velocity U_1 (e.g., in a duct) suddenly enters air moving at a velocity U_2 (e.g., the duct suddenly contracts or expands). In this case, the particle velocity will also change from U_1 to U_2 in roughly 3τ sec.

10.8 PARTICLE AERODYNAMIC DIAMETER

We have previously defined the aerodynamic diameter of a particle in Chapter 9 as the equivalent diameter of a sphere with the density of water (ρ_w = 1000 kg/m^3), which settles with the same velocity under the effect of gravity as the particle under consideration. Thus, if a spherical particle has a density of ρ_p and a diameter of d, then it will have the same settling velocity as a spherical droplet of water with diameter d_{ae} and density ρ_w if

$$V_{TS} = \frac{\rho_p d^2}{18\mu} g = \frac{\rho_w {d_{ae}}^2}{18\mu} g \quad (10.22)$$

Here, d_{ae} is the aerodynamic diameter of the particle in question and is equal to

$$d_{ae} = d\sqrt{\frac{\rho_p}{\rho_w}} \quad (10.23)$$

Thus, a particle that has greater density than water will have an aerodynamic diameter larger than its physical diameter and vice versa.

Again, we should bear in mind that this definition of aerodynamic diameter should be appropriately corrected for particle slip, non-Stokesian flow, and particle shape. Thus,

$$d_{ae} = d_V \sqrt{\frac{\rho_p}{\rho_w} \frac{C_c}{C_{c(w)}} \frac{C_{D(w)} \operatorname{Re}_{p(w)}}{C_D \operatorname{Re}_p} \frac{1}{\phi}} \quad (10.24)$$

where d_V is the volume equivalent diameter of a nonspherical particle with shape factor ϕ, and the subscript w indicates that the quantities are for the water droplet.

10.9 INSTRUMENTS BASED ON PARTICLE SETTLING

Several instruments for aerosol sampling are based on particle settling under the action of gravity. The *vertical elutriator* is a vertical cylindrical duct of a given height in which air, containing particles, flows upward at a low velocity. Thus, the duct air velocity and the settling velocity of the particles are opposite in direction. Particles that have a terminal settling velocity greater than the air velocity (i.e., particles that have an aerodynamic diameter greater than a given value) cannot be carried out of the duct and are therefore removed from the airstream. Particles with lower settling velocities (i.e., smaller aerodynamic diameters) stay in the airstream for sampling further downstream. Achieving a sharp cutoff, i.e., a clear separation of particles below and above a certain size, depends on a constant and uniform air velocity across the cross section of the duct. Most commercial instruments based on vertical elutriation do not achieve this and hence have a gradual cutoff. Vertical elutriators are used for cotton dust sampling, in which the aerosol enters the instrument through a conical inlet at the bottom. The instrument operates at a flow rate of 7.4 l/min, which provides an air velocity of 0.68 cm/sec at the widest section of the device. This corresponds to an aerodynamic cutoff size of 15 μm, i.e., particles below this size are sampled and those above are not. However, the nonuniform flow creates a more gradual cutoff such that particles twice this size are let in. The particles that stay in the airstream are collected on a standard 37-mm filter.

In a *horizontal elutriator*, the airstream containing suspended particles moves horizontally through a duct of a rectangular cross section. Here, the settling velocity of the particles and the horizontal air velocity are perpendicular to each other. In Figure 10.4, a horizontal elutriator is shown that has a length L, height H, and a gas velocity U. A particle entering the duct has a horizontal velocity of U (equal to the gas velocity) and a vertical velocity equal to its terminal settling velocity, V_{TS}. Thus, a particle starting at the very top of the duct (i.e., at height H) will settle out just as it reaches the end of the duct length of L if its settling velocity is given by

$$V_{TS} = \frac{HU}{L} \tag{10.25}$$

In the above equation, the ratio $\frac{L}{U}$ is the *residence time* of the air in the elutriator, and H is referred to as the *settling distance.*

Particles with settling velocities (and hence, aerodynamic diameters) greater than this will settle out earlier, whereas particles with settling velocities (and aerodynamic diameters) smaller than this will not be collected along the duct length. Again, the sharpness of the cutoff depends on the uniformity of the gas flow and the narrowness of the aerosol inlet.

In many cases, however, a gradual cutoff is desirable because it allows sampling of particles according to a specified sampling efficiency curve that may be derived using health-based criteria. Horizontal elutriators, for example, can be designed such

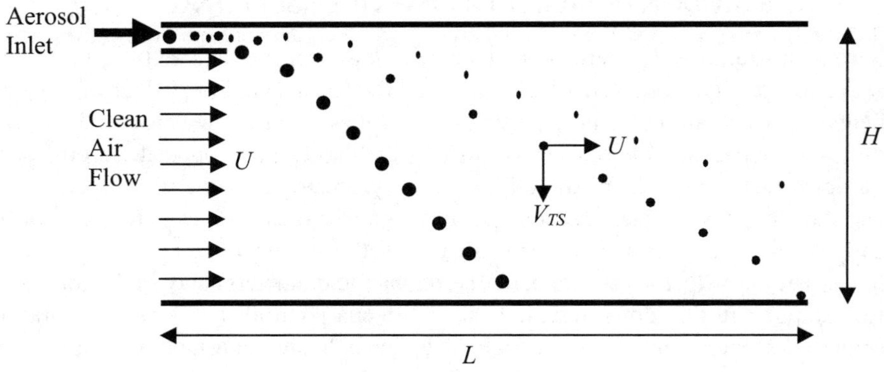

FIGURE 10.4 Schematic of a horizontal elutriator, the trajectories of particles with the critical terminal settling velocity to be just collected, and particles with velocities greater and lesser than the critical terminal settling velocity.

that their sampling efficiency matches the so-called respirable criterion (discussed in Chapter 11 and Chapter 12).

10.10 STOPPING DISTANCE

If there were no external force in Equation 10.14, then the equation reduces to

$$m\frac{dv}{dt} = -3\pi\mu dv$$

If the initial conditions are such that the particle has a velocity V_i at time $t = 0$, then the equation is easily solved to obtain

$$v(t) = V_i e^{\frac{-t}{\tau}} \tag{10.26}$$

The above equation describes the velocity of a particle projected with an initial velocity V_i into still air. The final velocity of the particle is asymptotically zero. Equation 10.26 can be integrated to calculate the distance traveled by the particle before it comes to rest. This distance S is called the *stopping distance* for the particle and is given by

$$S = V_i\tau \tag{10.27}$$

It is clear that small particles move a very small distance before coming to rest. For example, a particle with an aerodynamic diameter of 1.5 µm projected into still air with a velocity of 10 m/sec will travel 76.6 µm before coming to rest. Again, from our discussion of particle relaxation time, it is clear that although this distance is covered in infinite time, 95% of this distance is traveled in a time of 3τ. Equation 10.27 is derived assuming Stokes' formula, and thus appropriate corrections need to be made when the assumptions underlying Stokes' law do not hold.

In the absence of any external forces, the stopping distance is the distance that a particle with some initial velocity travels before coming to a stop due to drag forces. It is, therefore, a measure of the particle's inertia that makes it continue in its original direction before it is brought to a stop by the drag forces acting on it. An important application of stopping distance is when an airstream in which a particle is moving in a straight line takes a sudden turn. Whereas the streamline of air can make a sudden change in direction, the particle, due to its greater inertia, continues in its original direction for some distance.

10.11 STOKES NUMBER

When a particle is moving along a curved path, a dimensionless quantity called the *Stokes number* is useful to describe the particle. For example, when an airstream, containing aerosol particles, moving in a straight line with velocity U approaches an obstacle with a characteristic dimension D, the streamlines of air diverge around the obstacle. The particle, due to its inertia, cannot adjust its motion instantaneously to the distortion in the flow field. Stokes number is the ratio of the particle relaxation time (τ) to the time taken by a parcel of air to flow past the obstacle (D/U). Thus,

$$St = \frac{\tau U}{D} = \frac{d_{ae}^{\ 2}\rho_w U C_c}{18\mu D} \tag{10.28}$$

Thus, the ratio is a measure of how quickly a particle adjusts to a flow distortion. A particle that has a small Stokes number ($St \ll 1$) adjusts very quickly to changes in the flow field and follows the air streamlines closely. A particle with a large value of St ($St \gg 1$) takes a longer time to adjust to a change in the flow direction; it does not follow the air streamline faithfully and deviates from it. Thus, the Stokes number is a measure of the inertia of the particle.

Stokes number is a dimensionless number because it is a ratio of two timescales. For particle motion around obstacles of two widely different sizes to be geometrically similar, it is essential that the Stokes numbers for the particles in the two situations be equal. In addition, for the airflow to be geometrically similar, the flow Reynolds number for the two situations should be equal.

10.12 INERTIAL IMPACTION

When an aerosol changes direction suddenly due to an obstacle in the flow path, the particles, due to their inertia, cannot follow the air streamlines, and deviate from it. If the Stokes number of the particle is large enough, then the deviation is large enough for the particle to strike the obstacle and be "collected" by it (see Figure 10.5). Particles with smaller Stokes number values follow the flow streamlines closely and fail to be collected by the obstacle. This principle underlies the operation

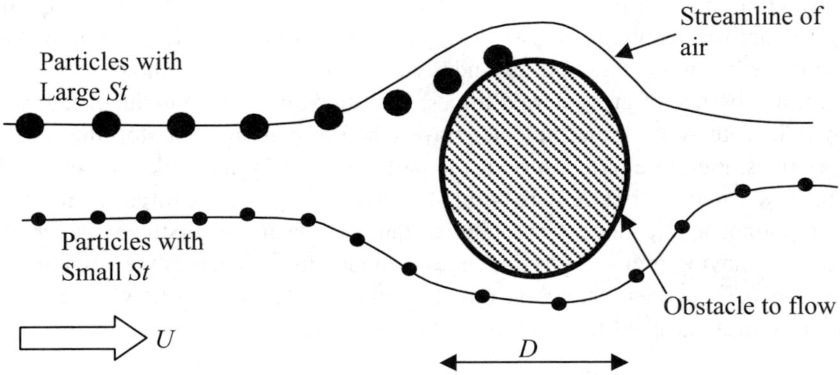

FIGURE 10.5 Particles with large Stokes numbers deviate from the air streamlines, whereas particles with small Stokes numbers closely follow the streamlines.

of one of most common methods of particle collection, i.e., impaction. A jet-and-plate impactor is the simplest configuration to achieve this. The aerosol emerges from a jet nozzle and moves toward a plate that is placed perpendicular to the jet. The streamlines of air make a sharp turn and move around the plate. The aerosol particles, depending on their Stokes numbers, either strike the plate and get collected or manage to move around the plate.

Figure 10.6 shows the arrangement of a nozzle-and-plate impactor. For a given flow rate, Q, through the nozzle, the air velocity through the nozzle is given by $U = \frac{4Q}{\pi W^2}$. If the number of particles of a given aerodynamic diameter (and hence a given Stokes number) is N_0, of which only N_i strike the plate and get collected, then the efficiency of the impactor is given by

$$E = \frac{N_i}{N_0} \tag{10.29}$$

Thus, particles with larger aerodynamic diameters (and thus, larger Stokes numbers) will have a greater collection efficiency than particles with smaller aerodynamic diameters. A plot of the collection efficiency of the impactor against Stokes number has a characteristic S-shaped curve as shown in Figure 10.7.

For particle size classification, it is preferable to have the collection efficiency curve as sharp as possible, the ideal being a step-function shape. Most commercially available impactors have a sharp S-shaped curve that is characterized by a single number, which could either be the *cutoff diameter* (the diameter at which collection efficiency is 50%, represented as d_{50}) or the *cutoff Stokes number* (represented as St_{50}). Empirical studies have determined that St_{50} for rounded and rectangular jets are 0.24 and 0.59, respectively. These values can then be used with Equation 10.28 to determine the cutoff aerodynamic diameter for the impactor.

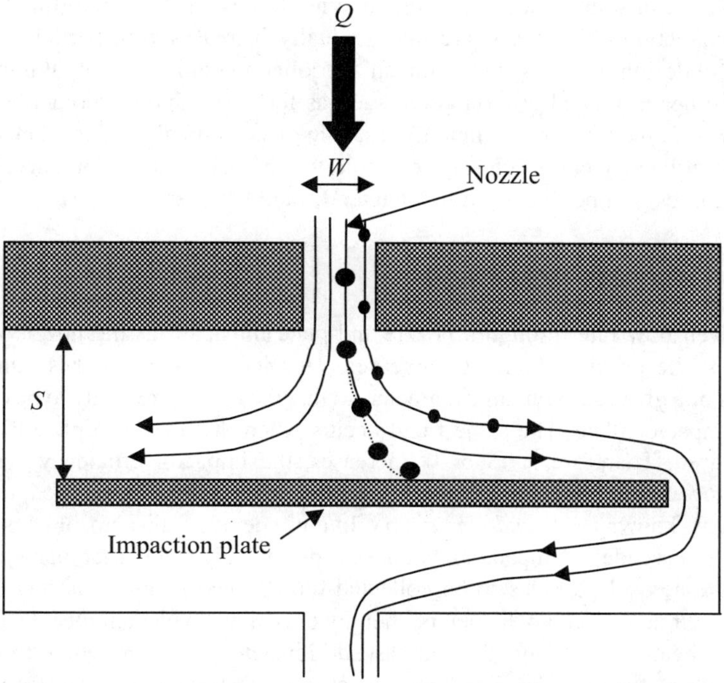

FIGURE 10.6 Nozzle jet and impactor plate. The jet has a nozzle width of W, the distance between the nozzle and the plate is S, and the flow rate through the nozzle is Q.

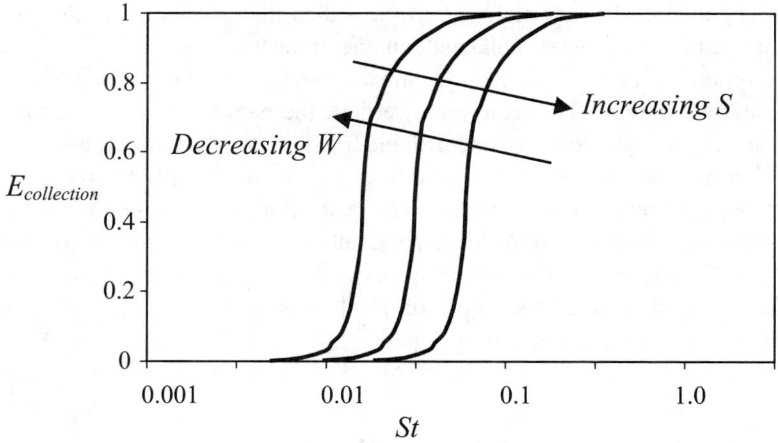

FIGURE 10.7 Collection efficiency as a function of Stokes number for an impactor, for different ratios of nozzle-to-plate distance, S, and jet diameter, W.

However, in some cases, it is preferable not to have a sharp cutoff and instead, have a collection efficiency curve that gradually increases with particle diameter. By careful design, it is possible to match the collection efficiency of an impactor to a specific health-related criteria curve such as the respirable or thoracic criterion. *Respirable impactors* are commonly used in occupational hygiene, and *PM-10 impactor* efficiency curves closely resemble the thoracic penetration curves. These criteria curves will be discussed in Chapter 11 and Chapter 12.

10.13 CASCADE IMPACTORS

For a given flow rate through a nozzle-and-plate impactor, as the nozzle width W decreases, the jet air velocity U increases. This increases the Stokes number for particles of a given aerodynamic diameter, so that they are more likely to be collected by the impactor plate. The same trend occurs when the nozzle-to-plate distance S is decreased. Therefore, as S or W increases, the impactor efficiency curves get shifted toward the right, as shown in Figure 10.7. This idea is used to design instruments known as *cascade impactors*. In these devices, the aerosol goes through a series (or cascade) of impactors that have progressively smaller jet diameters. This causes the aerosol particles to be collected on a series of impactor stages on the basis of their aerodynamic diameters, thereby providing an elegant means of particle size classification. In Figure 10.8, a cascade impactor is shown where the aerosol enters through the top. The nozzle jet diameters of each stage decrease from the top to the bottom. Because the same air flows through all the stages, this has the effect of increasing nozzle air velocities in successive stages, thereby reducing the cut size d_{50} for successive stages. Thus, successively smaller particles are collected on each stage from top to bottom. The last stage of the cascade impactor is followed by a filter that collects all the particles of size less than the cutoff size for that stage.

The particulate masses collected on the impactor stages, the entry section between the inlet orifice and the first impactor stage, and the backing filter of the instrument are the raw data required to retrieve the particle size distribution of the total aerosol in the ambient air, the inhalable fraction, and the thoracic and respirable subfractions. Also required is knowledge of the detailed, particle size–dependent collection characteristics of each stage. The reconstruction of the continuous aerosol size distribution from a set of N discrete measurements can be formulated as solving a system of equations. The relationship between the discrete set of measurements of mass on each stage of the impactor $\{M_k\}$ (in which $k = 1, 2, \ldots N$) and the unknown function $f(d_{ae})$ is given by

$$M_k = \int_a^b K_k(d_{ae}) \cdot f(d_{ae})\, dd_{ae} + \varepsilon_k;\ k = 1, 2 \ldots\ldots N \tag{10.30}$$

where $f(d_{ae})$ is the particle aerodynamic size distribution for the aerosol in the ambient air, K_k is the efficiency with which particles of a given size deposit on the kth stage after penetrating through all the preceding stages, a and b define the range within

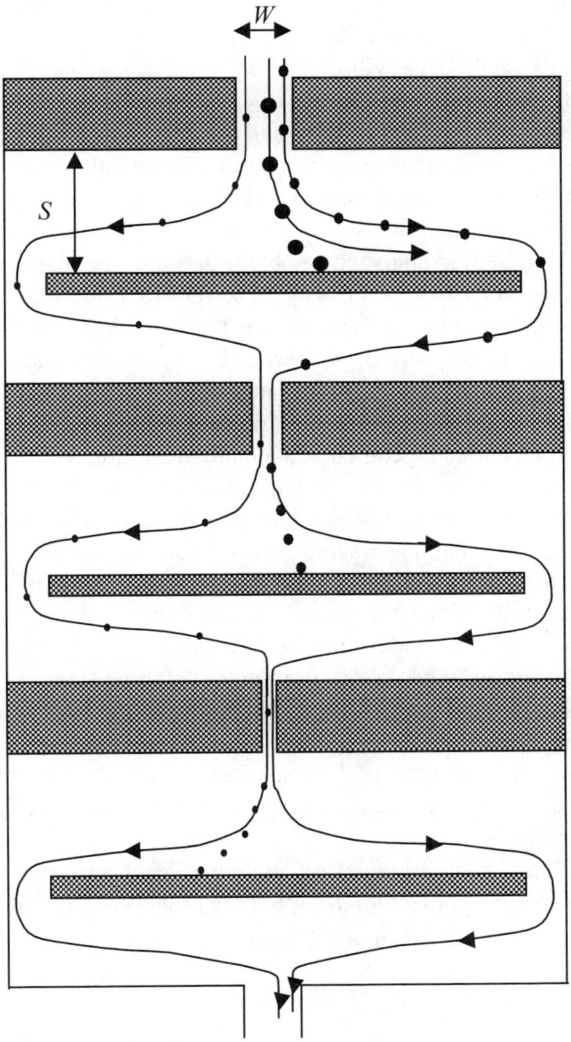

FIGURE 10.8 A three-stage cascade impactor. Note that the nozzle width decreases in each successive stage from the top to the bottom.

which the particle size distribution lies, and ε_k is the measurement error in that channel. K_k describes the instrument response and is determined from design and experimental calibration data.

Each stage of the cascade impactor contains a removable plate or substrate on which the particles are collected. The plates or substrates can be removed and analyzed gravimetrically or chemically for mass, or microscopically for particle count. The standard method of analyzing cascade impactor data is to assume that the collection efficiency curves have ideally sharp cutoffs. Thus, each stage is assumed to collect all the particles in the aerosol reaching that stage which are above the cutoff size for that stage.

For example, if a cascade impactor has five stages with cutoff d_{50}'s of 12, 9, 6, 3, and 1 μm, respectively, then the first stage will collect all the particles greater than 12 μm, the second stage will collect all particles between 9 and 12 μm, the third stage will collect all particles between 6 and 9 μm, the fourth stage will collect all particles between 3 and 6 μm, and the fifth stage will collect all particles between 1 and 3 μm. Particles less than 1 μm will be collected on a filter that is downstream of the lowest impactor stage. Thus, the instrument provides mass or count measurements divided into several classes on the basis of particle size. These measurements can then be analyzed to obtain particle size distributions using the methods described in Chapter 9. For example, Table 9.7 and Figure 9.12 illustrate the calculations that need to be carried out to obtain the cumulative mass size distribution of the aerosol. In this scenario, the cumulative masses on the stages may therefore be considered as representative of the cumulative particle size distribution from which, when plotted on log-probability axes, the median particle aerodynamic diameter and geometric standard deviation may be estimated by direct visual inspection (under the assumption that the distribution is lognormal).

Although the above method of data analysis is commonly used, it rests on the assumption that each stage has a sharp cutoff, and that there is no overlap of the collection efficiency curves of successive stages. This assumption is typically not true. In reality, the collection characteristics of each impactor stage are not perfectly sharp, so that there is substantial overlap between the stage collection curves, causing particles of a given size to be collected on more than one stage. In addition, many possible size distributions would be consistent with the observed masses. This problem derives in part from the fact that we are trying to recover a continuous size distribution from a small number of discrete pieces of information. The mathematical analysis of the data, referred to as *data inversion*, becomes complicated, and is an active area of research.

One of the simpler algorithms that attempt to deal with this problem uses a weighted least squares optimization to fit bimodal lognormal distribution functions. The optimization routine itself minimizes the expression

$$\sum_{k=1}^{n}\left(\frac{M_k - \int_a^b K_k(d_{ae})\cdot f(d_{ae})\,dd_{ae}}{E(\varepsilon_k)}\right)^2 - N \qquad (10.31)$$

where N is the number of measurements and $E(\varepsilon_k)$ is the expected value of the measurement error. Thus, the optimization procedure finds a solution for the particle size distribution of the total aerosol in the ambient air that satisfies the measurements to just within experimental error. For aerosols encountered in the industrial workplace environment, it is reasonable (from previous experience) to assume that the basic form of the distribution is lognormal. The solution is sought for a unimodal lognormal distribution that is described by two parameters (i.e., the mass median

TABLE 10.1
Results from a Personal Cascade Impactor for Lead-Containing Aerosol for the Milling Area of a Primary Lead Smelter, Showing the Mass of Lead Collected on Each Stage of the Instrument

Stage	d_{50} (μm)	Mass of lead (μg)
Entry	26.0	154.0
1	18.2	25.0
2	14.4	14.0
3	10.6	13.0
4	6.0	20.0
5	4.8	8.2
6	3.3	5.5
7	1.7	6.5
8	0.9	2.8
Filter	0.0	2.8

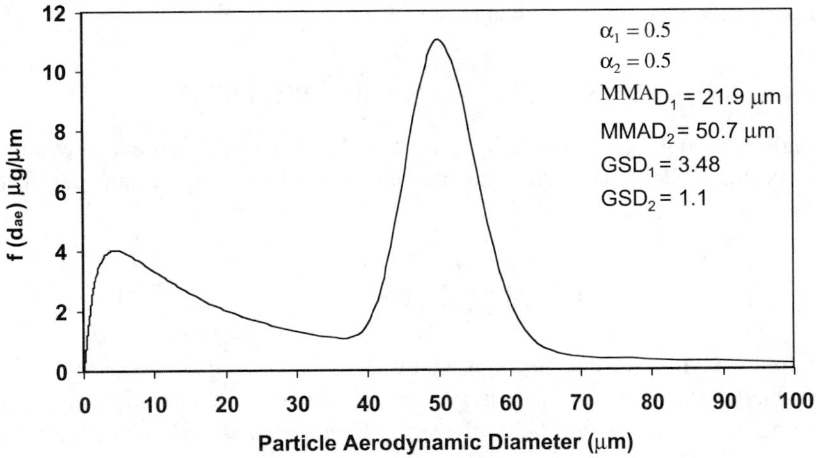

FIGURE 10.9 Particle size distribution for airborne lead for one sample obtained at a milling operation in a primary lead smelter.

particle aerodynamic diameter and the geometric standard deviation) or a bimodal lognormal distribution that may be described by five parameters (i.e., the mass median particle aerodynamic diameters, the geometric standard deviations of the two modes, and the relative weighting of the masses between the two modes).

Table 10.1 shows raw data of mass of lead-containing aerosol collected using a personal cascade impactor in the milling area of a primary lead smelter. The cut sizes of the different stages of the impactor are given to show the range of the instrument. However, the data were used to estimate the size distribution by using the collection efficiency characteristics of each impactor stage and by using the algorithm described by Equation 10.31. Figure 10.9 shows the size distribution retrieved using this approach, as well as the parameters of the bimodal lognormal distribution.

Another departure from ideal behavior is that solid particles might strike an impactor stage plate, bounce off, and get reentrained in the airflow. They may subsequently be collected on a lower stage or clog the nozzles of subsequent stages. Thus, the measured size distribution might be different from the true size distribution. This distortion can be somewhat prevented by using a sticky surface, e.g., by coating the collection surfaces with a thin film of grease that is dissolved in a solvent. However, this does not completely solve the problem, because once a layer of particles has been deposited on the sticky surface, subsequent particles will impact on particles already collected and be more likely to bounce.

Particles can also deposit on surfaces other than the impaction plate, e.g., on the walls of the impactor. These wall losses are more likely to occur for larger particles due to their larger inertia. Because the large particles collected on a wall would normally have been deposited on one of the impactor stages, their absence skews the measured size distribution toward smaller sizes. Typically, the wall loss as a fraction of the total mass collected on each stage is determined experimentally as a function of particle diameter. This correction factor is then applied to subsequent measurements using the instrument.

10.14 PARTICLE MOTION IN AN ELECTRIC FIELD

If a particle carries a charge q (in SI units of coulombs) in an electric field of strength $\vec{E}$ (a vector in SI units of V/m), then the electrical force F_E (in SI units of newtons) on the particle is given by

$$\vec{F_E} = q\vec{E} \tag{10.32}$$

This force on the particle is opposed by the drag force on the particle. Using arguments similar to that in the case of gravity, we obtain the steady state velocity of the particle in an electric field, called the *terminal electrical drift velocity*, as

$$V_E = \frac{qE}{3\pi\mu d} \tag{10.33}$$

A related quantity is the particle *electrical mobility, Z,* which is equal to the drift velocity when the applied field strength is unity.

$$Z = \frac{q}{3\pi\mu d} \tag{10.34}$$

The most common configuration for collectors is the parallel plate collector in which two conducting plates are held at different electric potentials. The electric field between the two plates is given by

$$E = \frac{V_2 - V_1}{X}$$

where V_2 and V_1 are the potentials (in units of volts) at which the two plates are held, and X is the spacing between the plates. Here, the electric field is constant at every point between the plates, and the field lines are parallel to each other and perpendicular to the plates. Another common configuration is a cylinder having a wire running down its axis. Here the electric field is has a radial direction and a magnitude given by

$$E = \frac{V_2 - V_1}{r \ln\left(\frac{r_2}{r_1}\right)}$$

where V_2 and V_1 are the potentials of the outer cylinder and the inner wire, respectively, and r_2 and r_1 are their respective radii. Equation 10.36 also shows that the electric field strength depends on the radial location r.

Electrostatic forces are particularly useful in collecting small aerosol particles (<1 μm) for which inertial forces might be negligible. In typical industrial hygiene applications (e.g., in electrostatic precipitators that are used for air cleaning or air sampling), the aerosol particles are charged artificially by collisions with ions or ion clusters. This can be accomplished by *diffusion charging*, in which the particles are charged by collisions with diffusing ions without an external electric field, or by *field charging*, in which particles collide with ions moving in an applied electric field. In field charging, the ions move rapidly in the direction of the applied electric field, and this increases the frequency of collisions between the ions and the particles. Therefore, field charging can achieve a significantly higher particle charge than diffusion charging for the same ion concentration. In both cases, as the charge on the particle increases, it repels and slows down further ions from approaching the particle, and thus decreases the charging rate. These methods require the production of ions of the same polarity using a corona discharge.

Even in the absence of active charging mechanisms, aerosol particles in workplaces (and elsewhere) tend to have one or more positive or negative charges due to random collisions with ions in air. Typically, there are ~10^9 ions per cubic meter of air, and these are evenly divided between positive and negative ions. Collisions may lead to the acquisition of one or more charges that may attract charges of opposite sign. Thus, further collisions might reduce the charge on the particle. Because the collisions of aerosol particles and the ions are random, the particles will also acquire positive and negative charges such that the aerosol as a whole is neutral. The aerosol thus attains an equilibrium charge state called the *Boltzmann equilibrium charge distribution*.

However, the median particle charge carried by a given particle is a nonlinear function of particle diameter ($\propto d^n$, in which n is an integer). Therefore, larger particles are likely to have much greater electrical drift velocities, and thus are more likely to be captured by electrostatic precipitators. Chapter 13 describes, in greater detail, instruments based on particle charge measurement.

10.15 PARTICLE DIFFUSION

In Chapter 2, we studied the random thermal motion of air molecules. When particles are suspended in air, they are subjected to constant collisions with the air molecules, resulting in random movement of the aerosol particles as well. This motion is referred to as *Brownian motion* and results in a net drift of particles from a region of higher concentration to a region of lower concentration. This transport mechanism is called *diffusion*. The mass transfer process is described by Fick's law:

$$J = -D_p \frac{dc}{dx} \tag{10.35}$$

where J is the mass flux in the x direction (the mass that is transported per unit area across a plane perpendicular to the concentration gradient in unit time, mg/m^2/sec), D_p is the particle diffusion coefficient (m^2/sec), c is the local concentration (mg/m^3), and $\frac{dc}{dx}$ is the local concentration gradient (mg/m^4). This is identical to the equation describing transport of gas molecules by diffusion, except that the diffusion coefficient is for particles and not gas molecules.

By equating the diffusion force to the drag force, we can obtain an expression for the diffusion coefficient as

$$D_p = \frac{kTC_c}{3\pi\mu d} \tag{10.36}$$

where k is the Boltzman constant (1.38×10^{-23} J/K), T the temperature in K, C_c the Cunningham correction factor, and d the particle diameter. Equation 10.36, referred to as the *Stokes–Einstein equation*, shows that the diffusion coefficient increases with temperature. For large particles, C_c can be neglected, and the diffusion coefficient is inversely proportional to particle diameter. Thus, the larger the particle, the less its transport will be driven by collisions with gas molecules. For small particles, C_c is significant (see Equation 10.8 and Equation 10.9), and thus the diffusion coefficient is roughly inversely proportional to d^2. The diffusion coefficients of even very small particles are much smaller than the diffusion coefficients of gas molecules. For example, the diffusion coefficients of particles with diameters of 0.01 μm, 0.1 μm, and 1 μm at 25°C are of the order of 10^{-8}, 10^{-10}, and 10^{-11} m^2/sec, respectively. The corresponding diffusion coefficient for an air molecule (which was calculated in Chapter 2) is of the order of 10^{-5} m^2/sec.

As in the case of electrical forces acting on a particle, particle mobility B can be defined as the velocity given to the particle by a unit driving force.

$$B = \frac{C_c}{3\pi\mu d} \tag{10.37}$$

which for a sphere of mass m and relaxation time τ becomes

$$B = \frac{\tau}{m} \tag{10.38}$$

Thus, the diffusion coefficient can be expressed as

$$D_p = \frac{\tau}{m} kT \tag{10.39}$$

During Brownian diffusion, each particle gets displaced by a small distance in a random direction. If we consider movement only along one axis, then the displacements are random, but only backward and forward along the axis. Using simple arguments, one can derive an expression for the root-mean-square displacement for an aerosol particle at time t:

$$s_{rms} = \sqrt{2D_p t} \tag{10.40}$$

If we consider motion in all three dimensions, then the expression is

$$s_{rms} = \sqrt{\left(\frac{4}{\pi}\right) D_p t} \tag{10.41}$$

This is indicative of the distance that a particle with diffusion coefficient D_p will travel in time t. For example, the alveoli in the human lung can be modeled as spherical chambers with a diameter of roughly 300 μm. A particle with diameter 0.01 μm at the center of an alveolus will have to travel 150 μm to get deposited on the alveolar wall. Using Equation 10.41, we can estimate the time for this to occur to be roughly 0.33 sec. A particle with diameter 0.1 μm will take roughly 25 sec to cover the same distance. Thus, for small particles, diffusion is a much more significant means of particle deposition in the alveoli than for larger particles.

11 Inhalation and Respiratory Tract Deposition of Aerosols

11.1 INTRODUCTION

Inhalation is the main route of human exposure to most aerosols. The transport of aerosol particles from the ambient environment into the respiratory tract through the nose and mouth depends on aerosol properties such as the Stokes number. Once the aerosol is inhaled, particles are deposited in different regions of the respiratory tract. This deposition depends on phenomena described in Chapter 10, such as inertial impaction, gravitational settling, and diffusion.

A healthy adult breathes in 10 to 20 m^3 of air every day. The *tidal volume* (the volume convected in and out during each breathing cycle) is ~0.7 l at rest, whereas it increases to greater than 2 l during heavy work. The breathing rates at rest and during heavy work are ~10 breaths/min and ~30 breaths/minute, respectively. Around 2.4 l of air is not exhaled, but is retained in the deepest region of the lung. This is referred to as *reserve air*. Table 11.1 shows the values of respiratory parameters for a "representative worker" as defined by the International Commission on Radiological Protection (ICRP, 1975).

11.2 THE HUMAN RESPIRATORY TRACT

Whereas the human respiratory tract is a complex structure, we can use a simplified model of it to understand aerosol deposition. This simplified model divides the respiratory tract into three regions as shown in Figure 11.1. The air enters through the nose and mouth and goes into the upper airways of the head. This region is called the *extrathoracic* or *nasopharyngeal region*. It includes the airways of the nose, the mouth, and the throat (the nasopharynx) where air becomes humidified after entry. The nasal passages are referred to as *turbinates* and provide a winding and twisting path for the entering air. Some of the nasal passages are covered with hair-like projections called *cilia*. The rhythmic beating of these cilia is an important means of removal of deposited particles by transporting them to the pharynx. The transported particles then enter the gastrointestinal tract by swallowing. For a steady breathing rate of 1 l/sec, the air velocity in this region can be as high as 3 to 5 m/sec.

Below the larynx (or the voice box) is the *thoracic region* or the lung. Air moves into the *trachea* or windpipe. The trachea then branches repeatedly into a series of airways referred to as *bronchi* and *bronchioles*. The trachea is referred to as generation 0. This divides into two bronchi (generation 1). Each airway in one generation

TABLE 11.1
Values of Respiratory Parameters for a Reference Worker

Parameter	Value
Weight	70 kg
Height	175 cm
Lung weight	1000 g
Lung surface area	80 m^2
Total lung capacity	5.6 l
Vital capacity	4.3 l
Functional residual capacity	2.2 l
Breathing rate	15 breaths/min
Tidal volume	1450 ml
Inspiratory flow rate	43.5 l/min
Inspiratory period	2 sec
Expiratory period	2 sec

Source: From International Commission on Radiological Protection (ICRP) (1975), *Reference Man*, ICRP Publication 23, Pergamon, Elmsford, NY, pp. 122–124.

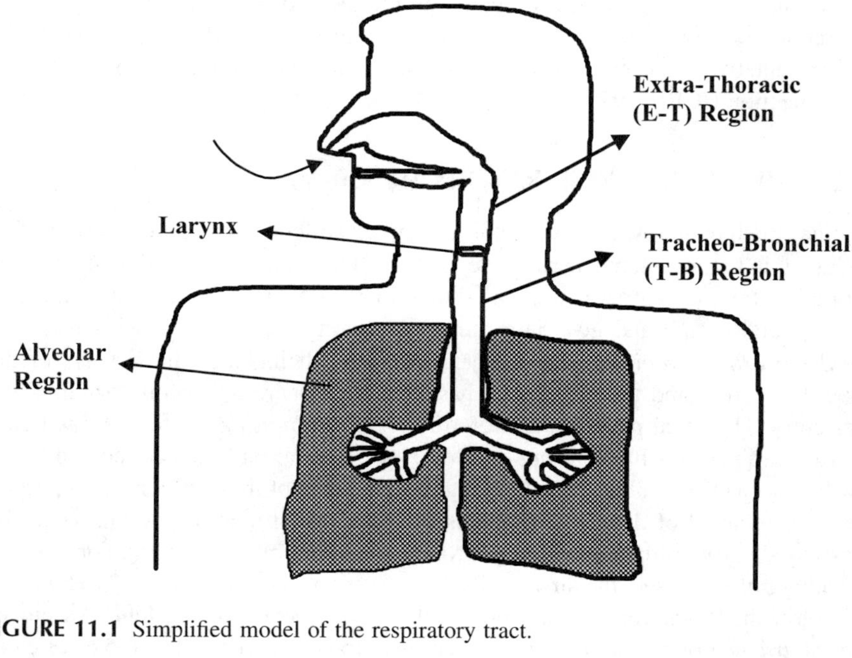

FIGURE 11.1 Simplified model of the respiratory tract.

gives rise to two branches in the next generation. Generations 1 through 11 are bronchi, whereas the rest, up to generation 16, are bronchioles and *terminating bronchioles*. The airways in the generations 0 through 16 are together referred to as the *tracheobronchial region* of the lung. These airways are covered with hair-like

TABLE 11.2
Physical Dimensions of Various Regions of the Thoracic Region According to the Weibel Model

Region	Airway	G	N_G	D_G	L_G	A_G	V_G	t_G
Tracheobronchial	Trachea	0	1	18	120	2.5	3.9	30
	Bronchi	1	2	12	48	2.3	4.3	11
		11	2×10^3	1.1	3.9	20	0.52	7.4
	Bronchioles	14	16×10^3	0.74	2.3	69	0.14	16
		16	66×10^3	0.60	1.6	180	0.05	31
Alveolar	Respiratory bronchioles	18	26×10^4	0.50	1.2	530	0.03	60
	Alveolar ducts	21	2×10^6	0.43	0.7	3×10^3	0.003	210
	Alveolar sacs	23	8×10^6	0.41	0.5	1×10^4	0.001	550
	Alveoli		300×10^6	0.28	0.2			

Note: G: generation number; N_G: number per generation; D_G: diameter of duct at generation G (mm); L_G: length of duct at generation G (mm); A_G: total cross sectional area of generation G (cm^2); V_G: air velocity at generation G (m/s); t_G: residence time in generation G (ms). Velocity and residence times are calculated assuming a flow rate of 1 l/sec.

Source: From Hinds, W.C. (1999), *Aerosol Technology: Properties, Behavior, and Measurement of Airborne Particles*, 2nd ed. John Wiley & Sons, New York.

ciliary projections and a mucus layer (the mucociliary escalator). As in the case of the nasopharyngeal region, the rhythmic beating of the cilia moves deposited particles on the mucus layer toward the larynx, where the action of swallowing transports them into the gastrointestinal tract. Due to the presence of the ciliary projections, these airways are also called *conducting airways*.

From generation 16 to generation 23 are the respiratory bronchioles, alveolar ducts, alveolar sacs, and the alveoli. This region is called the *alveolar region* of the lung. Thus the thoracic region comprises the tracheobronchial and alveolar regions. The exchange of oxygen and carbon dioxide occurs in the alveolar region. There are no cilia or mucus in the alveolar region, because these would diminish the gas exchange capacity of the alveoli. However, *alveolar macrophages* patrol the alveolar surfaces, and these cells scavenge any foreign objects, including aerosol particles that get deposited on the surfaces. The particles are engulfed by these cells, which then move toward the mucociliary escalator for ultimate removal.

Table 11.2 provides the number and dimensions of the airways in each generation and the average air velocity in those airway generations for a steady inhalation rate of 1 l/sec. Although regular breathing is not steady, but exhibits cyclical changes in direction, these calculations are useful approximations. We see that the air velocity is several meters per second in the trachea and the first few generations. The flow is turbulent in this region. The velocity falls rapidly thereafter due to the increase in the total cross-sectional area caused by the large number of small ducts. The Reynolds number is sufficiently reduced so that the flow is laminar in this region. In the alveolar sacs, the velocity drops to 1 mm/sec and the residence time is 550 ms. This is the region occupied by the reserve air. Molecular and convective diffusion between the tidal air and the reserve air leads to transport of gases into the alveolar region. The individual alveoli are spherical, closed-ended structures roughly 300 μm in diameter. The 300 million alveoli thus provide a surface area of roughly 75 m^2 for gas exchange.

As mentioned earlier, the main mechanisms of particle deposition in the respiratory tract are inertial impaction, gravitational settling, and diffusional deposition. The ideas discussed in Chapter 10 are used in estimating the relative importance of these mechanisms in different regions of the respiratory tract, and the results are shown in Table 11.3. In the upper airways, the air has to negotiate a winding path with many direction changes. Aerosol particles, depending on their Stokes number (i.e., their inertia), will deviate from the streamlines of air, impact on the walls of the airways, and get deposited. This deposition by inertial impaction is more pronounced for larger particles than for smaller particles. Table 11.3 uses the ratio of the particle stopping distance (calculated using Equation 10.27) to the airway diameter as a measure of the probability of deposition by inertial impaction. This is the dominant deposition mechanism for larger particles in the trachea up to generation 11 (terminal bronchus). As the air moves into the lower respiratory tract, its velocity decreases dramatically. This increases the particle residence time in the lower airways. Therefore, particles now have sufficient time to settle due to gravity. The ratio of particle settling distance (calculated using Equation 10.25) to the airway diameter is a measure of the probability of deposition by gravitational settling. This effect is greater for larger particles (that have larger settling velocities) than for smaller particles. Diffusion is an important mechanism of motion for small particles. In the lower airways, the small airway diameters and the comparatively long residence times lead to a greater probability of deposition of small particles by diffusional deposition. The ratio of particle root-mean-square displacement (calculated using Equation 10.41) to the airway diameter is a measure of the probability of deposition by diffusional deposition.

11.3 PENETRATION AND DEPOSITION EFFICIENCY

Figure 11.2 shows the inhaled particles penetrating and depositing in different regions of the respiratory tract. The ability of particles to penetrate beyond the nose and mouth is called the *inhalation efficiency* or *inhalability.* If there are N_0 particles in the ambient air per unit volume, and N_{inh} particles enter through the nose and mouth, then the inhalation efficiency is given by

$$I = \frac{N_{\text{inh}}}{N_0} \tag{11.1}$$

TABLE 11.3
Relative Importance of Inertial Impaction, Gravitational Settling, and Diffusion for Particle Deposition in Different Regions of the Respiratory Tract

Airway (Generation)	Stopping Distance / Airway Diameter (%)			Settling Distance / Airway Diameter (%)			RMS Distance / Airway Diameter (%)		
	0.1 µm	1 µm	10 µm	0.1 µm	1 µm	10 µm	0.1 µm	1 µm	10 µm
Trachea (0)	0	0.08	6.8	0	0	0.52	0.04	0.01	0
Main bronchus (1)	0	0.13	10.9	0	0	0.41	0.03	0.01	0
Terminal bronchus (11)	0	0.17	14.9	0	0.02	2.1	0.29	0.06	0.02
Terminal bronchiole (16)	0	0.03	2.8	0	0.18	15.6	1.1	0.22	0.06
Alveolar duct (21)	0	0	0.23	0.04	1.7	150	3.9	0.79	0.23
Alveolar sac (23)	0	0	0.07	0.12	4.7	410	6.7	1.3	0.40

Note: The particle diameters refer to aerodynamic diameters in the case of impaction and settling and geometric diameters in the case of diffusion. All calculations were performed using a steady breathing rate of 60 l/min.

Source: From Hinds, W.C. (1999), *Aerosol Technology: Properties, Behavior, and Measurement of Airborne Particles*, 2nd ed. John Wiley & Sons, New York.

Of the N_{inh} particles entering the respiratory tract, D_{ET} get deposited in the extrathoracic region and N_{thor} particles penetrate into the thoracic region. Therefore, the efficiency of deposition in the extrathoracic region is given by

$$E_{\text{ET}} = \frac{D_{\text{ET}}}{N_{\text{inh}}} = 1 - \frac{N_{\text{thor}}}{N_{\text{inh}}} = 1 - T \qquad (11.2)$$

Equation 11.2 shows that the efficiency of deposition in the extrathoracic region is also equal to 1 minus the penetration into the thoracic region (T).

The efficiency of deposition in the tracheobronchial region is given by

$$E_{\text{TB}} = \frac{D_{\text{TB}}}{N_{\text{inh}}} = \frac{N_{\text{thor}} - N_{\text{Alv}}}{N_{\text{inh}}} = T - R \qquad (11.3)$$

where D_{TB} is the number of particles deposited in the tracheobronchial region, N_{Alv} is the number of particles penetrating into the alveolar region and R is the fractional penetration into the alveolar region. Thus, the efficiency of deposition in the tracheobronchial region is the difference between the penetration into the thoracic region and the penetration into the alveolar region.

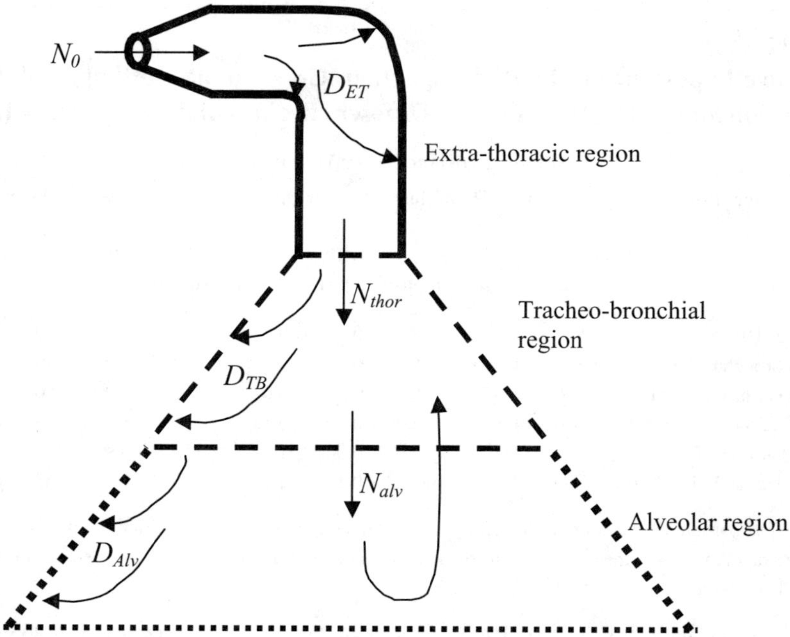

FIGURE 11.2 Schematic diagram defining various fractions of the inhaled aerosol that penetrate and get deposited in various regions of the respiratory tract (Vincent, J.H., 1995, *Aerosol Science for Industrial Hygienists*, Pergamon, Elsevier Science, New York.)

The efficiency of deposition in the alveolar region is given by

$$E_{\text{Alv}} = \frac{D_{\text{Alv}}}{N_{\text{inh}}} = \frac{N_{\text{Alv}} - N_{\text{exh}}}{N_{\text{inh}}} = R - \frac{N_{\text{exh}}}{N_{\text{inh}}} \tag{11.4}$$

where N_{exh} is the number of particles exhaled out. Thus, the efficiency of deposition in the alveolar region is the difference between the penetration into the alveolar region and the fraction of inhaled particles that are exhaled without being deposited.

The *thoracic penetration*, also called the *thoracic fraction*, T is given by

$$T = \frac{N_{\text{Thor}}}{N_{\text{inh}}} = \frac{D_{\text{TB}} + D_{\text{Alv}} + N_{\text{exh}}}{N_{\text{inh}}} \tag{11.5}$$

and the *alveolar penetration*, which is also called the *respirable fraction*, is given by

$$R = \frac{N_{\text{Alv}}}{N_{\text{inh}}} = \frac{D_{\text{Alv}} + N_{\text{exh}}}{N_{\text{inh}}} \tag{11.6}$$

The total respiratory tract deposition efficiency is given by

$$E_{\text{total}} = \frac{D_{\text{ET}} + D_{\text{TB}} + D_{\text{Alv}}}{N_{\text{inh}}} \tag{11.7}$$

11.4 INHALATION AND THE INHALABLE SAMPLING CRITERION

In terms of exposure, not all sizes of particles suspended in the air can be breathed in with 100% efficiency. Thus, any exposure assessment should focus on the particles that can actually enter the respiratory tract. The human head can be thought of as an aerosol sampler. The *inhalation efficiency* or the *aspiration efficiency* of the human head is defined by Equation 11.1. The breathing rate, the dimensions of the head, and the ambient air velocity, as well as the aerodynamic diameter of the particles, determine the fraction of ambient particles that enter the head through the nose and mouth. The *inhalable fraction* was experimentally determined in a number of studies conducted in the 1970s through the 1990s. These experiments were typically conducted in a wind tunnel where a full-size mannequin was placed and attached to a breathing machine. A test aerosol was generated that contained particles of known aerodynamic diameters up to 100 μm, under wind speeds relevant to workplace conditions. A filter placed just behind the mouth and nose of the mannequin collected the inhaled aerosol breathed in by the mannequin (N_{inh}), while a reference sampler upstream of the mannequin measured N_0. The inhalable fraction was then calculated using Equation 11.1. The sampling (or inhalation) efficiency results were reported for head orientations with respect to the wind averaged over 360° about a vertical axis. This was done for a wide range of particle aerodynamic diameters. Based on such data derived from several studies, standard-setting organizations such as the American Conference of Governmental Industrial Hygienists (ACGIH), the International Standards Organization (ISO), and the Comité Européen de Normalisation (CEN) have agreed upon a so-called inhalable fraction. For wind velocity less than 4 m/sec, the inhalable fraction is given by

$$I\left(d_{\text{ae}}\right) = 0.5\left(1 + \exp\left(-0.06\, d_{\text{ae}}\right)\right) \tag{11.8}$$

It is defined as the probability of particles of a given aerodynamic diameter entering through the nose or mouth (or both) during breathing. Equation 11.8 is valid for aerodynamic diameters up to 100 μm. Figure 11.3 shows the curve corresponding to Equation 11.8.

The shaded region contains greater than 90% of the experimental data for wind speeds less than 4 m/sec. The curve shown in Figure 11.3 is applicable for most indoor workplaces. However, some studies have shown that for very low wind speeds, the sampling efficiency is significantly higher than the curve. However, for outdoor situations, wind speeds greater than 4 m/sec are common. In such cases, the inhalable

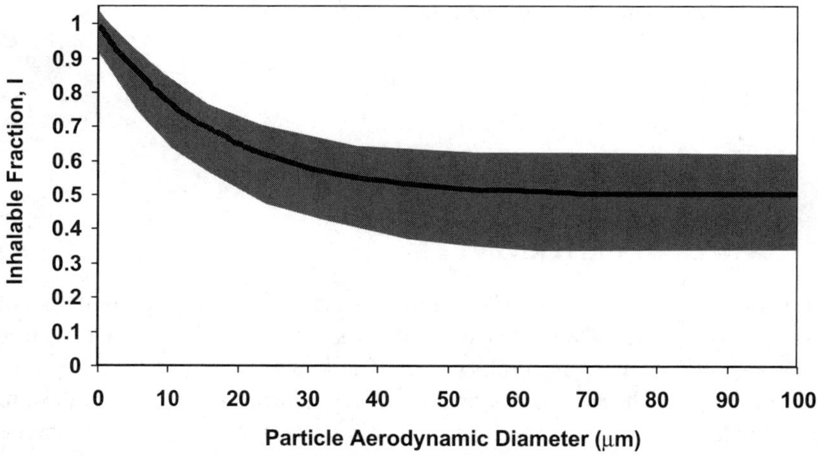

FIGURE 11.3 Inhalable curve as adopted by ACGIH. The shaded area represents the envelope of experimental data using mannequins in wind tunnels.

curve deviates significantly from that defined by Equation 11.8. A modified expression is recommended in such situations (Vincent, 1999), and is given by

$$I\left(d_{ae}\right) = 0.5\left(1 + \exp\left(-0.06\, d_{ae}\right)\right) + 10^{-5}\, U^{2.75} \exp\left(0.055\right) \tag{11.9}$$

where U is the wind speed in meters per second.

There are several practical benefits of defining the inhalable fraction mathematically. First, it serves as a reference against which the efficiency of a sampler can be compared. The idea is that if the sampling efficiency of an aerosol sampler matches the inhalable curve, then it is behaving like the human head, and therefore a sample obtained by such a sampler is representative of human exposure to inhaled particles. Second, if we know the size distribution (by mass) of an aerosol to be $m(d)$, then we can easily calculate the total inhaled mass to be

$$Inhaled\ mass = \int_0^{\infty} m\left(d_{ae}\right) I\left(d_{ae}\right) dd_{ae} \tag{11.10}$$

11.5 EXTRATHORACIC DEPOSITION

Aerosol deposition in this region occurs primarily by inertial impaction. Due to their inertia, particles are unable to follow the rapidly changing directions of airflow around the nasal turbinates and nasal hairs, and may collide with airway walls and be collected. The deposition efficiency for a given particle size depends on the breathing flow rate

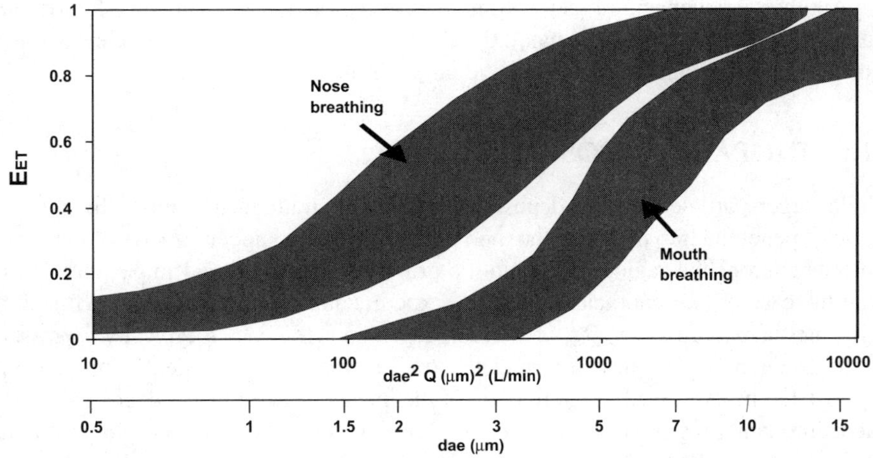

FIGURE 11.4 Deposition efficiency in the extrathoracic region as a function of the inertial parameter $d_{ae}^2 Q_{inh}$. The aerodynamic diameters on the secondary horizontal axis are calculated assuming a breathing rate of 43.5 l/min for a reference worker. Based on data from several studies summarized by Raabe, O.G., and Stuart, B.O. (1999), Sampling criteria for the thoracic and respirable fractions, in *Particle Size Selective Sampling for Particulate Air Contaminants*, Vincent, J.H., Ed., ACGIH, Cincinnati, OH.

and whether breathing is through the nose or the mouth. Thus, Stokes number is an important parameter affecting deposition in this region. Experimental results have, therefore, been reported as a function of $d_{ae}^2 Q_{inh}$, where Q_{inh} is the average inhalation flow rate (that depends on air velocity). The deposition efficiency is defined according to Equation 11.2. Figure 11.4 shows the envelopes of data for deposition in the extrathoracic region. These envelopes are based on the data from several studies summarized by Raabe and Stuart (1999). It is clear that as particle inertia (represented here by $d_{ae}^2 Q_{inh}$) increases, the deposition efficiency increases. Larger particles get deposited more efficiently in the extrathoracic region. It is also clear from Figure 11.4 that nasopharyngeal deposition from nose breathing is greater for all particle sizes than oropharyngeal deposition from mouth breathing. Thus, for nose breathing, less of these particles are available for deposition in the small airways of the thoracic region. The deposition efficiency for nose breathing is given by

$$E_{ET} = -0.62 + 0.475 \log_{10}\left(d_{ae}^2 Q_{inh}\right) \tag{11.11}$$

whereas the deposition efficiency for mouth breathing is given by

$$E_{ET} = -1.4 + 0.6 \log_{10}\left(d_{ae}^2 Q_{inh}\right) \tag{11.12}$$

Another mechanism of deposition in this region is by diffusion of ultrafine particles (with diameters less than 0.01 μm). However, this is of little relevance for most aerosols encountered in occupational environments.

11.6 THORACIC DEPOSITION

While larger particles tend to deposit more in the extrathoracic region, the smaller particles penetrate into the lung (the thoracic region). In the upper airways of the lung, the tracheobronchial region, deposition is primarily due to inertial impaction. Thus, as in the case of extrathoracic deposition, experimental data are shown as a function of the inertial parameter, $d_{ae}^2 Q_{inh}$. However, deposition efficiency is typically expressed as the fraction of the mass entering the trachea that gets deposited. This can be converted to be expressed as the fraction of the inhaled aerosol that is deposited in the tracheobronchial region as in Equation 11.3. Figure 11.5 shows the envelope of data for deposition in the tracheobronchial region. The envelope is based on the data from Lippmann (1977). For smaller particles, deposition efficiency increases with inertial parameter, as expected. For larger particles, deposition efficiency decreases with particle size (or inertial parameter). This is because these particles have already been preferentially removed by deposition in the extrathoracic region. A simple calculation illustrates this point. Consider 100 particles of aerodynamic diameter 15 μm being inhaled. Roughly 90 of these will be deposited in the extrathoracic region (from Figure 11.4) and 10 particles will enter the tracheobronchial region. About 8 of these particles get deposited in the tracheobronchial region. Therefore, the efficiency of deposition as a fraction of particles being inhaled is 8%, whereas the efficiency of deposition as a fraction of particles entering the thoracic region is 80%.

The inhaled air mixes with the reserve air in the tracheobronchial region by turbulent eddy diffusion. This mixing transfers particles into the reserve air that occupies the alveolar region. Particles that penetrate through the tracheobronchial region enter the alveolar region, or the gas-exchange region of the lung. Here, the air velocities are very low (see Table 11.2), and therefore residence times are long. The settling distances are of the order of 300 μm (the diameter of an alveolus) and particles with large enough aerodynamic diameters can settle down on the alveolar walls rapidly. For very small particles, diffusion is the primary deposition mechanism.

The efficiency of alveolar deposition is defined by Equation 11.4. Figure 11.6 shows the envelope of experimental data from several studies summarized by Raabe and Stuart (1999). For particles larger than 10 μm, the alveolar deposition is close to zero due to the efficient filtration of the particles by the extrathoracic region. For sizes between 2 μm and 10 μm, the deposition efficiency decreases with particle diameter due to filtration of particles in the extrathoracic and tracheobronchial region. For sizes between 0.5 and 2 μm, the deposition efficiency increases with particle size due to sedimentation by gravity. At 0.5 μm, there is a minimum in the deposition efficiency curve, and deposition efficiency increases with decreasing particles below ~0.5 μm. This is due to diffusional deposition.

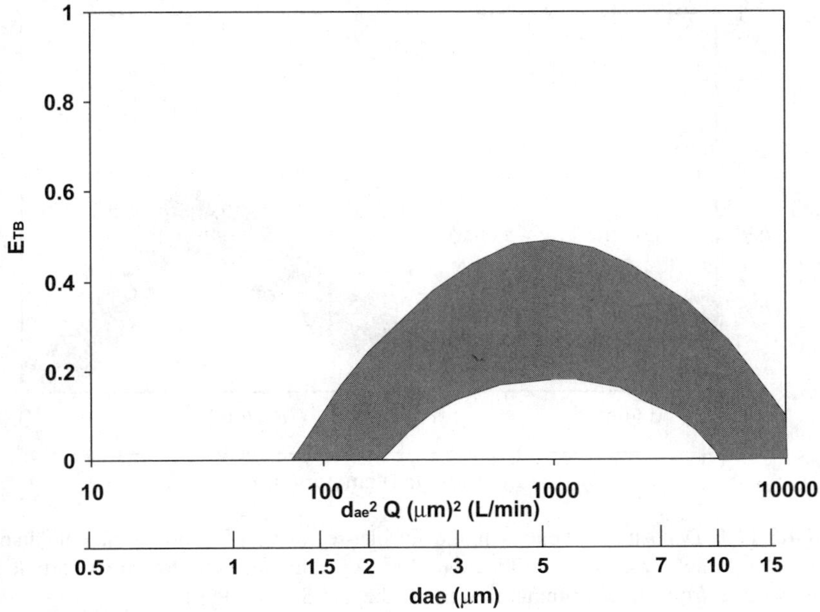

FIGURE 11.5 Deposition efficiency in the tracheobronchial region as a function of the inertial parameter $d_{ae}^2 Q_{inh}$. The aerodynamic diameters on the secondary horizontal axis are calculated assuming a breathing rate of 43.5 l/min for a reference worker. Based on data from studies summarized by Lippmann (1977).

11.7 TOTAL DEPOSITION

Total deposition is the combined deposition in all regions of the respiratory tract. This is determined by carefully measuring the total inhaled and exhaled aerosol from human subjects. Figure 11.7 shows the envelope of experimental data.

Figure 11.7 shows that particles greater than ~10 µm are completely deposited in the respiratory tract. Smaller particles are not completely deposited and get exhaled. From Figure 11.2 and Equation 11.7, we can infer that the fraction of aerosol exhaled is $(1–E_{total})$.

11.8 DEPOSITION MODELS

Based on the available experimental data and theory, several mathematical models have been developed to predict aerosol deposition in the respiratory tract. The most widely used model is that developed by the International Commission on Radiological Protection (ICRP, 1994). It is complex and takes into account the level of activity, gender, breathing rate, tidal volume, breathing frequency, and functional reserve capacity, among other parameters. Regional deposition is calculated for an average-sized person for a breathing rate of 15 breaths/min via the nose for three tidal volumes, 0.75 l ("at rest"), 1.45 l ("moderate activity"), and 2.15 l ("at work"). Hinds

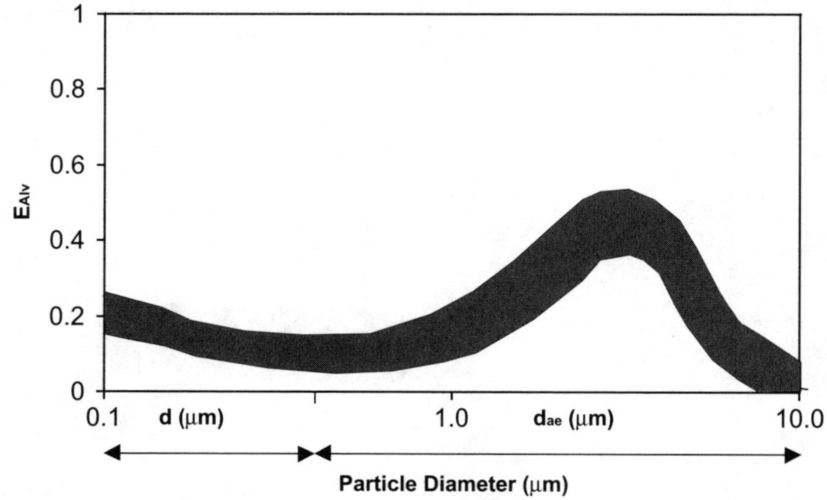

FIGURE 11.6 Deposition efficiency in the alveolar region as a function of particle diameter for smaller particle sizes and as a function of aerodynamic diameter for larger particle size. Based on data from studies summarized by Raabe and Stuart (1999).

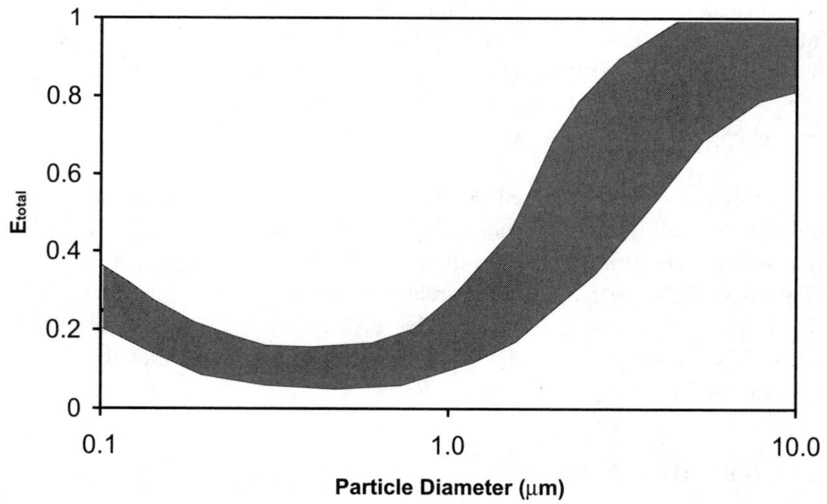

FIGURE 11.7 Total deposition in the respiratory tract as a function of particle diameter. Based on data from studies summarized by Raabe, O.G. and Stuart, B.O. (1999), Sampling criteria for the thoracic and respirable fractions, in *Particle Size Selective Sampling for Particulate Air Contaminants*, Vincent, J.H., Ed., ACGIH, Cincinnati, OH.

(1999) has obtained simple expressions for deposition efficiencies in different regions of the respiratory tract that are averaged for these levels of activity and averaged for men and women. The deposition efficiency in the extrathoracic region is given by:

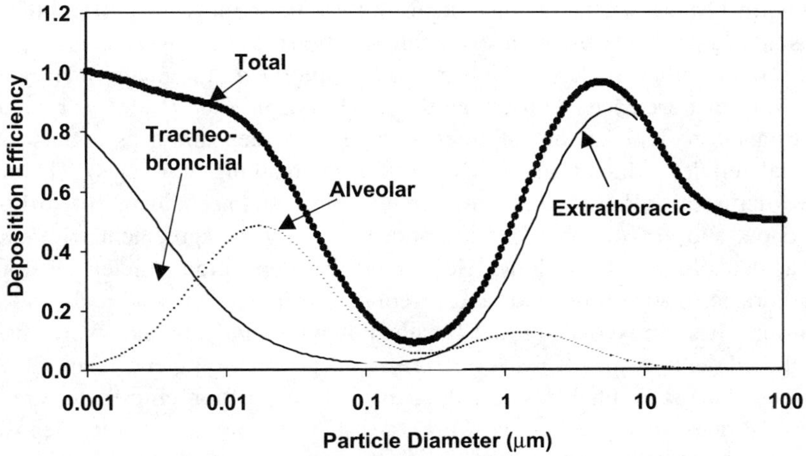

FIGURE 11.8 Deposition efficiency in the extrathoracic, tracheobronchial, and alveolar regions of the respiratory tract according to an approximation of the ICRP model. (Hinds, W.C. (1999), *Aerosol Technology: Properties, Behavior, and Measurement of Airborne Particles,* 2nd ed. John Wiley & Sons, New York.)

$$E_{ET} = IF \times \left(\frac{1}{1 + \exp(6.84 + 1.183 \ln d)} + \frac{1}{1 + \exp(0.924 - 1.885 \ln d)} \right) \tag{11.13}$$

where *IF* is the inhalable fraction as defined by ICRP and is given by

$$IF = 1 - 0.5 \left(1 - \frac{1}{1 + 0.00076\, d^{2.8}} \right) \tag{11.14}$$

The deposition efficiency in the tracheobronchial region is given by:

$$E_{TB} = \left(\frac{0.00352}{d} \right) \left[\exp\left(-0.234 (\ln d + 3.40)^2\right) + 63.9 \exp\left(-0.819 (\ln d - 1.61)^2\right) \right] \tag{11.15}$$

The deposition efficiency in the alveolar region is given by:

$$E_{Alv} = \left(\frac{0.0155}{d} \right) \left[\exp\left(-0.416 (\ln d + 2.84)^2\right) + 19.11 \exp\left(-0.482 (\ln d - 1.362)^2\right) \right] \tag{11.16}$$

Figure 11.8 shows the regional deposition for these three regions and the total deposition as predicted by the above approximations to the ICRP model.

There are other models as well in the literature, e.g., the model of Heyder et al. (1986), that are easier to use than the ICRP model. Such models can be used, for instance, to look at the differences in regional deposition as a function of physical activity (which translates into different breathing flow rates). The model of Heyder et al. (1986) takes into account physical mechanisms of diffusion, impaction, and gravitational settling, and provides good agreement with experimental data. Figure 11.9 shows Heyder et al.'s deposition efficiencies for the extrathoracic, tracheobronchial, and alveolar regions for "at rest" and "at work" conditions that corresponded to 7.5 breaths/min with 1 l/breath and 15 breaths/min with 1.5 l/breath, respectively. As before, all deposition efficiencies are given as fractions of what is inhaled. Clear differences in deposition efficiencies are with breathing rate corresponding to work rate. Upper respiratory tract deposition increases with the breathing rate, owing to the increase in contributions from impaction. On the other hand, deposition in the lower respiratory tract decreases, owing to the decreased availability of particles (since more are deposited higher up) and the decreased breathing cycle residence time during which gravity (and, for the smaller particles, diffusion) can bring about deposition. The differences are most marked for the extrathoracic and alveolar regions and the least so for the tracheobronchial region.

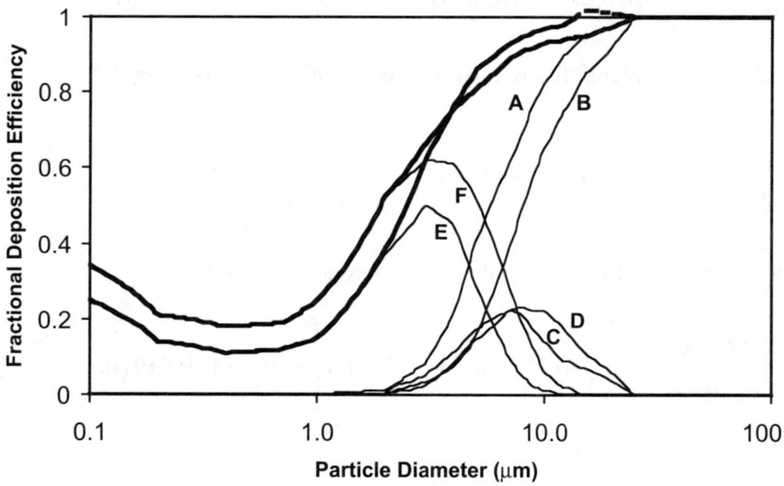

FIGURE 11.9 Regional respiratory tract deposition efficiencies for inhaled particles (Heyder et al., 1986). Curves A, C, and E are for breathing conditions corresponding to "at work" for the extrathoracic, tracheobronchial and alveolar regions, respectively. Curves B, D, and F are for breathing conditions corresponding to "at rest" for the same regions.

The mass deposited in a particular region r is given as

$$\textit{Deposited mass} = \int_0^\infty m\left(d_{ae}\right) \times I\left(d_{ae}\right) \times DE_r \, \mathrm{d}d_{ae} \tag{11.17}$$

where r refers to the extrathoracic, tracheobronchial, or alveolar region; $m(d_{ae})$ is the total mass size distribution of the ambient aerosol; $I(d_{ae})$ is, the inhalable fraction; and DE is the deposition efficiency.

11.9 THORACIC AND RESPIRABLE CRITERIA FOR SAMPLING

Equation 11.8 provides the inhalable criterion for sampling, and it is the fractional penetration of the ambient aerosol into the respiratory tract through the nose or mouth (or both) during breathing. As mentioned earlier, the curve serves as a reference against which the efficiency of a sampler that purports to sample the inhalable fraction can be compared. In a similar vein, two other criteria curves can be defined that reflect the size-selective particle collection of the lung airways. These size-selective curves do not indicate the deposition of particles in the lung, but provide a measure of the aerosol mass available to the lung.

Thus, the thoracic fraction of the aerosol contains particles of those aerodynamic sizes that can penetrate the head airways beyond the larynx and enter the lung airways (the thoracic region). This fraction can be thought of as the greatest potential exposure of the whole lung to inhaled particles. Sampling using this criterion is appropriate when the adverse health outcome arises from aerosol deposition in this region, e.g., bronchoconstriction and bronchogenic carcinomas. The thoracic criterion, as adopted by ACGIH, ISO, and CEN, is based on a cumulative lognormal function with a median of d_{ae} = 10 μm and a geometric standard deviation of 1.5. Thus, expressed as a fraction of the total aerosol, it is given as

$$T = 1 - \int_0^{d_{ae}} \left[\frac{1}{x\sqrt{2\pi}\,\ln 1.5} \exp\left\{ -\frac{1}{2} \left(\frac{\ln(x/10)}{\ln 1.5} \right)^2 \right\} \right] \mathrm{d}x \tag{11.18}$$

It can also be expressed as a subfraction of the inhalable fraction as:

$$T = I(d_{ae}) \left[1 - \int_0^{d_{ae}} \left[\frac{1}{x\sqrt{2\pi}\,\ln 1.5} \exp\left\{ -\frac{1}{2} \left(\frac{\ln(x/11.64)}{\ln 1.5} \right)^2 \right\} \right] \right] \mathrm{d}x \tag{11.19}$$

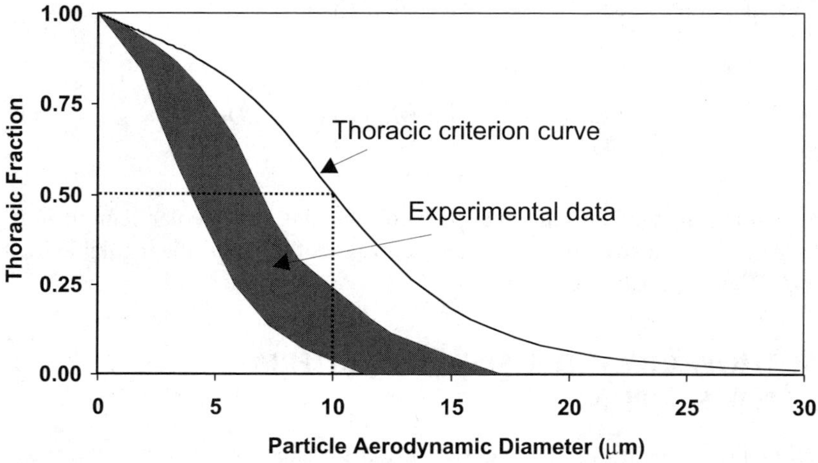

FIGURE 11.10 Thoracic criterion curve (as a fraction of the total) as adopted by ACGIH, ISO, and CEN. Also shown is the envelope of experimental penetration data of Lippmann, M. (1977), Regional deposition of particles in the human respiratory tract, in *Handbook of Physiology, Section 9, Reactions to Environmental Agents,* Lee, D.H.K., Falk, H.L., and Murphy, S.D., Eds., American Physiological Society, Bethesda, MD, pp. 213–232; Stahlhofen et al. (1980); Chan and Lippmann (1980). The point of 50% efficiency of penetration occurs at 10 μm aerodynamic diameter.

where now the cumulative lognormal function has a median of 11.64 μm. Therefore, expressed as a fraction of the total aerosol, this curve has a median diameter of 10 μm, whereas expressed as a fraction of the inhalable aerosol, the curve has a median diameter of 11.64 μm.

A computationally easier expression for calculating the thoracic fraction as a subfraction of the inhalable fraction is given by

$$T = I\left(d_{ae}\right)\left(1 - \frac{\exp\left(-10.0366 + 4.0891\ln d_{ae}\right)}{1 + \exp\left(-10.0366 + 4.0891\ln d_{ae}\right)}\right) \tag{11.20}$$

where $I(d_{ae})$ is the inhalable fraction.

As seen in Figure 11.10, the envelope of the experimental data obtained by Lippmann (1977), Stahlhofen et al. (1980), and Chan and Lippmann (1980) lies to the left of the thoracic curve and shows that the actual penetration to the lung is typically less than the thoracic criterion. Thus, the curve tends to overestimate the amount of exposure of the lung and provides a conservative estimate.

Given the size distribution of an aerosol, the thoracic curve can be used to determine the amount of aerosol penetrating to the lungs, as

$$\textit{Thoracic mass} = \int_0^\infty m\left(d_{ae}\right)T\left(d_{ae}\right)\mathrm{d}d_{ae} \tag{11.21}$$

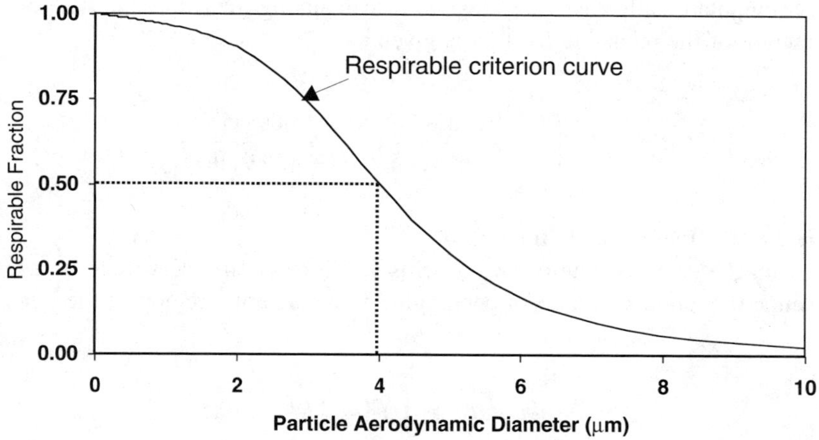

FIGURE 11.11 Respirable criterion curve (as a fraction of the total) as adopted by ACGIH, ISO, and CEN.

The respirable fraction of the aerosol contains particles of those aerodynamic sizes that can penetrate to the gas exchange region of the lungs (the alveolar region). As in the case of the thoracic fraction, the respirable fraction represents the highest possible exposure to the aerosol in the alveolar region. It does not represent deposition in the alveolar region, but, rather, penetration into the alveolar region. From Equation 11.6, the mass penetrating into this region is the sum of the mass deposited and the mass exhaled. Sampling using this criterion is appropriate when the adverse health outcome arises from aerosol deposition in this region, e.g., pneumonitis, emphysema, and fibrotic diseases such as silicosis, asbestosis, and coal workers' pneumoconiosis. The respirable criterion, as adopted by ACGIH, ISO, and CEN, is based on a cumulative lognormal function with a median of d_{ae} = 4 μm and a geometric standard deviation of 1.5 (see Figure 11.11). Thus, it is given as

$$R = 1 - \int_0^{d_{ae}} \left[\frac{1}{x\sqrt{2\pi}\ln 1.5} \exp\left\{ -\frac{1}{2}\left(\frac{\ln(x/4)}{\ln 1.5} \right)^2 \right\} \right] dx \tag{11.22}$$

It can also be expressed as a subfraction of the inhalable fraction as:

$$R = I(d_{ae}) \left[1 - \int_0^{d_{ae}} \left[\frac{1}{x\sqrt{2\pi}\ln 1.5} \exp\left\{ -\frac{1}{2}\left(\frac{\ln(x/4.25)}{\ln 1.5} \right)^2 \right\} \right] \right] dx \tag{11.23}$$

We again note that expressing this curve as a fraction of the total or inhalable aerosol changes its median diameter from 4.0 μm to 4.25 μm.

A computationally easier expression for calculating the respirable fraction as a subfraction of the inhalable fraction is given by

$$R = I\left(d_{ae}\right)\left(1 - \frac{\exp\left(-5.9164 + 4.0891\ln d_{ae}\right)}{1 + \exp\left(-5.9164 + 4.0891\ln d_{ae}\right)}\right) \tag{11.23}$$

where $I(d_{ae})$ is the inhalable fraction.

Given the size distribution of an aerosol, the respirable curve can be used to determine the amount of aerosol penetrating to the alveolar region of the lungs, as

$$\textit{Respirable mass} = \int_0^\infty m\left(d_{ae}\right) R\left(d_{ae}\right) \mathrm{d}d_{ae} \tag{11.24}$$

11.10 APPLICATION OF DEPOSITION CURVES AND CRITERIA CURVES TO ESTIMATING EXPOSURES

In Chapter 10, we considered the example of a personal cascade impactor data set obtained from a primary lead smelter, and obtained the particle size distribution by mass from the data (see Table 10.1 and Figure 10.9). The total air volume sampled was 1.72 m^3. The aerosol had a bimodal lognormal distribution which may be described by six parameters, namely, the mass median particle aerodynamic diameters of the two modes ($MMAD_1$ and $MMAD_2$), the geometric standard deviations of the two modes (σ_{g1} and σ_{g2}), and the relative weighting of the masses between the two modes (α_1 and α_2). For the data set in Table 10.1, the parameters were determined to be $MMAD_1$ = 21.9 μm, $MMAD_2$ = 50.7 μm, σ_{g1} = 3.48, σ_{g2} = 1.1, α_1 = 0.5, and α_2 = 0.5. Because the size distribution, as well as the three criteria curves, can be expressed as analytic functions, we can easily calculate the amounts of the inhalable, thoracic, and respirable masses by integration using Equations 11.10, 11.21, and 11.24.

For this aerosol sample, the inhalable, thoracic, and respirable fractions were 251 μg (57.7%), 56.2 μg (12.8%), and 20.7 μg (4.7%), respectively, where the numbers in parentheses show them as percentages of the total mass. Because we also know that the volume of air sampled was 1.72 m^3, we can obtain the inhalable, thoracic, and respirable concentrations as 146 μg/m^3, 32.7 μg/m^3, and 12.0 μg/m^3, respectively. Figure 11.12 shows the size distributions of the three fractions as well as the total aerosol.

Using the size distribution information, we can estimate the masses deposited in the extrathoracic, tracheobronchial, and alveolar regions of the respiratory tract for "at rest" (7.5 breaths/min with 1 l/breath) and "at work" (15 breaths/min with 1.5 l/breath) conditions using the curves proposed by Heyder et al. (1986). To carry out the calculations easily, we use a discretized form of Equation 11.17. For this size distribution, the amounts of aerosol mass deposited (per unit volume of air inhaled) in the three regions are:

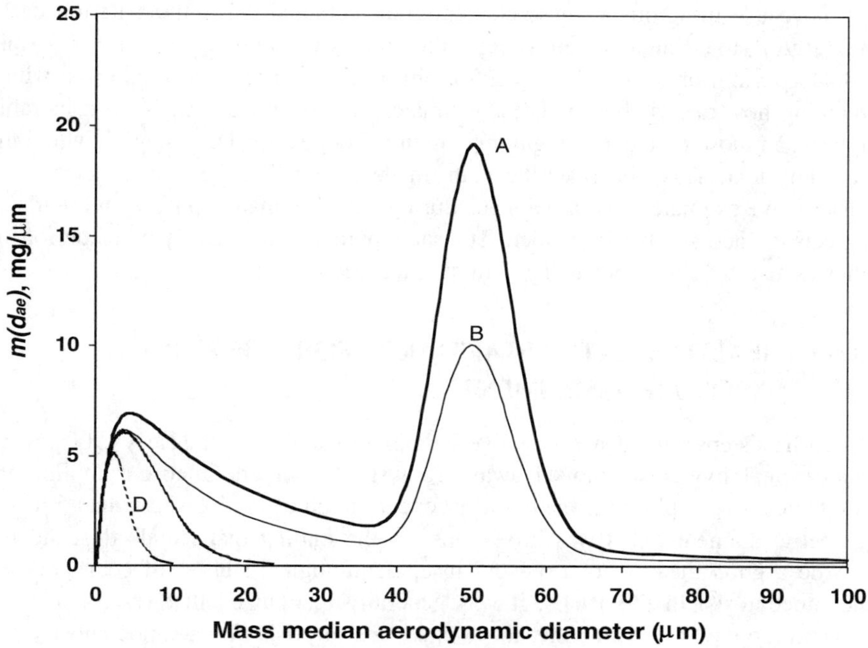

FIGURE 11.12 Particle size distribution for airborne lead obtained using a personal cascade impactor. The curves show the size distributions for A, total airborne lead; B, the inhalable fraction; C, the thoracic fraction; and D, the respirable fraction.

$$A_{E\text{-}T} = 114.5\ \mu g/m^3;\ A_{T\text{-}B} = 6.2\ \mu g/m^3;\ A_{alv} = 11.3\ \mu g/m^3;$$
for "at rest" conditions, and

$$A_{E\text{-}T} = 121.3\ \mu g/m^3;\ A_{T\text{-}B} = 5.2\ \mu g/m^3;\ A_{alv} = 6.7\ \mu g/m^3;$$
for "at work" conditions.

The mass deposited in the lungs (thoracic mass) is the sum of the tracheobronchial and alveolar masses. Thus, it is equal to 17.5 μg/m^3 (6.2 + 11.3) for the "at rest" condition and 11.9 μg/m^3 (5.2 + 6.7) for the "at work" condition. We see the interesting result that the concentration of the relevant depositing aerosol is greater for "at rest" than for "at work." However, the index more relevant to health is the rate of mass deposition, and this involves the inspiration flow rate for the two conditions. For the above example, we have

$$\text{Mass deposition "at rest"} = 17.5\ \mu g/m^3 \times 7.5\ l/min = 0.131\ \mu g/min, \text{ and}$$

$$\text{Mass deposition "at work"} = 11.9\ \mu g/m^3 \times 22.5\ l/min = 0.267\ \mu g/min.$$

Thus, although the concentration of relevant depositing aerosol is greater for "at rest" than for "at work," this is more than offset by the increased rate of inspiration during the "at work" conditions.

If we use the thoracic mass concentration obtained using the criterion curve (32.7 μg/m^3) to calculate the mass deposition rate, we obtain 32.7 μg/m^3 × 7.5 l/min = 0.245 μg/min or 32.7 μg/m^3 × 22.5 l/min = 0.735 μg/min, depending on which breathing flow rate is chosen. These estimates of deposition rates are considerably higher than those obtained using human regional deposition curves, as shown in the preceding text. This illustrates the point made earlier that the thoracic curve is a conservative estimate of what happens during actual human exposure and that also neglects the aerosol that is exhaled. The same point can also easily be made for the other two aerosol fractions using similar calculations.

11.11 HEALTH-RELATED STANDARDS FOR AEROSOL EXPOSURE ASSESSMENT

The earliest steps toward size-selective sampling took place in the early 1900s, when occupational hygienists moved away from short-term gravimetric sampling for "total" dust to sampling for the number concentration of particles less than 5 μm in geometric diameter. This was in response to the finding that "total" dust did not provide a good measure of exposure in epidemiological studies of coal workers' pneumoconiosis. In the 1960s, it was generally recognized that respirable mass concentration was a better metric of exposure for risk of pneumoconiosis than number concentration. Since the 1970s, time-weighted average (TWA) personal sampling for mass concentration has been considered the most relevant metric of worker exposure. There has also been a concerted international effort to emphasize the fact that particles deposited in different parts of the respiratory tract control the risk of disease. For instance, deposition in the extrathoracic region (the head airways) is associated with nasal cancer in wood workers and nickel primary production workers; deposition in the tracheobronchial region is associated with bronchitis and bronchial cancer; and deposition in the alveolar region can cause fibrotic diseases such as emphysema, silicosis, and asbestosis.

The discussion in this chapter so far presents our current understanding of the regional deposition of aerosols in the respiratory tract and the sampling criteria that have been developed based on this understanding. The sampling criteria refer to the three progressively finer aerosol fractions, i.e., the inhalable, thoracic, and respirable fractions. They reflect an understanding that the most appropriate metric of exposure should consider particle size distribution characteristics that influence where they deposit in the respiratory tract. The criteria curves do not attempt to match particle deposition curves in specific regions but, rather, match particle penetration curves to those specific regions. This choice not only makes the task of designing samplers much easier but also provides a more conservative estimate of exposure, as calculations in the previous section have shown.

Thus, the choice of sampler for measuring exposures to a particular toxicant depends on the health effect it causes. For materials that cause adverse health effects when deposited in the head airways, it is appropriate to use samplers that follow the inhalable criterion, i.e., the sampling efficiency curve matches the inhalable curve (within some specified tolerance). The inhalable criterion should also be used for substances that cause systemic toxic effects when deposited anywhere in the respiratory tract, i.e., they can be absorbed into the blood and transported to other organs. For materials that are hazardous when deposited in the lungs (the thoracic region), samplers that follow the thoracic criterion should be used. For materials that are hazardous only when deposited in the alveolar region of the lungs, samplers that follow the respirable criterion should be used. Chapter 12 discusses various samplers whose particle collection characteristics match one or the other of these three criteria. Many of them are integrating mass-collection devices that obtain a time-weighted average.

The previous sections make it clear that the deposition region is primarily governed by particle size. However, the biological response may be a function of particle size, number, surface area, mass, morphology, chemical composition, and surface chemistry. Therefore, it is critical that the biologically relevant dose be measured in terms of the most appropriate standard of measurement or metric. In practice, it is more convenient to measure penetration to the relevant areas of the respiratory system rather than the dose. This approach results in a measure of the *potential* dose, and provides an indicator of the maximum potential risk. Although mass concentration is now widely accepted as the predominant metric for characterizing occupational exposure to aerosols, notable exceptions include fibrous aerosols (such as asbestos and man-made vitreous fibers (MMVF)) and viable bioaerosols. With these two latter types, the association between respiratory disease and exposure is closely linked to their particle number and (in the case of fibers) shape. In both cases, number concentration provides a better indicator of the hazard associated with exposure. Recent studies have suggested that the biological response may be associated with the number of deposition sites within the lungs, leading to the conclusion that particle number concentration is a more relevant exposure metric (Donaldson et al., 2001). There is also increasing evidence that the surface area of low-solubility particles plays a key role in triggering biological responses in the lungs. A number of studies indicate response vs. aerosol surface area to be independent of particle size for low-solubility materials, suggesting that surface area may be a more appropriate exposure metric. Using surface area rather than mass concentration to measure exposure will be particularly important for aerosols with a high specific surface area (surface area to mass ratio) if these results are found to be applicable to occupational aerosols. Examples within this category include aerosols resulting from combustion (such as diesel exhaust particulates) and metal and metal oxide particles from hot processes such as smelting and welding.

12 Sampling of Aerosols

12.1 INTRODUCTION

Sampling for aerosols is done to identify and quantify the airborne particles in an environment. As in the case of sampling for gases and vapors, the reasons for obtaining a sample may be to assess compliance with an occupational exposure limit (OEL), to assess the health risk posed by the pollutant, to determine the efficacy of control measures, to minimize exposures, or for an epidemiological study. Aerosol concentrations can be expressed as the mass of aerosol particles per unit volume of the air in which it is dispersed, e.g., $\mu g/m^3$. Other metrics can include the number of particles per unit volume of air (e.g., particles per cubic centimeter, ppcc) or the surface area of particles per unit volume of air (e.g., $\mu m^2/m^3$).

Chapter 11 laid out the rationale for sampling size-selective, health-relevant aerosol fractions. Although much of this chapter will focus on the practical elements of sampling systems for aerosols, we should also be concerned with the duration and frequency of sampling for exposure assessment. For some aerosols, the health effects of exposures, even for short time periods, can be acute and rapid, and thus sampling should be for short durations. Other aerosols may cause health effects that become manifest after a long time and are chronic in nature, and in such instances sampling should be of longer duration (e.g., the traditional 8-h time-weighted average).

Another consideration is whether the best representation of actual worker exposures can be achieved using area samplers (in which the sampler is placed at some fixed point in the workplace environment) or using personal samplers (in which the sampler is placed on a worker's body and moves with him or her at all times for an entire work shift). Area samplers typically undersample compared with personal samplers, i.e., they yield a lower value of the aerosol concentration. This is due to the fact that they measure the average background concentration in a workplace, whereas personal samplers measure the concentration in the breathing zone around the worker (which is typically higher because the worker is usually working near contaminant sources). The advantage of area samplers is that, in some cases, a relatively small number of them can be used to survey a large workforce if the measurements can be shown to be valid and representative of worker exposures. They can be run at relatively high flow rates, which implies that even at very low concentrations, a relatively large mass of aerosol can be collected in a short sampling time. In other words, they provide much lower limits of detection. Personal samplers are more labor intensive, and require more instruments and the direct cooperation of workers. Because they need to be worn by workers, small pumps that provide relatively low flow rates are typically used. Despite these disadvantages, personal

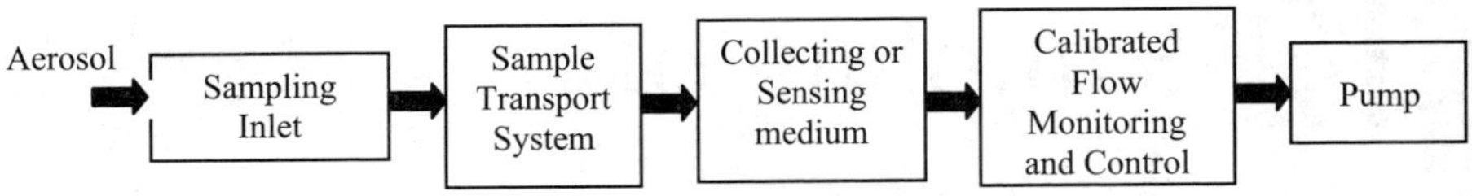

FIGURE 12.1 Schematic diagram showing elements of an aerosol sampling system.

aerosol sampling is generally accepted as the gold standard for assessing the true aerosol exposures of individual workers.

12.2 ELEMENTS OF AN AEROSOL SAMPLING SYSTEM

Figure 12.1 shows the essential elements of an aerosol sampling system. Air is drawn through the sampling inlet, which is designed specifically to sample a specific health-related aerosol fraction or particles within a given size range. The aerosol passes through a sample-transport section, where some of the aerosol may potentially be lost. The aerosol then enters a sensing zone or collection medium, which captures the particles and/or measures some relevant property. This could be a filter that collects airborne dust, which can be further analyzed by gravimetry, microscopy, or chemical means. It could also be a zone through which the aerosol moves and interacts with a light beam, some aerosol property getting measured in the process. The rest of the sampling train is similar to that for any sampling system and consists of a flow measurement device and a pump for drawing the air through the system. This chapter will discuss the nature of sampling inlets, the losses in the transport section, and the collection or sensing medium.

12.3 ASPIRATION EFFICIENCY

As mentioned earlier, in many occupational hygiene situations it is necessary to obtain an aerosol sample that mimics what would reach a particular region of the human respiratory tract during inhalation. In such a case, the sampler inlet should be designed such that its efficiency in sampling particles matches one of the three health-related criteria curves — inhalable, thoracic, or respirable — discussed in Chapter 11. In other situations, e.g., during sampling exhaust from smokestacks, we might want to obtain a representative sample of all particle sizes, i.e., the sampling efficiency should be 100% for all particle sizes.

We start by considering an aerosol sampler of arbitrary shape oriented such that its sampling orifice is at some angle with respect to the airflow outside the sampler. This general approach is useful because it encompasses all situations independent of the sampling configuration. These situations can range from a sampling probe inserted into a particle-laden stream of air to a worker wearing a personal aerosol sampler on his or her body so that the worker's torso becomes part of the aerosol sampler. Figure 12.2 shows such an arbitrarily shaped sampler. The airflow approaches the sampler from the left. As it nears the sampler, the flow streamlines begin to diverge to flow around the sampler. At the same time, some streamlines

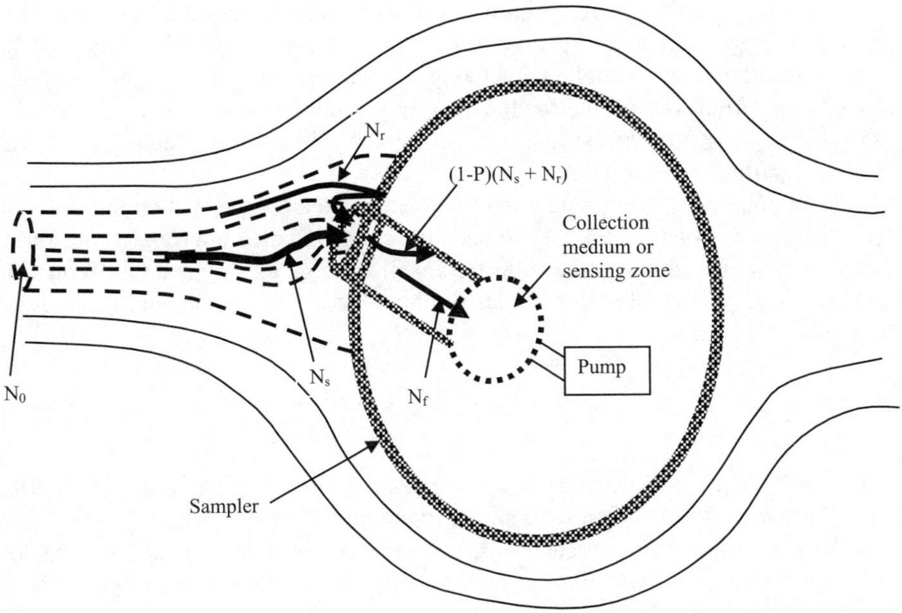

FIGURE 12.2 Schematic diagram illustrating the ideas of aspiration efficiency, sampling losses, and sampling efficiency. (Based on Vincent, 1989.)

converge to flow into the sampler orifice. This leads to what has been vividly described as the onion-peel shape of the air streamlines.

The dotted streamlines are the ones that are sampled by the aerosol sampler. All the streamlines outside this surface are not sampled. Thus, it is the air inside this tubular element that is sampled. Let N_0 be the number of particles per unit volume in the sampled air volume far upstream of the sampler, where the airflow is not affected by the presence of the sampling body. Of these N_0 particles, N_s particles directly enter the sampling inlet airborne (i.e., cross the inlet orifice plane). These two quantities define what is referred to as the *aspiration efficiency, A*.

$$A = \frac{N_s}{N_0} \tag{12.1}$$

This is conceptually identical to the inhalation efficiency (or the inhalability criterion) discussed in Chapter 11. In addition to the N_s particles entering the orifice directly, there are N_r particles that rebound from the sampler body and enter the orifice. The entry efficiency accounts for these particles and is defined as

$$A_{entry} = \frac{(N_s + N_r)}{N_0} \tag{12.2}$$

The entry efficiency can therefore potentially overestimate the aspiration efficiency, because it accounts for the particles that rebound from the sampler body. Careful design of the sampling inlet (e.g., by having an inlet lip that prevents rebounding particles from entering the inlet) or sampling practices (such as greasing the sampler body so that any particles striking it will remain attached to it) can minimize particle bounce effects.

Of the ($N_s + N_r$) particles entering the inlet, some are deposited on the walls of the transition section between the inlet and the collection medium (or sensing zone). These particles do not reach the collection medium (e.g., a filter) and thus represent particle losses. The number of particles reaching the collection medium is therefore N_f, where

$$N_f = P(N_s + N_r) \tag{12.3}$$

and P is the fractional penetration of particles through the transition section. The particles lost in the transition section are, therefore, $(1 - P)(N_s + N_r)$.

The overall sampling efficiency, $A_{overall}$, is therefore defined as the number of particles reaching the collection medium as a fraction of the number of particles in the undisturbed air.

$$A_{overall} = \frac{N_f}{N_0} = \frac{P(N_s + N_r)}{N_0} \tag{12.4}$$

12.4 SAMPLING INLETS

By proper design of the sampling inlet, one can selectively sample a size fraction of the aerosol that is of interest to us. In this section, we will consider samplers that have been specifically designed to sample either the health-relevant fractions (discussed in Chapter 11) or aerosols in ducts and smokestacks.

12.4.1 Sampling Using Thin-Walled Probes

Aerosol sampling systems such as those used in environmental and occupational hygiene have been defined as "blunt," acknowledging that the sampler body in all such cases provides significant blockage to the flow (Vincent, 1989; 1995). This applies also to the cylindrical thin-walled probes that have been the most widely studied and have many practical applications, for example, the representative sampling of particulates in stack gases and ducts. Even thin-walled probes must have finite tube thickness and so exhibit finite bluntness. However, thin-walled probes may usefully be described as a limiting case of a much wider family of blunt aerosol samplers of more complex geometry. With this in mind, knowledge gained from studies aimed at understanding the performance characteristics of thin-walled aerosol sampling probes has been useful to the understanding of the much more complex sampling systems, of wider interest to environmental and occupational hygienists. So, out of the theory for aspiration efficiency of thin-walled probes has grown a limited body of understanding of the factors controlling the aspiration efficiencies of blunt samplers.

In the simplest case, a cylindrical thin-walled tube faces the wind and samples the aerosol. The sampled air velocity is denoted by U_s and the wind velocity by U. The ratio $R = \frac{U}{U_s}$ is an important parameter determining the physics of particle entry into the probe.

If the sampled air velocity U_s is equal to the wind velocity U, then the streamlines of air approach the tube in straight lines (see Figure 12.3a). All the particles within the limiting stream surface are sampled, and no particle outside it is sampled. In this case, the aerosol concentration in the air entering the tube will be equal to the aerosol concentration in the outside air. This is called *isokinetic sampling.*

If the sampled air velocity U_s is greater than the wind velocity U, then the limiting stream surface contracts (i.e., the streamlines converge) as it approaches the tube entry (see Figure 12.3b). Particles inside this limiting stream surface may, due to their inertia, cross the limiting stream surface and not be sampled. Thus, the sampled air will have a lower particle concentration than the outside air. This situation is referred to as *superisokinetic sampling*.

If the sampled air velocity U_s is less than the wind velocity U, then the limiting stream surface expands (i.e., the streamlines diverge) as it approaches the tube entry (see Figure 12.3c). Particles even outside this limiting stream surface may, due to their inertia, cross the limiting stream surface and be sampled. Thus, the sampled air will have a higher particle concentration than the outside air. This situation is referred to as *subisokinetic sampling*.

Thus, if sampling is not done isokinetically, the true concentration is under- or overestimated by an amount related to the particle Stokes number and the velocity ratio R. The ratio of the concentration of particles just crossing the plane of the tube entry to the concentration of particles in the undisturbed air is the aspiration efficiency of the tube sampler $\left(A = \frac{C_s}{C_0}\right)$. The aspiration efficiency of the sampler is given by (Vincent, 1989)

$$A = \frac{C_s}{C_0} = 1 + (R-1)\left(1 - \frac{1}{1 + \left(2 + \frac{0.62}{R}\right) St}\right) \tag{12.5}$$

where $R = \frac{U}{U_s}$.

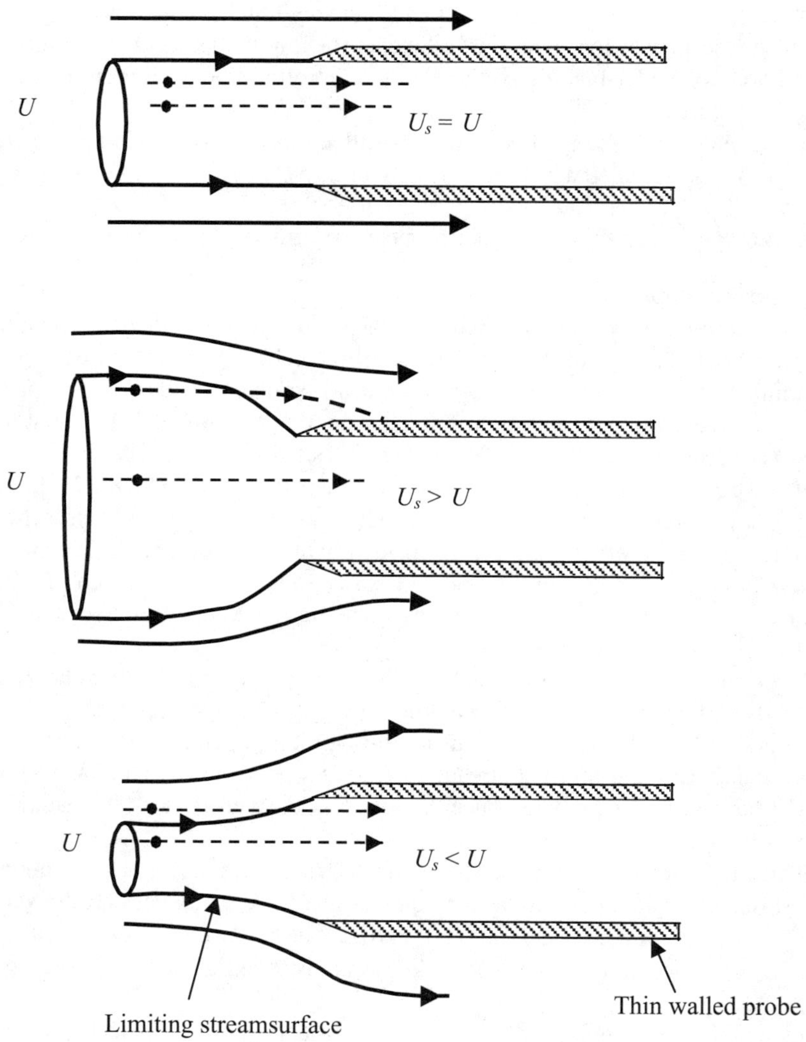

FIGURE 12.3 Schematic diagram showing (a) isokinetic sampling; (b) superisokinetic sampling; and (c) subisokinetic sampling. The solid lines are the streamlines of air and the dashed lines are particle trajectories. The streamlines that end on the probe tip form a boundary within which all air is sampled and outside which the air is not sampled. These streamlines together form a limiting stream surface.

Figure 12.4 shows the effect of the velocity ratio on the relationship between aspiration efficiency and particle aerodynamic diameter for a thin-walled probe facing the wind.

Although A is the most basic index of performance for the sampler, the actual performance in practice is complicated by the fact that the aspirated aerosol has to adjust to the new flow conditions inside the tube. This, in turn, means that there

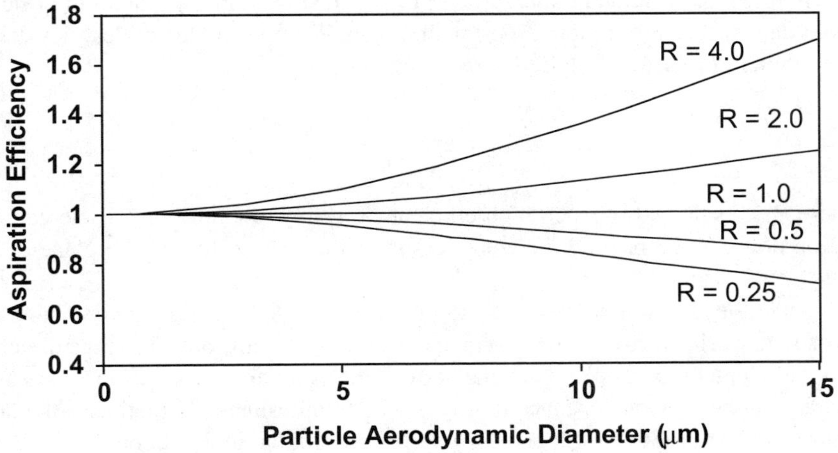

FIGURE 12.4 Aspiration efficiency of a thin-walled probe facing the wind at different values of the velocity ratio, *R*.

will be particle losses in the so-called entry region (within a few diameter lengths past the entry plane) directly as a result of this transition or "coupling" between the external and internal flows. The importance of internal entry loss was first noted in the early reports of Durham and Lundgren (1980) and Jayasekera and Davies (1980), where it was noted that a large fraction of the aspirated aerosol was deposited on the inner wall of the inlet. However, the only data currently available for quantifying internal entry loss comes from the body of work carried out by Willeke and his coworkers to determine the sampling efficiency of thin-walled probes oriented at angles up to 90° from the freestream (e.g., Okazaki et al., 1987a, 1987b, 1987c, and 1987d; Grinshpun et al., 1993). They reported that most of the loss occurs within 3 to 5 diameters downstream of the inlet, where the flow is very complex, most notably associated with the formation of the *vena contracta* region of separated flow region (including flow reversal), whose structure or properties are poorly understood. Willeke and his colleagues argued that contributions to internal entry loss for tubes oriented at an angle to the freestream come from a combination of gravitational settling, impaction onto inner walls, inward and outward bounce and blow-off, and the losses due to the presence of the *vena contracta*.

For the horizontal (i.e., perpendicular to gravity) sampler facing the wind, an inlet deposition parameter *K* was identified by Okazaki and Willeke (1987a) as:

$$K = \sqrt{\frac{Z \cdot St}{\sqrt{Re}}} \quad \text{or} \quad K = St\sqrt{\frac{g \cdot L \cdot R}{U^2 \cdot \sqrt{Re}}} \tag{12.6}$$

where *Z* is the gravitational deposition parameter, g is the acceleration due to gravity, *Re* is the Reynolds number for the airflow inside the tube, and *L* is the length of the tube. The parameter *K* reflects the roles of (1) inertia in decelerating the particles as they enter the tube from the external flow and encounter the more slowly moving air in the boundary layer inside the tube and (2) gravity in bringing about deposition. From their experimental data, Willeke and his colleagues developed the empirical relation

$$P_{\text{entry}} = \exp(-4.7K^{0.75}) \tag{12.7}$$

where P_{entry} is the entry penetration efficiency given by the ratio of particle concentration downstream beyond the entry region of the inlet to that in the plane of the entry.

When the thin-walled probe is oriented at an angle to the wind containing the aerosol, its performance is more complex. The sampled flow has to change direction in order to enter the sampler. Now the body of the sampler is "visible" to the aerosol, whereas in the previous instance it provided an infinitesimal obstruction to the flow. Vincent et al. (1986) developed an expression similar to Equation 12.5 for the aspiration efficiency of a thin-walled probe at an angle α to the freestream:

$$A = 1 + \left(R\cos\alpha - 1\right)\left(1 - \frac{1}{1 + G(\alpha)St\left(\cos\alpha + 4R^{1/2}(\sin\alpha)^{1/2}\right)}\right) \tag{12.8}$$

where $G(\alpha)$ is a function of R and α. The variation of aspiration efficiency with orientation is schematically depicted in Figure 12.5. A detailed analysis of the entry losses in such configurations is provided by Sreenath et al. (2001).

12.4.2 Sampling Using Blunt Samplers

In contrast to thin-walled tube samplers, blunt samplers are so characterized because the area projected by the sampler body is much greater than that projected by the

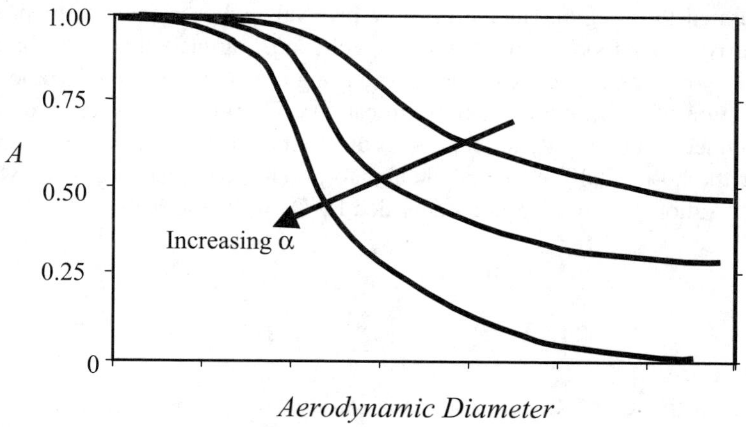

FIGURE 12.5 Aspiration efficiency of a thin-walled probe at different orientations to the wind.

sampler inlet. The airflow in the vicinity of such a sampler is complicated. This is especially relevant when the sampler is worn on the body of a worker. The torso of the worker, in effect, becomes an extension of the actual sampler, because it has a profound influence on particle behavior close to the body. The behavior of personal samplers, therefore, needs to be studied as worn on mannequins representing workers, rather than as isolated samplers suspended in the aerosol stream. Thus, consideration needs to be given to parameters that relate to the shape and magnitude of the distortion of the flow near the sampler due to its aspirating action. These are $R = \frac{U}{U_s}$ (where U_s is the mean air velocity at the sampling inlet and U is the mean freestream air velocity) and $r = \frac{\delta}{D}$ (where δ is the width of the sampling orifice and D is the characteristic dimension of the sampler), which together form the parameter $\phi = \frac{r^2}{R}$ describing the ratio of the sampled air volume to that which is geometrically incident on the sampler. The aerodynamic bluntness factor, B, as well as the orientation of the sampler inlet with respect to the freestream, α, also play an important role. The Reynolds number has usually not been regarded as a major influence, because it is considered to be large enough that inertial fluid forces predominate over viscous forces. Instabilities leading to vortex shedding are embodied in the Strouhal number $\left(Str = \frac{fD}{U}\right)$, where f is the frequency of vortex shedding. Sreenath et al. (1997) have shown that *Str* depends strongly on the sampling flow rate, wind speed, and sampling orientation, and that it can affect the size of the wake cavity. This, in turn, can affect the aspiration efficiency of samplers, especially when they are oriented away from the freestream and sampling from the wake. Several expressions have been developed for the aspiration efficiency as a function of *St*, *R*, *r*, ϕ, α, and *B*. However, these will not be discussed further. Interested readers can find more details in Vincent (1989) and Sreenath et al. (1999; 2001; 2002).

From the discussion in Chapter 11, it is clear that samplers need to be designed so that they collect health-relevant aerosol fractions. Unfortunately, aerosol science has not progressed to the point where new samplers can be designed from the outset with the desired performance. As a result, progress has been primarily achieved by the empirical testing of candidate samplers in wind tunnels, accepting only those that meet the required criteria.

12.4.3 Sampling for Inhalable Aerosols in Workplaces

Historically, the sampling of coarse particles has been based on the idea of the so-called total aerosol, which referred to all airborne particulate matter. However, most sampling instruments that purported to measure the total aerosol were developed without regard to their sampling efficiency characteristics. It was only in the 1970s that the concept of the human head as an aerosol sampler emerged, which in turn led to the idea of inhalability discussed in Chapter 11.

The most commonly used sampler in the U.S. and many other countries for measuring the total aerosol is a 37-mm plastic cassette that can be deployed in the open-faced or closed-faced mode and operated at a flow rate of 2 l/min. The aerosol enters the narrow inlet and is collected on the filter medium in the cassette. The filter is weighed before and after sampling to determine the amount of aerosol collected. However, there is always the possibility that some of the aspirated aerosol is not collected on the filter but on the walls of the cassette and is thus unaccounted for. In the open-faced mode, its performance is strongly dependent on ambient wind speed.

Most American Conference of Governmental Industrial Hygienists (ACGIH) threshold limit values (TLVs) and Occupational Safety and Health Administration (OSHA) permissible exposure limits (PELs) are based on measurements made by the 37-mm cassette. However, a number of mannequin studies performed in wind tunnels have shown that this sampler significantly undersampled with respect to the inhalable criterion curve (and, thus, also with respect to the IOM sampler) for particles greater than 20 μm in aerodynamic diameter (see Figure 12.6).

Mark and Vincent (1986) proposed an inhalable aerosol sampler that matches the inhalable curve quite closely. The sampler, now commonly referred to as the "IOM sampler," also uses a sampling flow rate of 2 l/min and has a 15-mm-diameter circular entry that faces directly outward when worn on the torso. The entry is incorporated into a lightweight collection capsule, which ensures that the entire aspirated aerosol is weighed and there are no sampling losses. Also, the lips of the entry protrude outward slightly to prevent oversampling through particle rebound from the walls of the sampler body. Early experiments by Vincent (1989) showed good agreement between measured sampling efficiencies and the inhalable criterion for wind speeds ranging between 0.5 m/sec and 2.6 m/sec. More recent studies by

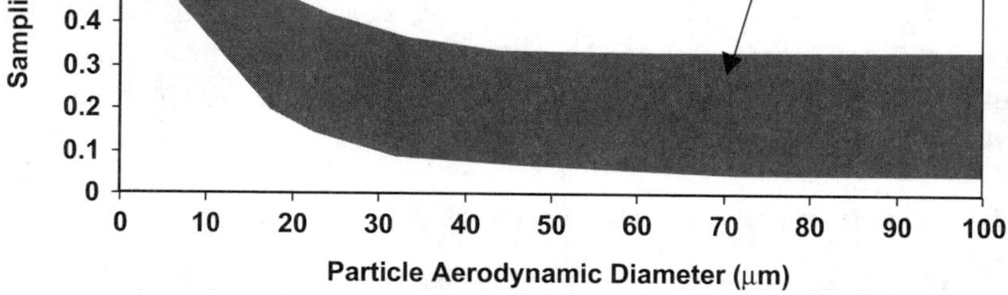

FIGURE 12.6 Envelope of sampling efficiency data for the 37-mm cassette (Kenny, L.C. et al., 1997, A collaborative European study of personal inhalable aerosol sampler performance, *Ann. Occup. Hyg.*, 41: 135–153.) shows that it significantly undersamples with respect to the inhalable curve.

Kenny et al. (1997) show that at wind speeds less than 0.5 m/sec, the sampling efficiency is significantly above the inhalable curve (see Figure 12.7). However, these results are in agreement with the inhalability measurements made at very low wind speeds with mannequins in wind tunnel experiments.

A number of side-by-side comparison studies of the IOM sampler and the 37-mm cassette show that the degree of undersampling varies with industrial operation. The 37-mm cassette undersamples, on average, by a factor of 2.5 in mining, ore and rock handling, textiles, and flour and grain handling, by a factor of 2.0 in oil mist and machining fluids, paint sprays, and electroplating, and by a factor of 1.5 in metal smelting and refining operations. Sampling of welding and smoke and fume aerosols does not appear to result in any such biases.

The Button Sampler (SKC, Inc., Pennsylvania) consists of a 25-mm filter holder with a hemispherical perforated screen covering the sampling inlet. The screen serves a threefold purpose — reduction of aspiration dependency on wind speed, formation of a uniform deposit on the filter, and exclusion of large projectiles from the sample. This sampler also shows good agreement with the inhalable convention (Aizenberg et al., 2000). Various other inhalable samplers are in use, including the GSP inhalable sampler, the conical inhalable sampler, and the PAS-6 inhalable sampler. These three samplers use conical inlets and appear not to be as susceptible to external wind speed as other devices (Kenny et al., 1997).

12.4.4 Sampling for Thoracic and Respirable Aerosols in Workplaces

Chapter 11 presented the criteria curves for the thoracic and respirable aerosol fractions, which were defined as the aerosol fractions that could penetrate into the

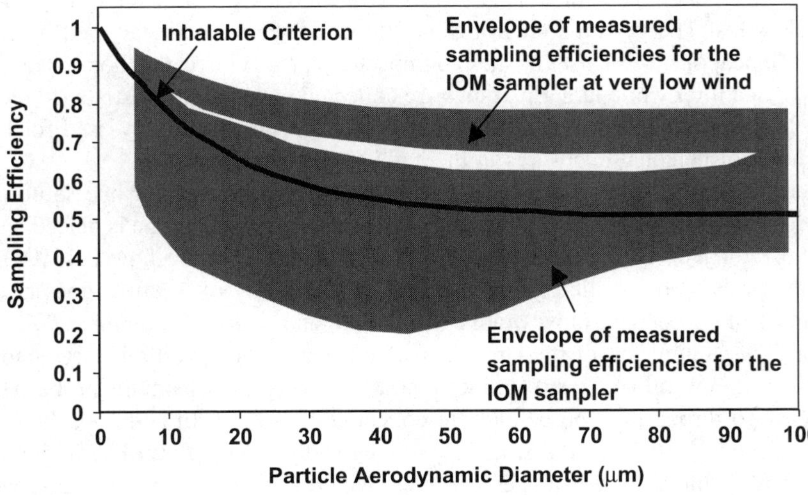

FIGURE 12.7 Envelope of sampling efficiency data for the IOM sampler. (Vincent, 1989; Kenny, L.C. et al., 1997, A collaborative European study of personal inhalable aerosol sampler performance, *Ann. Occup. Hyg.*, 41: 135–153.)

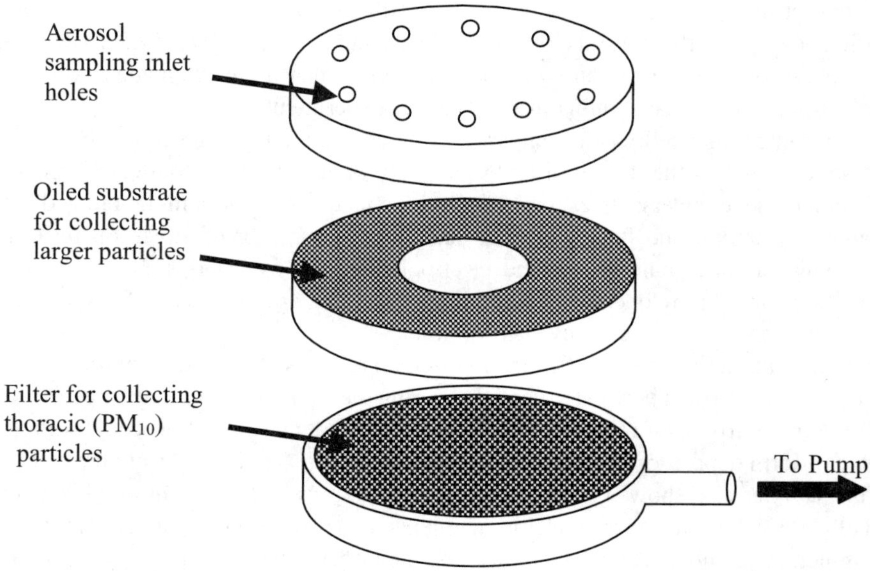

FIGURE 12.8 Schematic diagram of thoracic (PM_{10}) sampler used for personal exposure monitoring. Particle collection is achieved using inertial impaction.

thoracic (the lung) and alveolar regions, respectively, of the human respiratory tract. Thoracic and respirable aerosol samplers therefore have to possess sampling efficiency curves that match these criteria curves.

The thoracic criterion curve is very similar to the PM_{10} criterion curve, which is the basis of ambient environmental particle sampling by the U.S. Environmental Protection Agency. The biases between the two curves are significant only at larger particle sizes. The personal environmental monitor (PEM) manufactured by MSP, Inc. (Minneapolis, MN), uses an inertial impactor plate to collect the thoracic fraction (PM_{10}) on a filter while larger particles are collected on an oiled substrate (to reduce particle bounce) — see Figure 12.8. This device has been primarily used for measurements of personal exposures in the ambient environment.

Virtual impactors do not have a collection plate and thus offer one solution to the problem of particle bounce. Instead of a collection plate, a probe is placed below the impactor jet (see Figure 12.9). Only a small portion of the flow (~10%) goes into the probe and is called the *minor flow.* The majority of the flow goes around the tip of the probe and moves radially outward, and is called the *major flow.* The minor flow contains all of the larger particles because their inertia is large enough that they cannot follow the streamlines that turn sharply away from the probe. These particles go through the probe and are collected on a filter. In addition, there is a small amount (~10%) of the smaller particles in the minor flow. The major flow carries away most of the smaller particles, which can be collected on a separate filter. Thus, both the small and large particle fraction (albeit with some contamination by the small particles) are collected separately. A cascade virtual impactor that collects the inhalable, thoracic, and respirable fractions, called the Respicon, is available from TSI, Inc. (Dunkhorst et al., 1995).

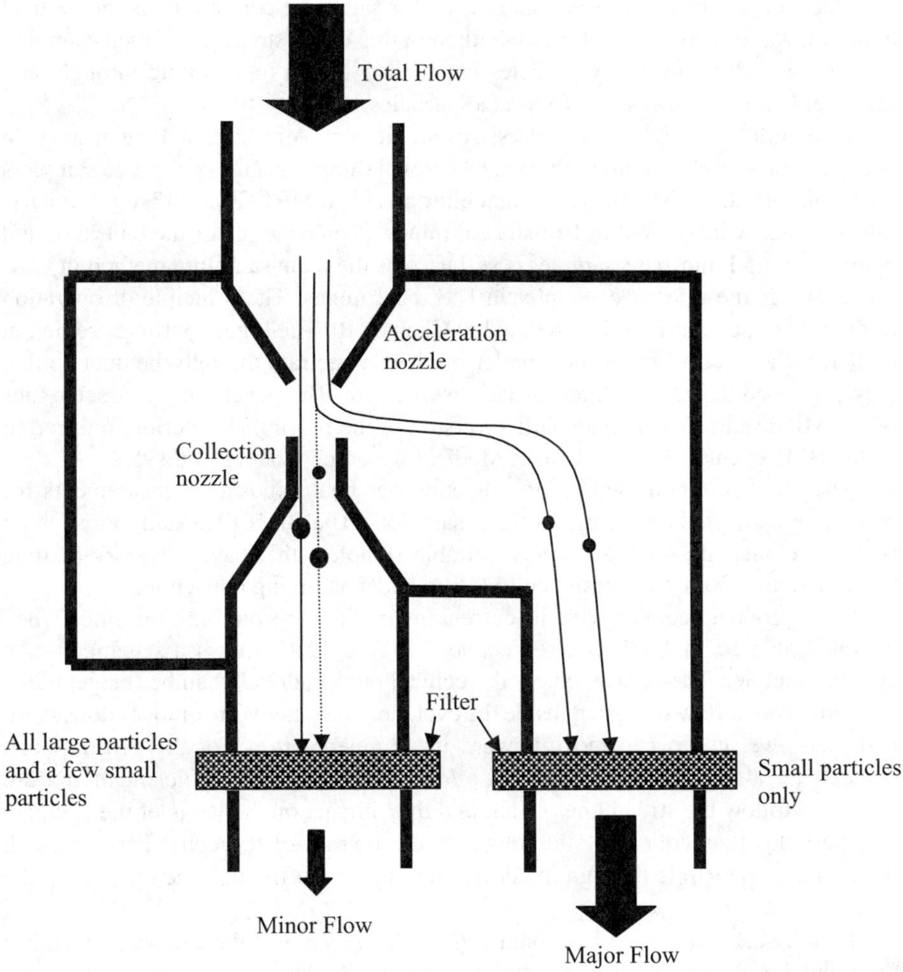

FIGURE 12.9 Virtual impactor showing major and minor flows.

The French CIP10 sampler can measure the thoracic fraction (Fabries et al., 1989) by using a porous foam. Vincent et al. (1993) used porous polyurethane foam (PUF) media whose penetration characteristics were carefully tailored to match the thoracic criterion curve. The IOM thoracic sampler uses a 24-mm length of 30 pores/in. (ppi) PUF behind an inhalable inlet, collecting the penetrating aerosol onto a 37-mm filter. When operated at 2 l/min, sampling efficiency is close to the thoracic convention (Maynard, 1999). The IOM inhalable sampler has been modified by placing a foam plug (17.5-mm diameter, 10-mm deep, 45 ppi) in the inlet (Stancliffe and Kenny, 1997). The modified sampler follows the thoracic convention reasonably well (Maynard, 1999). None of these samplers have found widespread use in occupational settings. A more comprehensive list of thoracic samplers is presented by Baron and John (1999).

One sampler that has been widely used for sampling cotton dust is the vertical elutriator (described in Chapter 10). Although this is not strictly a thoracic sampler, the elutriator does not allow particles larger than 15 μm to penetrate through, and thus yields a rough measure of thoracic particles.

In contrast to thoracic samplers, respirable samplers have a long history in occupational sampling both for area and personal sampling. One of the area samplers for respirable aerosols is the horizontal elutriator. The MRE Type 113A gravimetric dust sampler, widely used in British coal mines, is an example of the elutriator and operates at 2.5 l/min. This sampler is still used as the main sampling method in U.K. mines and is the reference sampler in U.S. coal mines. The principle of operation of the horizontal elutriator is discussed in Chapter 10. The bigger particles settle out earlier in the duct, whereas the smaller particles penetrate through the duct so that they can be collected on a filter further downstream. The penetration characteristics of the MRE sampler match an earlier version of the respirable criterion, referred to as the BMRC curve (for the British Medical Research Council) of 1952.

The most common method of collecting personal exposure measurements for respirable aerosols is by using cyclone samplers. The SIMPEDS and Dorr–Oliver (U.S.) cyclones are both personal respirable samplers that have a history of long continued use. Both were designed to follow older sampling conventions. However, both show good agreement with the current international respirable convention when operated at 2.2 and 1.7 l/min, respectively. Figure 12.10 shows a schematic of a cyclone sampler. The aerosol enters the conical or cylindrical chamber tangentially. A double vortex flow is created inside the cyclone. The outer vortex moves downward and then reverses flow to move upward in an inner vortex. For this reason, such devices are also called *reverse flow cyclones*. Particles with sufficient inertia are unable to follow the streamlines of air, and they impact on the walls of the cyclone. The particles thus collected slide down to the bottom of the cone. Particles with lesser inertia penetrate through the device and move out through the opening at the top.

Figure 12.11 shows the fractional *collection efficiency* of the cyclone, which has the typical S-shaped curve characteristic of inertial impaction. As the airflow rate through the cyclone increases, the diameter of 50% collection efficiency (i.e., the cut size) decreases. Thus, smaller and smaller particles can be collected with greater efficiency by increasing the sampling flow rate. However, this also increases the pressure drop across the cyclone, necessitating bigger pumps. The dimensions of the cyclone (e.g., the inlet and outlet diameters, the diameter of the cylindrical main body, and the height of the conical section) also affect the collection efficiency characteristics. The penetration P through the cyclone is defined as $P = 1–E$, where E is the collection efficiency. Thus, the penetration characteristics can be adjusted by designing the cyclone dimensions and the flow rate through it so that it matches the respirable criterion curve. The most commonly used cyclone is the 10-mm nylon cyclone that operates at a flow rate of 1.7 l/min to provide a good match with the respirable criterion curve.

Another method is to use impactors to collect the respirable fraction. The principle of operation of impactors has been described in Chapter 10. Larger particles are collected on an oil-coated porous plate, whereas the respirable particles are

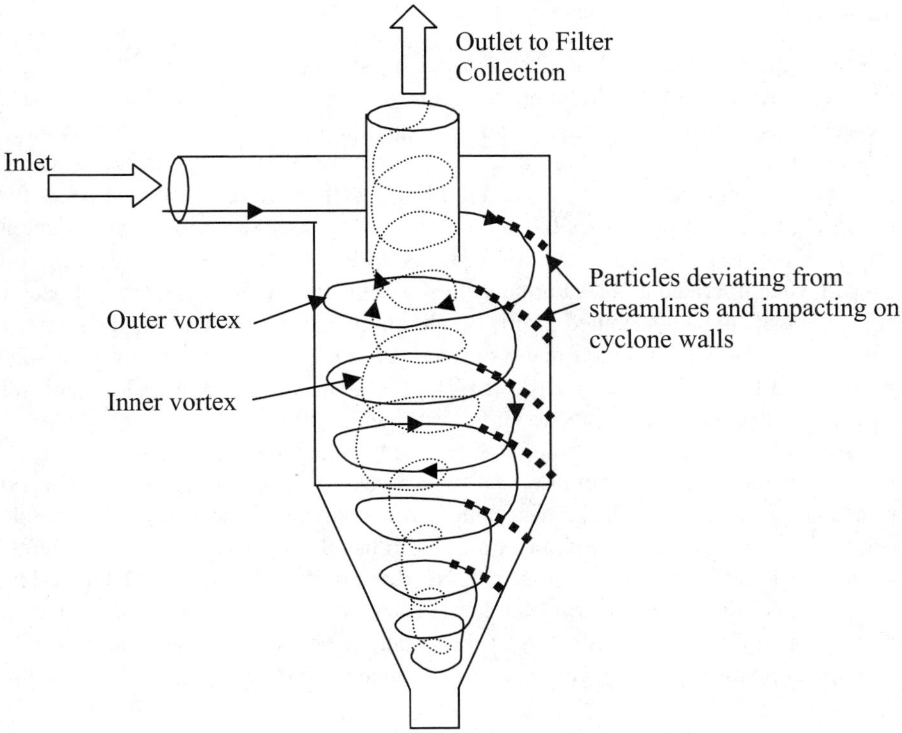

FIGURE 12.10 Schematic of a reverse flow cyclone.

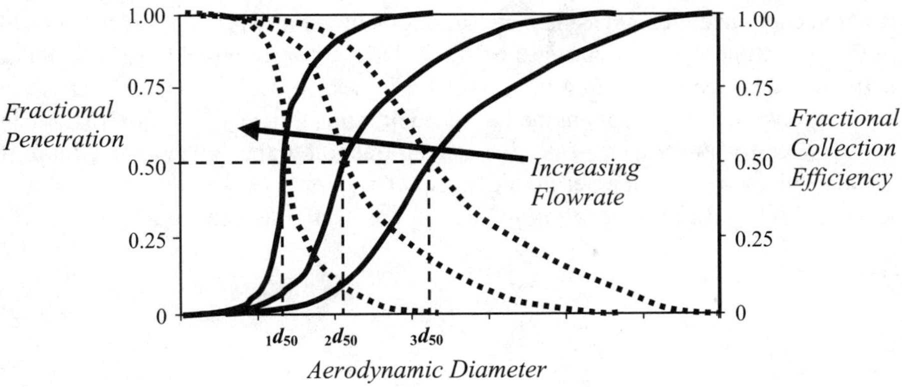

FIGURE 12.11 Fractional collection efficiency of cyclone (solid curves) and fractional penetration through it (dotted curves). Increasing the flow rate decreases the 50% cut diameter of the cyclone.

collected on a filter downstream (Marple and Rubow, 1983). The use of the oil-coated plate is to prevent particle bounce and overloading, which are drawbacks of most impactor designs. Virtual impactors have been used for sampling the respirable aerosol fraction (e.g., the Respicon sampler mentioned earlier).

12.4.5 Cascade Impactors

These impactors, discussed in Chapter 10, can be used to obtain particle size distributions from which the three aerosol criteria fractions can be estimated. These are generally capable of giving the size distribution of an aerosol between around 0.1-μm and 15-μm aerodynamic diameter and above. Cascade impactors such as the Anderson eight stage impactor and the Multi Orifice Uniform Deposit Impactor (MOUDI, MSP, Inc., Minneapolis) are widely used for area sampling. The Anderson impactor consists of eight multiorifice stages with cut points between 10 μm and 0.4 μm when operated at 28.3 l/min (1 CFM). The multiple orifices in this impactor allow deposits to be distributed evenly on aluminum substrates. This is taken further within the MOUDI, in which many orifices per stage, together with rotating substrates, lead to highly uniform deposits. The MOUDI is capable of making aerosol size distribution measurements down to 0.056 μm at 30 l/min.

Aerosol size distributions within the breathing zone are generally of greater relevance to health than static samples, and two cascade impactors have been developed to enable personal aerosol size distribution measurements to be made. The Marple personal cascade impactor (Rubow et al., 1987) has 8 stages and can provide information on particle size distribution down to 0.5 μm at a flow rate of 2 l/min. The personal inhalable dust spectrometer (PIDS) has an inhalable entry, allowing it to directly obtain the size distribution of the inhalable aerosol fraction (Gibson et al., 1987). Cut points in the 8 stages of the PIDS range from 0.9 μm to 19 μm at 2 l/min.

12.5 SAMPLE-TRANSPORT SYSTEM

The sample-transport system consists of the section between the sampling inlet and the collection medium or sensing zone, and its main purpose is to convey the aerosol to the collection medium. This section might have elbows, constrictions, and tubes in most cases, that cause unwanted particle losses. In some cases, the transport section consists of porous foam media whose filtration efficiency characteristics can be exploited to deliver a size-selective aerosol fraction to the collection medium. If the aerosol concentration entering the transport system is C_1, and the concentration leaving it is C_2, then the *penetration* through this section is defined as

$$P = \frac{C_2}{C_1} \tag{12.9}$$

The *loss* or *deposition efficiency* to the surface is then defined as

$$E = 1 - P = 1 - \frac{C_2}{C_1} \tag{12.10}$$

Deposition on surfaces of the transport system (e.g., the walls of the tubing and elbows) may occur due to a variety of mechanisms. These include the phenomena discussed in Chapter 10, i.e., gravitational settling, inertial impaction, diffusion, and electrostatic deposition. Other mechanisms can include interception and thermophoresis. The losses due to these mechanisms can be combined by assuming that each mechanism operates independently of the others, and sequentially. Thus,

$$E = 1 - P_{\text{gravitaton al}} P_{\text{inertial}} P_{\text{diffusion}} P_{\text{electrosta tic}} \cdots \tag{12.11}$$

The following equations present expressions for the losses due to some of these mechanisms (expressed as penetrations).

Particle losses can occur because the particles are large enough that they settle down in the tube by gravity. For gravitational settling in laminar flow in a circular tube at an angle θ to the horizontal, the penetration is given by

$$P_{\text{tube,grav}} = 1 - \frac{2}{\pi}\left[2\kappa\sqrt{1-\kappa^2} - \kappa^{1/3}\sqrt{1-\kappa^{2/3}} + \arcsin\left(\kappa^{1/3}\right)\right] \tag{12.12}$$

where $\kappa = (3/4)Z\cos\theta$, and Z is the gravitational settling parameter given by

$$Z = \left(\frac{L}{d}\right)\left(\frac{V_{\text{TS}}}{U}\right) \tag{12.13}$$

L is the length of the tube, d the inside diameter of the tube, V_{TS} the terminal settling velocity of the particles, and U the gas velocity in the tube (Heyder and Gebhart, 1977).

For gravitational settling in turbulent flow in a circular tube at an angle θ to the horizontal, the penetration is given by

$$P_{\text{tube,grav}} = \exp(-4Z\cos\theta/\pi) = \exp(-dLV_{\text{TS}}\cos\theta/Q) \tag{12.14}$$

where Q is the volumetric flow rate.

Small particles can diffuse onto the walls of the tube and get attached. The loss due to diffusional deposition is expressed as:

$$P_{\text{tube,diff}} = \exp(-\pi dLV_{\text{diff}}/Q) = \exp(-\xi Sh) \tag{12.15}$$

where V_{diff} is the deposition velocity due to diffusion onto the walls, and Sh the Sherwood number that is defined for laminar flow as

$$Sh = 3.66 + \frac{0.0668(d/L)Re\,Sc}{1 + 0.04\left[(d/L)Re\,Sc\right]^{2/3}} = 3.66 + \frac{0.2672}{\xi + 0.10079\xi^{1/3}} \tag{12.16}$$

$$\xi = \frac{\pi D L}{Q} \tag{12.17}$$

where *Re* is the Reynolds number for the flow $\left(\frac{\rho U d}{\mu}\right)$, *Sc* the Schmidt number $\left(\frac{\mu}{\rho D}\right)$, ρ the density of air, μ the viscosity of the air, D the particle diffusion coefficient, and Q the volumetric flow rate (Holman, 1972).

For turbulent flow, the Sherwood number is given by Friedlander (1977) as

$$Sh = 0.0118\, Re^{7/8}\, Sc^{1/3} \tag{12.18}$$

Thus, Equation 12.18, along with Equation 12.15, can be used to determine diffusional deposition in turbulent flow. The loss due to turbulent inertial deposition is given by

$$P_{\text{inertial turbulence}} = \exp\left(-\pi\, d\, L\, V_t / Q\right) \tag{12.19}$$

where V_t is the turbulent inertial deposition velocity (Liu and Agarwal, 1974).

The loss due to inertial deposition in a tube bend of angle ϕ (in radians) for laminar flow is given by

$$P_{\text{bend inertial}} = 1 - St\,\phi \tag{12.20}$$

where *St* is the Stokes number (Crane and Evans, 1977). For turbulent flow, we use the formula by Pui et al. (1987):

$$P_{\text{bend inertial}} = \exp\left(-2.823\, St\,\phi\right) \tag{12.21}$$

Electrostatic losses in a tube can be obtained using

$$P_{\text{electrostatic}} = \exp\left(-\frac{V_{\text{TE}}\, A_c}{Q}\right) \tag{12.22}$$

Here, A_c is the curved surface area of the tube ($A_c = 2\pi RL$) where R is the radius of the tube, L the tube length, Q the volumetric flow rate, and V_{TE} the terminal electrical drift velocity, given by

$$V_{\mathrm{TE}} = \frac{n\,e\,E\,C_{\mathrm{c}}}{3\pi\mu\,d} \tag{12.23}$$

where n is the number of units of charge on the particle with diameter d, E is the electric field strength, and C_c is the Cunningham slip correction factor. It is clear that in most sampling situations, the electric field and particle charge are unknown, and therefore loss calculations are difficult to carry out. It is therefore prudent to avoid electrostatic losses by grounding all sampling lines and using metal tubing (or Tygon). Teflon tubing is to be avoided for sampling of aerosols.

The preceding discussion presents expressions for transport losses in a tube under laminar and turbulent flow conditions due to gravitational settling, inertial deposition, diffusional deposition, and electrostatic deposition. There are several other mechanisms that can also lead to settling losses; for example, thermophoresis (whereby airborne particles move along a thermal gradient from higher to lower temperatures) and diffusiophoresis (whereby particles suspended in a mixture of gases move in the direction of diffusion of the heavier molecules). Losses due to thermophoresis are difficult to quantify because of the difficulty in estimating temperature gradients and lack of knowledge of the thermal conductivity of the particles. It is best to avoid thermophoretic losses by heating or cooling the transport tubes so that their temperature is equal to the gas temperature.

12.6 FILTER COLLECTION

Once the sampled aerosol passes through the transport section, it enters the collection or sensing zone. In this section, we will discuss collection of the aerosol using filter media. The filter media usually are supported using a wire mesh screen or other backing media to hold the filter in place. An O-ring or gasket is used to provide a seal so that air moves only through the filter and does not leak around the sides. The filters and their physical supports are held in place by various types of filter holders. Both in-line and cassette-type holders are used in occupational hygiene. The bottom layer in Figure 12.8 shows an in-line filter that uses a wire screen mesh for support. The material used for the construction of the filter holders should be chosen carefully to minimize the potential for losses due to electrostatic and other mechanisms discussed in the previous section.

12.6.1 Theory of Filtration

The theory of filtration is well established for fibrous filters, i.e., filters composed of a mat of individual cylindrical fibers. The efficiency of particle collection by an individual fiber is used along with the more macroscopic parameters of the filter mat or bed to determine the collection efficiency of the entire filter. It is assumed that the single fiber has its axis perpendicular to the airflow. The single-fiber efficiency, η, is the fraction of particles geometrically approaching the filter laterally that strike the filter and get collected (Figure 12.12).

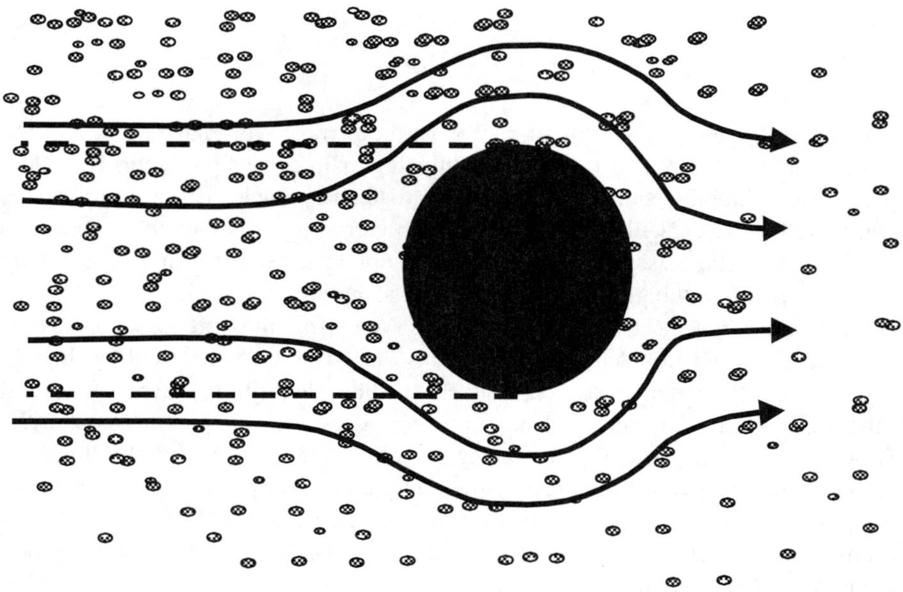

FIGURE 12.12 Particle-laden air approaching a single fiber of circular cross section. The streamlines of air move around the fiber. Particles that are within the dashed lines are geometrically approaching the fiber, but only a fraction of them actually deposit on the fiber.

The collection efficiency for a filter is defined as the fraction of the particles entering the filter bed that are collected in it.

$$E = \frac{C_{in} - C_{out}}{C_{in}} \tag{12.24}$$

where C_{in} is the concentration of particles entering the filter bed and C_{out} is the concentration of particles exiting it.

This collection efficiency of a filter composed of many fibers that are randomly oriented in a mat can also be expressed in terms of the physical parameters of the filter as

$$E = 1 - \exp\left(\frac{-4\,\eta\,\alpha\,L}{\pi\,d_f\,(1-\alpha)}\right) \tag{12.25}$$

Here, α is the packing density (the ratio of the volume of the fibers in a mat to the total volume of the mat), L is the filter mat thickness, d_f is the diameter of the filter, and η is the single-fiber efficiency. Equation 12.25 shows that the filter efficiency can be increased by increasing the thickness of the mat, the packing density, or the single-fiber efficiency.

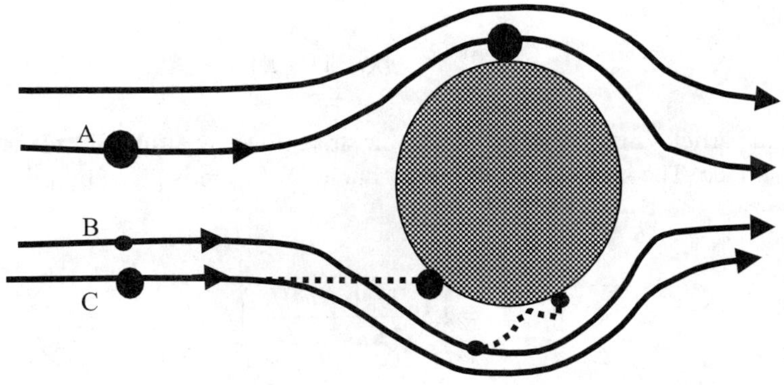

FIGURE 12.13 Particle A is collected by interception; particle B is collected by diffusion; and particle C is collected by inertial impaction.

Particles collect on filters by the same mechanisms that we have studied earlier — *inertial impaction*, *diffusion*, *electrostatic forces*, *gravity*, and *interception*. Figure 12.13 shows a schematic diagram of particles being collected on a single fiber by impaction, interception, and diffusion. Equations have been developed from theoretical and empirical considerations for the single-fiber collection efficiency of each of these mechanisms.

Inertial impaction occurs when the particles are unable to follow the air streamlines, and they deviate from them due to their inertia and strike a fiber. The single-fiber efficiency due to inertial impaction is given by

$$\eta_{\text{inertia}} = \frac{1}{\left(2\,Ku^2\right)}\left[\left(29.6 - 28\,\alpha^{0.62}\right)R^2 - 27.5\,R^{2.8}\right]St \qquad (12.26)$$

where Ku is the Kuwabara hydrodynamic factor $\left(Ku = -\frac{1}{2}\ln\alpha - \frac{3}{4} + \alpha - \frac{\alpha^2}{4}\right)$, which accounts for the flow distortion in the field around a fiber caused by the presence of neighboring fibers, R is the interception parameter, which is the ratio of particle diameter to fiber diameter $\left(R = \frac{d_p}{d_f}\right)$, St is the Stokes number $\left(St = \frac{\tau U_0}{d_f}\right)$, U_0 is the face velocity of the gas entering the filter mat, and τ is the particle relaxation time.

Even if particles do not deviate from the streamlines, they may come close enough to the fiber (less than one particle radius) to be collected by interception. The single-fiber efficiency due to interception is given by Lee and Ramamurthi (1993) as:

$$\eta_{\text{interception}} = \frac{1-\alpha}{Ku}\frac{R^2}{(1+R)} \tag{12.27}$$

Small particles may move away from air streamlines by diffusion and may strike a fiber surface. The single-fiber efficiency due to diffusion is given by Lee and Liu (1982) as:

$$\eta_{\text{diffusion}} = 2.58\frac{1-\alpha}{Ku}\left(\frac{d_f\,U_0}{D}\right)^{2/3} \tag{12.28}$$

where D is the diffusion coefficient of the particle. The term within brackets is called the *Peclet number*, and it is dimensionless.

Collection may also occur due to gravitational settling. A dimensionless parameter, G, is defined as the ratio of particle settling velocity and gas velocity $\left(G = \frac{V_{TS}}{U_0}\right)$, and the single-fiber efficiency is given by

$$\eta_{\text{gravity}} = \frac{G}{1+G} \tag{12.29}$$

Aerosol particles can acquire an electrostatic charge either during their generation or during flow through a gas stream. Likewise, the filter fibers can acquire a charge due to the friction caused by a gas stream passing over them. Some filters are designed to have a permanent charge. The following three cases can occur:

1. Charged particle–charged fiber

$$\eta_{\text{electrostatic}} = \frac{4Qq}{3\mu\,d_p\,d_f\,U_0} \tag{12.30}$$

where Q is the charge per unit length of the fiber, q the charge on the particle, and μ the viscosity of the medium.

2. Charged fiber–neutral particle

$$\eta_{\text{electrostatic}} = \frac{4}{3}\left(\frac{\varepsilon-1}{\varepsilon+1}\right)\left(\frac{d_p^2\,Q^2}{d_f^3\,\mu\,U_0}\right) \tag{12.31}$$

where ε is the dielectric constant of the particle.

3. Charged particle–neutral fiber

$$\eta_{\text{electrostatic}} = \sqrt{\frac{\varepsilon - 1}{\varepsilon + 1}} \left(\frac{q^2}{3\pi \mu d_p d_f U_0 (2 - \ln Re)} \right)^{1/2} \tag{12.32}$$

where Re is the Reynolds number given by $\frac{d_f U_0 \rho_g}{\mu}$.

By assuming that each of these mechanisms acts independently, we can use Equation 12.11 and calculate the total single-particle efficiency as

$$\eta = 1 - (1 - \eta_{\text{inertia}})(1 - \eta_{\text{interception}})(1 - \eta_{\text{diffusion}})(1 - \eta_{\text{gravity}})(1 - \eta_{\text{electrostatic}}) \tag{12.33}$$

Because the efficiencies due to each of the individual mechanisms are very small, this expression can be approximated as

$$\eta \approx \eta_{\text{inertia}} + \eta_{\text{interception}} + \eta_{\text{diffusion}} + \eta_{\text{gravity}} + \eta_{\text{electrostatic}} \tag{12.34}$$

Figure 12.14 shows a schematic diagram of particle collection mechanisms that are dominant for different particle sizes. As one might expect, diffusion is the primary mechanism for very small particle sizes and increases with decreasing particle size, whereas inertia, interception, and gravitational settling are the primary mechanisms for larger particles and increase with increasing particle size. A point of minimum collection efficiency is reached between these two regimes. The corresponding particle size is referred to as the most penetrating particle size and is ~0.3 μm. Filter testing is typically carried out at this particle size, and commercial filters are usually rated by their efficiency at this particle size.

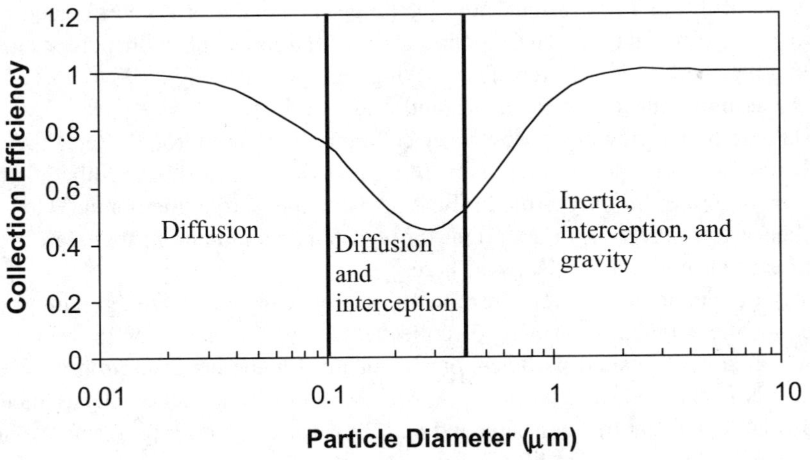

FIGURE 12.14 Particle collection mechanisms in filter collection, which are dominant for different particle sizes.

The airflow through the filter is resisted by the fiber elements. This resistance leads to a pressure drop across the filter. The pressure drop across a fibrous filter is given by

$$\Delta P = \frac{16\,\eta\,\alpha\,U_0\,L}{(Ku)\,d_f^2} \qquad (12.35)$$

12.6.2 Filter Selection and Gravimetry

A variety of filter media are available for aerosol sampling, and the choice of a particular medium should be dictated by the following criteria:

1. The particle size collection efficiency characteristics of the filter.
2. The pressure drop across the filter. A higher pressure drop leads to higher energy consumption for a given flow rate.
3. The analytical procedures that will follow sample collection.

Fibrous filters, as the name suggests, are composed of a mat of fibers that are made of cellulose, quartz, glass, or polymer. Fiber sizes range from less than 1 μm to several hundred micrometers. Packing densities range from 1 to ~30%, and filter thicknesses range from 0.1 to 0.5 mm. Particle collection occurs in the matrix of the fibers. They require low gas velocities for higher collection efficiency and have relatively low pressure drops.

Porous membranes are made of cellulose esters, Teflon, and polyvinyl chloride. They have packing densities between 10 and 50% and thicknesses between 0.05 to 0.2 mm. They have a complicated microstructure of pores, which provides a very irregular path for the aerosol particles, and the particles collect in this microstructure. Collection efficiency is very high, but comes at the cost of high pressure drop.

Straight-through or capillary pore membranes have uniform pores etched into a polycarbonate membrane. The membranes are ~10 μm thick with pore diameters ranging between 0.1 and 10 μm. The packing density is very high (90 to 95%). They also have high collection efficiencies and pressure drops.

Although the previously described equations are for fibrous filters, they can easily be extended to porous membrane filters by assuming an effective fiber diameter that can describe the microstructural elements of the porous membrane. However, the theory for collection in a straight-through pore membrane requires a different treatment that will not be discussed here.

After collection on a filter substrate, the sample can be analyzed gravimetrically to obtain the total mass of aerosol collected, microscopically for the number or surface area of deposited particles, or chemically for the concentration of specific chemicals in the collected particles. A wide variety of chemical analysis methods are available, e.g., atomic emission and mass spectroscopy, high-performance liquid chromatography, and x-ray diffraction analysis.

The accuracy of gravimetric samples may be affected by water adsorption onto substrates and filter cartridges. Cellulose ester membrane filters, polyurethane foams, and conducting plastic filter cassettes are particularly prone to weight changes following water uptake. It is, therefore, advisable to weigh a number of field blank filters with each set of sample filters (typically one blank per ten samples, with a minimum of three blanks). The field blanks should be transported with the sample substrates and exposed to the same conditions to minimize bias resulting from handling, transport, and changes in environment. Filters should be conditioned in a temperature- and humidity-controlled environment for up to 24 h before weighing to allow them to reach an equilibrium weight. Desiccation is generally not advisable prior to filter weighing, as weight changes after removal of the filter can be sufficiently rapid and can lead to significant weighing errors. Electrostatic attraction where substrates are highly charged can also lead to substantial biases during weighing. Electrostatic charge buildup may be significant for substrate materials such as PVC, particularly when working at low relative humidities. In all instances, samples should be neutralized using a source of bipolar ions. A common approach is to place samples close to a radioactive antistatic source prior to weighing. Readers should review Chapter 4, which provides a detailed description of limits of detection and quantitation (LOD and LOQ) that is especially relevant for gravimetric measurements.

12.7 SPECIAL SAMPLING PROBLEMS: VAPOR-PARTICLE PARTITIONING AND MEASUREMENT OF SEMIVOLATILE AEROSOLS

Semivolatile organic compounds (SOCs) have vapor pressures between 10^4 and 10^{11} atm over the ambient temperature range and can exist simultaneously in both gas and particle phases. Such compounds include alkanes, alkenes, aldehydes, acids, polychlorinated biphenyls, polycyclic aromatic hydrocarbons (PAHs), Nitro-PAHs, polychlorinated dibenzo-*p*-dioxins, and dibenzofurans. At equilibrium, the distribution of mass between the gaseous and condensed states can be described by a dimensionless partitioning ratio, K_p,

$$K_p = \frac{c_p}{c_g} \tag{12.36}$$

where c_p is the concentration of condensed SOCs in air and c_g is the concentration of SOC in the gas phase. Sampling of such aerosols and the determination of the partitioning ratio present an interesting challenge. One method that has been used is to place a vapor trap (e.g., a sorption tube containing activated charcoal) behind the sample filter. Ideally, this allows the particles to be captured on the filter and the vapors to be collected on the sorption material, thus allowing total aerosol and vapor concentration to be measured. However, filter sampling of SOCs can result in evaporative sampling artifacts that may underestimate K_p. For example, metal-working fluids contain SOCs that may not evaporate as pooled liquids but may show significant evaporation when aerosolized due to the increased surface area of the

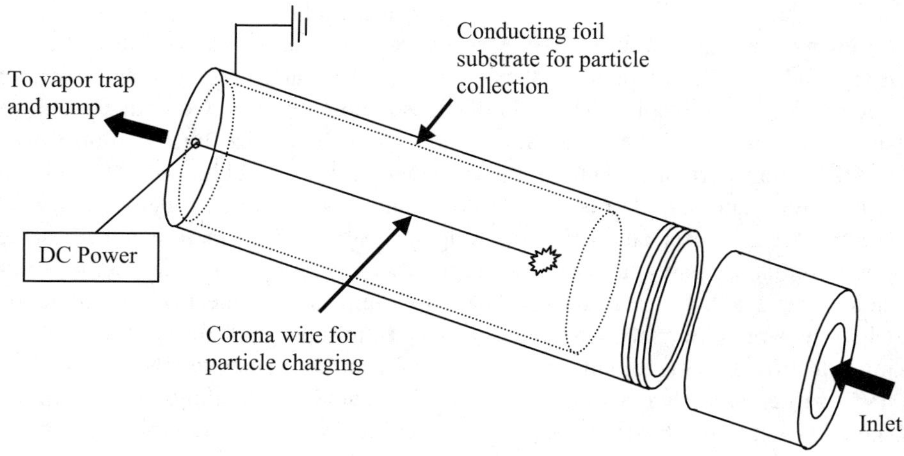

FIGURE 12.15 Schematic of an electrostatic sampler.

particles. Thus, if such aerosols are collected using a filter, deposited particles may evaporate during and following the sampling process if the vapor pressure of the material and the surface area of the particles are sufficiently high. This has been illustrated in laboratory and field studies by Volckens et al. (1999). Particle evaporation occurs whenever the gas-phase concentration surrounding a particle drops below the equilibrium level dictated by K_p. It is also possible that, in some instances, gas-phase semivolatiles may adsorb to the filter during sampling, resulting in an overestimation of K_p. Thus, both evaporative and adsorptive artifacts are important. In such situations, filter sampling does not provide information on the exact partitioning of the airborne contaminant between the particle and vapor phase in the workplace atmosphere.

One solution proposed to collect volatile aerosols while minimizing evaporative losses has been to use a coaxial electrostatic precipitator (Volckens and Leith, 2002a; 2002b). The sampler consists of a central positive electrode and an outer casing that is grounded, thus creating a strong electric field between the two electrodes (see Figure 12.15). Particles entering the sampler are first charged using a corona discharge and then deposited on the outer electrode. Particles collect at the flow boundary on a conductive foil substrate, where they aggregate. This aggregation reduces exposed particle surface area and thus should lower the rate of particle evaporation as well as gas-phase adsorption of SOCs onto the particles. After sampling, the sampler is sealed at both ends to prevent vapor release and the component of interest removed by washing out with a suitable solvent. One drawback of electrostatic precipitators is that the corona discharge produces ozone, which can potentially react with some of the components of the aerosol material. Therefore, such samplers are not useful for chemical speciation of highly reactive chemicals. However, because such reactions do not change the total amount of organic carbon, such samplers are useful in determining gravimetric concentrations. They are also useful in sampling more persistent SOCs such as PAHs.

13 Direct Reading Instruments for Aerosols

13.1 INTRODUCTION

Time-integrated samples obtained by the type of instruments described in Chapter 12 are usually sufficient in most cases. However, it is sometimes necessary to obtain measurements rapidly to estimate hazard levels or to evaluate control systems. Such measurements can also help in determining how the time-integrated measurements can be obtained optimally to provide the most useful information. Direct reading instruments can be used to determine a variety of aerosol properties. In some cases, the inertial properties of the aerosol are relevant, and hence it becomes important to measure the particle aerodynamic diameter. The mass concentration of a health-relevant aerosol fraction is clearly of interest, and hence several instruments have been developed for such measurements. In recent years, the surface area concentration and the number concentration of aerosol particles have also been thought to be relevant to human exposures that can cause health effects.

13.2 INSTRUMENTS BASED ON INERTIAL PROPERTIES OF PARTICLES

Instruments based on inertial properties of particles are used to measure the aerodynamic diameter of particles. Air containing particles is accelerated through a nozzle to a very high velocity. The velocity of each particle is determined using the time it takes to pass between two laser beams that are placed just downstream of the nozzle exit (see Figure 13.1). As the particle passes through each light beam, it creates a pulse of scattered light, and the time between the two pulses of light is determined electronically. Knowing the distance between the laser beams and the time taken by a particle to traverse the distance between them, the particle velocity is determined. The particles, due to their inertia, have velocities that lag behind the air velocity. The greater the particle inertia (i.e., the particle aerodynamic diameter), the greater the velocity lag (i.e., the lower the particle velocity between the two laser beams). This velocity lag is related to the particle's aerodynamic diameter (Wang and John, 1987). By sampling a large number of particles, the size distribution of the particles is obtained rapidly.

The most commonly used example of this type of instrument is the aerodynamic particle sizer (APS Model 3300, TSI, Inc.). This instrument can size particles between 0.5 and 30 μm. There are several limitations to this instrument. The particles are accelerated to a sufficiently high velocity in the nozzle that they are no longer in the Stokes regime, and therefore appropriate corrections need to be made (as

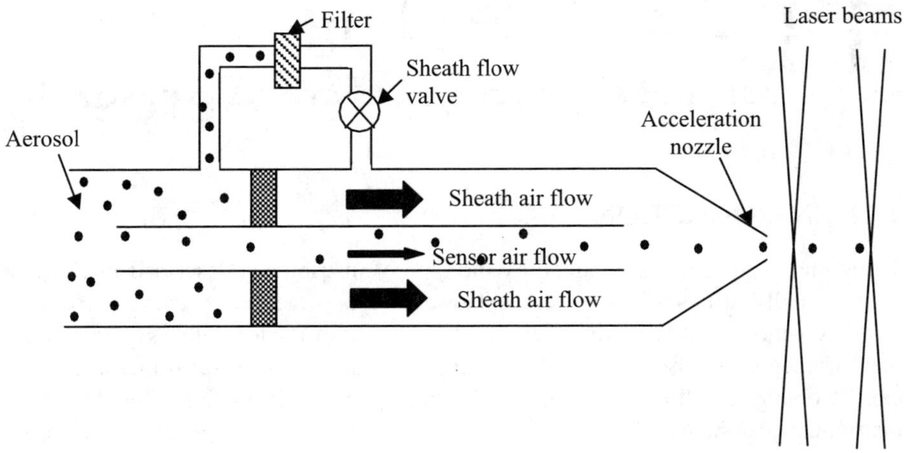

FIGURE 13.1 Schematic of aerodynamic particle sizer.

described in Chapter 10). Liquid particles may get distorted due to the high velocities and may appear smaller. At high concentrations, if more than one particle is present in the sensing zone at the same time (i.e., they go through the laser beams together), they may be sized as one larger particle. This is referred to as a *coincidence error*, and may be rectified by diluting the aerosol being sampled to a low enough concentration that such errors can be minimized. Another type of error that can occur is when a larger particle just grazes the edge of the laser beams and gets counted as a smaller particle. Interested readers can find more detailed descriptions of this instrument by Wang and John (1987), Baron (1986), Chen et al. (1985, 1989), and Chen and Crow (1986).

13.3 INSTRUMENTS BASED ON MASS MEASUREMENTS

The piezoelectric balance consists of a piezoelectric crystal that oscillates when an alternating electric field or electric potential is applied across the crystal. The resonant or natural frequency of the oscillation depends, among other things, on the mass of the crystal. The resonant frequency decreases in direct proportion to the increased mass. This property provides the basis of aerosol mass measurement using quartz crystal microbalances. A change in mass Δm will produce a change Δf in the resonant frequency, in which the two are related by

$$\Delta f = K f_o^2 \Delta m \tag{13.1}$$

where f_o is the fundamental frequency of the crystal and K is a constant. Thus, if f_o and Δf can be measured electronically, and K is obtained through calibration, then

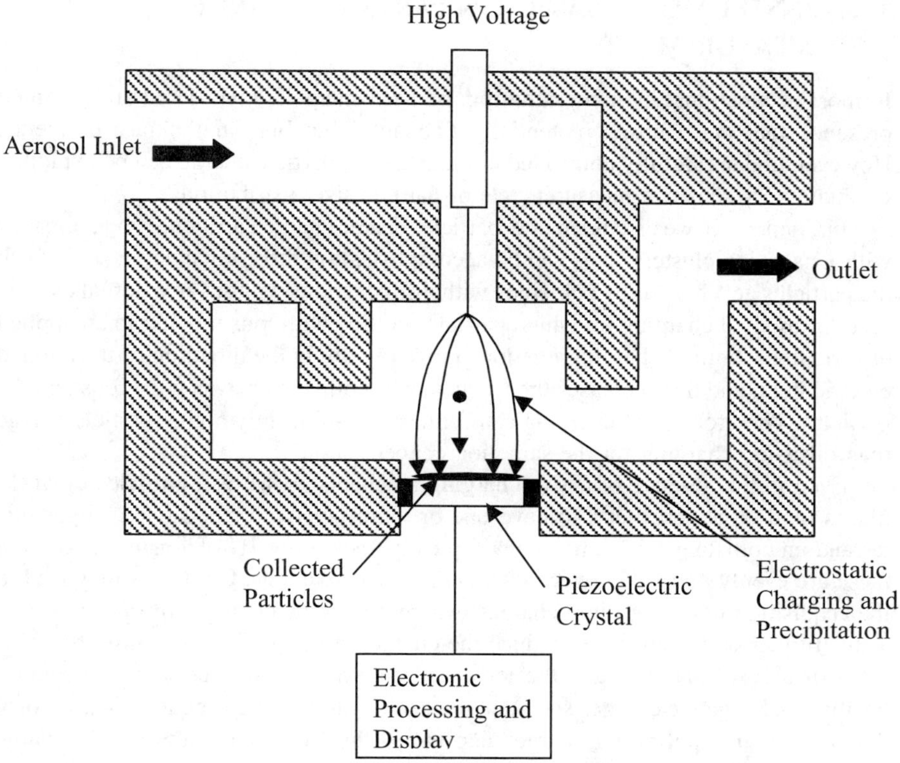

FIGURE 13.2 Piezoelectric sensor with electrostatic precipitation for particle collection.

Δm can be determined using such an instrument. The change in mass occurs due to particle deposition on the crystal surface.

The particles need to be accurately deposited onto the crystal surface. This is typically achieved using electrostatic precipitation (e.g., in Figure 13.2), although other methods, such as inertial impaction, can also be employed. The particles should be attached securely to the surface even during the rapid vibrations of the crystal. Thus, although the method works better for fine particles such as the respirable fraction, some particles may not bind well to the surface. For instance, one end of a fiber may attach to the crystal while the other end may flap around freely, or a large particle may not adhere sufficiently strongly to the crystal. If the crystal becomes overloaded with particles, the relationship between the change in frequency and the change in mass may become nonlinear and deviate from Equation 13.1. A more detailed description is provided by Williams et al. (1993).

Such instruments have been used in occupational hygiene for real-time monitoring of aerosol fractions of health relevance. This has been accomplished with partial success by passing the aerosol through an inlet that has been designed with a predetermined sampling efficiency.

13.4 INSTRUMENTS BASED ON PARTICLE CHARGE MEASUREMENT

In most occupational hygiene sampling, particle charge is considered an unwanted presence that can cause a potentially unquantifiable bias in the measurements. However, under carefully controlled circumstances, particle charge can be exploited to obtain very sensitive measurements of particle size distributions.

In Chapter 10, we discussed how particles can be charged artificially by collisions with ions or ion clusters. This can be accomplished by diffusion charging, in which the particles get charged by collisions with diffusing ions without an external electric field, or by field charging, in which particles collide with ions moving in an applied electric field. In field charging, the ions move rapidly in the direction of the applied electric field, and this increases the frequency of collisions between the ions and the particles. Therefore, field charging can achieve a significantly higher particle charge than diffusion charging for the same ion concentration.

Even in the absence of active charging mechanisms, aerosol particles in workplaces (and elsewhere) tend to have one or more positive or negative charges due to random collisions with ions in air. Typically, there are ~10^9 of ions/m^3 of air, and these are evenly divided between positive and negative ions. Collisions may lead to the acquisition of one or more charges, which may attract charges of opposite sign. Thus, further collisions might reduce the charge on the particle. Because the collisions of aerosol particles and the ions are random, the particles will also acquire positive and negative charges such that the aerosol as a whole is neutral. The aerosol thus attains an equilibrium charge state called the Boltzmann equilibrium charge distribution. This charge distribution is expressed as

$$f_n = \frac{\exp(-n^2/2\sigma^2)}{\sum_{-\infty}^{+\infty} \exp(-n^2/2\sigma^2)} \tag{13.2}$$

where

$$\sigma^2 = \frac{d_p \mathrm{k} T}{2\mathrm{e}^2} \tag{13.3}$$

and f_n is the fraction of particles of size d_p having n elementary units of charge (one elementary unit of charge is the charge on an electron, e = 1.6×10^{-19} C), and k is Boltzmann's constant (1.38×10^{-16} erg/K). For particles larger than 0.01 μm, Equation 13.2 can be approximated as

$$f_n = \frac{\exp(-n^2/2\sigma^2)}{\sqrt{2\pi\sigma^2}} \tag{13.4}$$

TABLE 13.1
Boltzmann Charge Distribution on Particles of Different Sizes

	Number of Charges on Particles								
d (μm)	0	1	2	3	4	5	6	7	8
0.01	0.994	0.006	—	—	—	—	—	—	—
0.02	0.948	0.052	—	—	—	—	—	—	—
0.05	0.606	0.380	0.012	—	—	—	—	—	—
0.1	0.428	0.479	0.084	0.005	—	—	—	—	—
0.2	0.303	0.453	0.190	0.045	0.006	—	—	—	—
0.5	0.191	0.341	0.241	0.135	0.060	0.021	0.006	0.001	—
1	0.135	0.256	0.215	0.161	0.107	0.064	0.034	0.016	0.007
2	0.096	0.186	0.171	0.148	0.120	0.093	0.067	0.046	0.030
5	0.061	0.120	0.116	0.109	0.101	0.091	0.080	0.069	0.058

Note: The numbers represent the fraction of charges of either sign. Thus, for 0.05 μm particles 60.6% of the particles are uncharged, 19% of the particles have one positive charge, 19% have one negative charge, 0.6% of the particles have two positive charges, and 0.6% have two negative charges.

which is the form of the normal Gaussian distribution. Table 13.1 shows the Boltzmann charge distribution, as given by Equation 13.4. The overall aerosol has an equal number of positive and negative charges, and thus is electrically neutral.

The charge distribution of an aerosol can be determined by measuring the distribution of electrical mobility of particles. In Chapter 10, we introduced the concept of the terminal electrical drift velocity, defined as $V_E = \frac{qE}{3\pi\mu d}$, where q is the charge on the particle of diameter d, and E is the electric field strength. Based on this idea, we can define a particle electrical mobility Z that is equal to the drift velocity when the applied field strength is unity, i.e., $Z = \frac{q}{3\pi\mu d}$, where μ is the viscosity of the medium. The first instrument based on this idea is the *Electrical Aerosol Analyzer* (EAA). The aerosol enters the instrument through an outer annular slit, while clean air (sheath air) is introduced into the inner core. The outer electrode is grounded while an adjustable voltage is applied to the inner electrode. Particles that have a sufficiently high mobility will be collected on the inner electrode, and particles with smaller mobility will penetrate through the cylindrical column and be detected by a downstream particle sensor. Figure 13.3 shows a schematic diagram of such an instrument. Thus, for a monodisperse aerosol that has a certain charge distribution, one can vary the voltage between the two electrodes and measure the particle penetration through the instrument at different voltages. From measuring the particle penetration at two different voltages, the number of particles in the mobility range defined by these voltages can be determined. From such measurements, the electrical mobility distribution can be determined. Now, if the particle

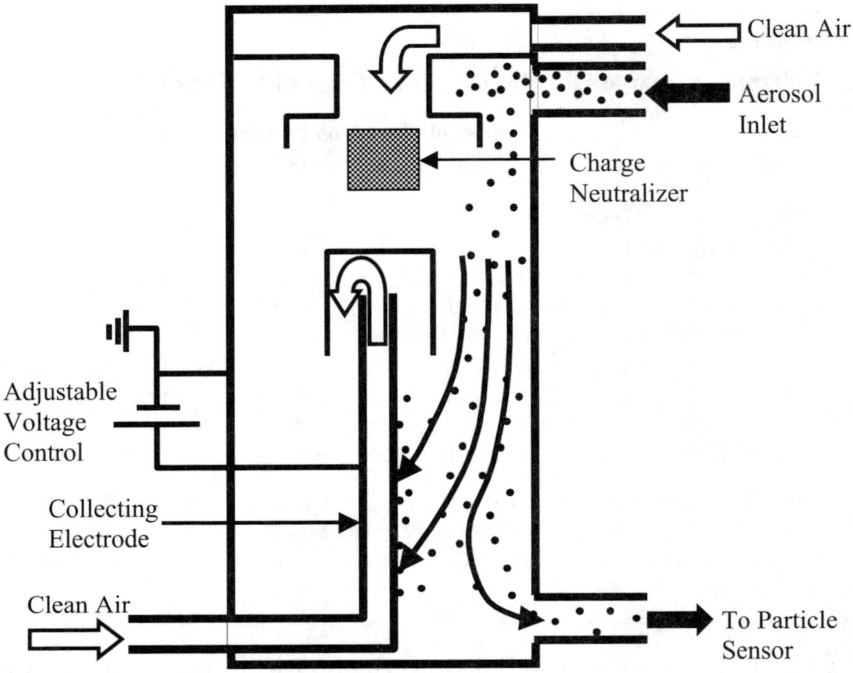

FIGURE 13.3 Schematic diagram of the Electrical Aerosol Analyzer (EAA).

size of the monodisperse aerosol is also known, the charge distribution can be ascertained.

Conversely, if the particles are charged under very controlled circumstances, then the particle size distribution can be determined. For example, under diffusion charging, there is a one-to-one monotonic relationship between particle size and particle charge, and thus each value of electrical mobility corresponds to a unique value of particle size. Therefore, if we know the distribution of particle electrical mobilities, we can determine the particle size distribution. The EAA manufactured by TSI, Inc. (St. Paul, MN) can size particles between 0.003 μm and 1 μm. The one-to-one relationship between mobility and particle size exists only for particles less than 1 μm, and therefore larger particles should be prevented from entering the instrument by means of an impactor-based preselector.

The *Differential Mobility Analyzer* (DMA) operates on a very similar principle. Here, a small slit is present at a specific location on the inner electrode through which aerosol can be drawn (Figure 13.4). Particles with higher electrical mobility are collected above this slit, whereas particles with lower electrical mobility are collected below this slit. Particles with a narrow range of electrical mobilities pass through the slit and are detected by a downstream aerosol sensor. The narrow slit results in a very high size resolution, and by gradually stepping through a range of voltages, the particle size distribution can be obtained for particles between 0.005 and 1 μm.

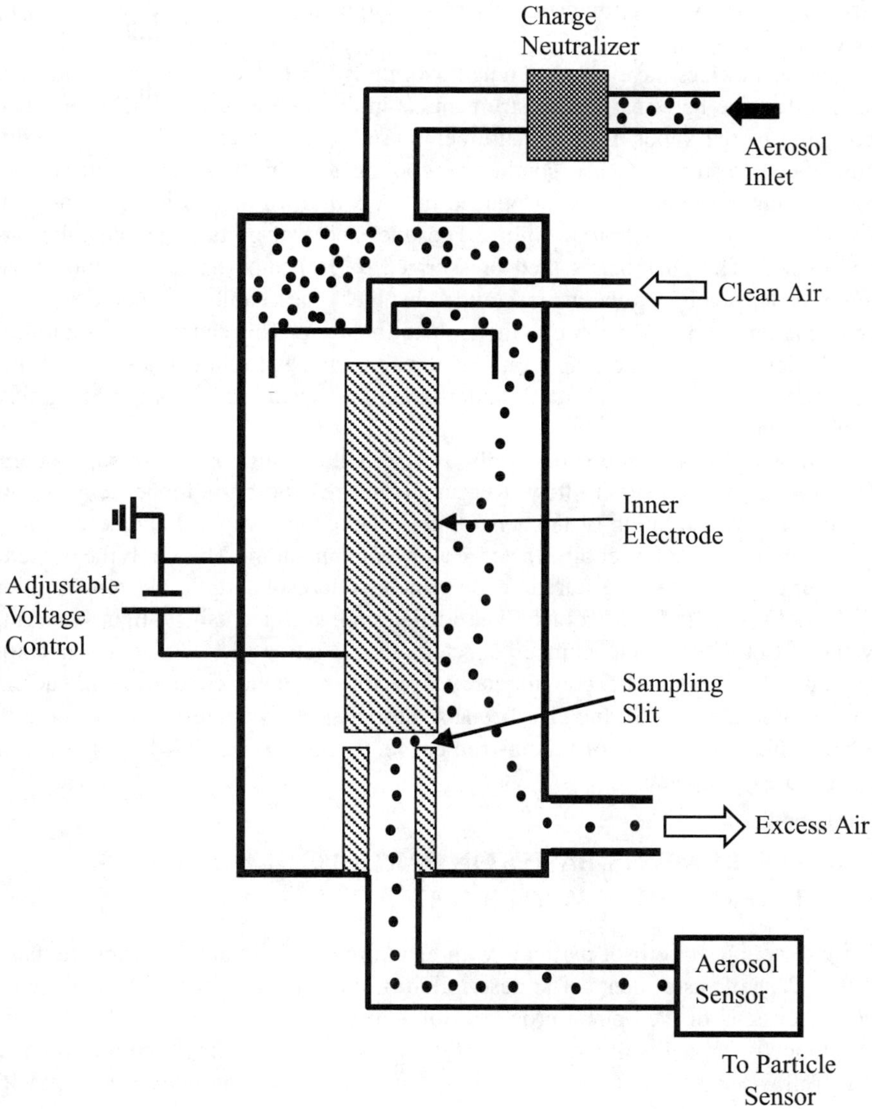

FIGURE 13.4 Schematic diagram for the Differential Mobility Analyzer.

13.5 CONDENSATION NUCLEI COUNTERS

Very small particles (less than 0.2 µm) can be detected using condensation nuclei counters (CNCs). In these instruments, the aerosol is first saturated with a vapor of water or alcohol and then cooled to supersaturation (i.e., the vapor pressure is greater than the saturation vapor pressure at that temperature). This causes condensation of the vapor onto the aerosol particles, resulting in the formation of liquid droplets between 5 and 15 μm in diameter. These are large enough to be detected easily by optical methods.

Several devices have been designed over the years based on this principle. The main difference between these instruments is in the method used to achieve supersaturation of the vapor. Earlier instruments used adiabatic expansion whereas the more recent instruments use conductive cooling to achieve supersaturation. In a Pollak counter, the aerosol is introduced into a cylindrical expansion chamber that has a water-saturated ceramic lining. The inlet and exit ports to the chamber are then closed. The chamber is then pressurized to 160 mm Hg above atmospheric pressure. This saturates the air inside the chamber. The chamber is then depressurized, leading to an expansion into the ambient pressure. This causes supersaturation and condensation of water vapor on the aerosol particles. Light extinction measurements are made before and after condensation has occurred, to determine particle number concentration.

Nowadays, CNCs more commonly use thermal cooling to achieve supersaturation. The aerosol is made to flow over an alcohol reservoir at a higher temperature that causes the saturation of the aerosol with the alcohol vapors. The aerosol then passes through a condenser tube that is at a lower temperature. This cools the particle-laden air and causes supersaturation and growth of aerosol particles by condensation of alcohol vapors to form droplets. The particles are detected using a light scattering system to obtain particle number concentration. Figure 13.5 shows a schematic diagram of a CNC. The commercially available portable condensation nucleus counter (Portacount, TSI, Inc.) has been used for quantitative fit testing of respirators. Other miniature versions of this instrument (e.g., the P-Trak, TSI, Inc.) have been used as area samplers.

13.6 INSTRUMENTS BASED ON PARTICLE INTERACTIONS WITH LIGHT

The interaction of aerosol particles with electromagnetic radiation forms the basis of this class of instruments. The description of these instruments will be preceded by a discussion of the optical properties of aerosols.

Optically, an aerosol particle is distinct from its surrounding medium in terms of its refractive index. The refractive index of a material is the ratio of the velocity of light in vacuum to the velocity of light in that material $\left(m = \frac{C_{vacuum}}{C_m}\right)$. For many materials, this is a complex number with a real and an imaginary component,

$$m = a + b\mathrm{i} \tag{13.5}$$

where a is the real part and b is the imaginary part of the refractive index. The real and imaginary parts are related to the different ways in which light interacts with matter. Some of the light is reflected, another fraction is diffracted, and yet another

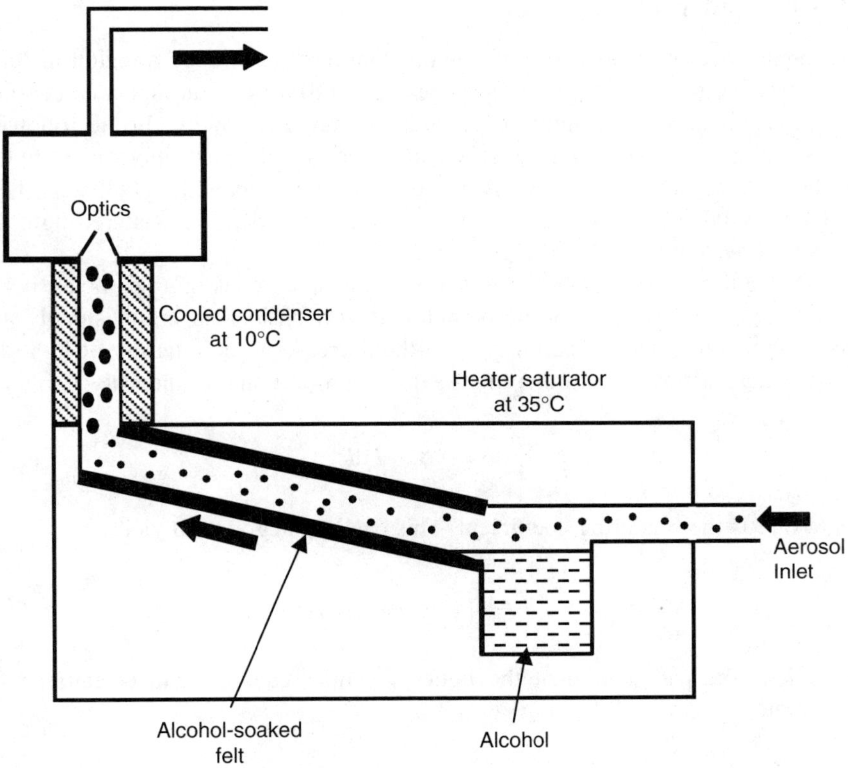

FIGURE 13.5 Schematic diagram of a condensation nucleus counter.

portion is refracted. These three phenomena are collectively referred to as scattering, and the real portion of the refractive index is related to light scattering. A portion of the light is absorbed by the material (similar to absorption of light by gas molecules), and the imaginary component of the refractive index is related to light absorption. Transparent particles have a small (or zero) imaginary component, whereas colored particles have a substantial imaginary component. Thus, glass particles can have a refractive index between 1.5 and 2.0, whereas carbon particles have a refractive index of 2 i.

Although most instruments use visible electromagnetic radiation only, i.e., radiation between wavelengths of 0.4 μm and 0.7 μm, the physics of light scattering and absorption are the same for larger and smaller wavelengths. The important parameter is the relative magnitude of the particle diameter (d) with respect to the wavelength of light (λ), and is referred to as the *size parameter*, α, where

$$\alpha = \frac{\pi d}{\lambda} \tag{13.6}$$

13.6.1 Light Extinction

The intensity (or radiation flux) of a light beam passing through a region in space is expressed as the radiant power (energy per second) passing through a unit surface area perpendicular to the light beam. Thus, its units are W/m^2. In the following discussion, it will be assumed that each aerosol particle interacts only with light that has directly been emitted by the source and does not interact with light that has been scattered by other particles. The second assumption is that the scattered light has the same wavelength as the incident light.

When a light beam passes through a region in space containing particles, it will be scattered and absorbed by the particles. If we consider an infinitesimally thin slice dl containing aerosol particles, then the decrease in the intensity of light due to scattering as it passes through this section is proportional to intensity:

$$dI = -\sigma_{scat} I \, dl \tag{13.7}$$

where σ_{scat} is the scattering coefficient. This can be integrated to yield

$$I = I_0 \exp(-\sigma_{scat} L) \tag{13.8}$$

where L is the path length of the light. A similar equation can be derived for absorption:

$$I = I_0 \exp(-\sigma_{abs} L) \tag{13.9}$$

where σ_{abs} is the absorption coefficient.

The scattering and absorption coefficients can be combined into a so-called extinction coefficient or attenuation coefficient or turbidity coefficient, σ_{ext}, so that

$$I = I_0 \exp(-\sigma_{ext} L) \tag{13.10}$$

Equation 13.10 is called *Bouguer's law.* Thus, σ_{ext} is the fraction of the light intensity that is lost per unit length traveled by the beam and has units of per unit length.

If we consider only one aerosol particle, then the extinction due to it can be described by a particle extinction efficiency, Q_{ext}, which is defined as

$$Q_{ext} = \frac{\textit{Power scattered and absorbed by the particle}}{\textit{Power geometrically incident on the particle}} \tag{13.11}$$

The power geometrically incident on a particle is equal to the product of the light intensity (radiant power per unit area) and the cross-sectional area of the particle. If we consider a beam of unit intensity incident on a spherical particle of diameter d, then the power scattered and absorbed by the particle is $Q_{ext}A$ or $\left(Q_{ext}\frac{\pi d^2}{4}\right)$. Because σ_{ext} is the fraction of the light intensity that is lost per unit length traveled by the beam, for n particles per unit volume that are all of the same diameter, σ_{ext} is given by

$$\sigma_{ext} = n Q_{ext} \frac{\pi d^2}{4} \tag{13.12}$$

Q_{ext} can be partitioned into its scattering and absorption components as

$$Q_{ext} = Q_{scat} + Q_{abs} \tag{13.13}$$

Therefore, σ_{ext} can also be partitioned into its scattering and absorption components as

$$\sigma_{ext} = \sigma_{scat} + \sigma_{abs} \tag{13.14}$$

For a polydisperse aerosol with n_i particles of cross-sectional areas A_i, we need to sum over all particle sizes, and hence

$$\sigma_{ext} = \sum_{i=1}^{\infty} n_i Q_{ext,i} A_i = \sum_{i=1}^{\infty} n_i Q_{ext,i} \frac{\pi d^2}{4} \tag{13.15}$$

If the size distribution is assumed to be a continuous function $n(d)$, then there are $n(d)dd$ particles per unit volume having diameters in the size interval d to $d+dd$. Then, the integral form of Equation 13.15 can be written as

$$\sigma_{ext} = \int_0^{\infty} n(d) Q_{ext}(d, \lambda, m) \frac{\pi d^2}{4} \mathrm{d}d \tag{13.16}$$

where the total number of particles per unit volume, N, is given as

$$N = \int_0^{\infty} n(d)\, dd \tag{13.17}$$

Equations similar to 13.16 can be written for σ_{scat} and σ_{abs}.

Equation 13.15 or Equation 13.16 can be simplified by assuming that the polydisperse aerosol can be represented by the diameter of the average projected surface area, d_A. Then,

$$\sigma_{ext} = N\left(\frac{\pi d_A^{\,2}}{4}\right)Q_{ext} = C_p\,Q_{ext} \tag{13.18}$$

where C_p is the projected surface area concentration (in units of particle area per volume of air). Now, using Bouguer's law, we can measure C_p as

$$C_p = \frac{-4\ln\left(\dfrac{I}{I_0}\right)}{Q_{ext}\,L} \tag{13.19}$$

The projected area concentration (C_p) and total surface area concentration (C_A) for spherical (or near spherical) particles are related by $C_A = 4C_p$. Thus, Equation 13.19 can be used to determine the projected surface area concentration and surface area concentration, if Q_{ext} is known.

13.6.2 Calculation of Particle Extinction Efficiency, Q_{EXT}

Q_{ext} is a function of particle diameter, the wavelength of light, and the refractive index of the particle. For particles that are very small compared with the wavelength of light (i.e., the size parameter $\alpha << 1$), Q_{ext} is given by the Rayleigh scattering formula, which is valid for particles less than 0.05 μm:

$$Q_{ext} = \frac{8}{3}\left(\frac{\pi d}{\lambda}\right)^4\left(\frac{m^2-1}{m^2+1}\right)^2 \tag{13.20}$$

We see from Equation 13.20 that Q_{ext} is proportional to the fourth power of the size parameter. Thus, as particle diameter decreases, Q_{ext} decreases; and as the wavelength decreases, Q_{ext} increases. For visible light, wavelengths near the blue end of the spectrum (smaller λ) will be scattered more than wavelengths near the red end of the spectrum (larger λ). The very small particles in the atmosphere scatter more blue light, leading to the sky appearing blue. Conversely, the red components of light are not scattered but are transmitted instead, which explains the reddish nature of sunsets. The same phenomenon explains the bluish appearance of ultrafine aerosols such as welding fumes and even cigarette smoke.

For large particles ($\alpha >> 1$), Q_{ext} asymptotically reaches a value of 2. This implies that each particle removes twice as much light as it would by merely blocking the light geometrically. This is because for such particles, diffraction (the bending of waves around corners) is the main contributor to scattering. Therefore, in addition to the geometrical blocking of the light, an equal amount is removed because light

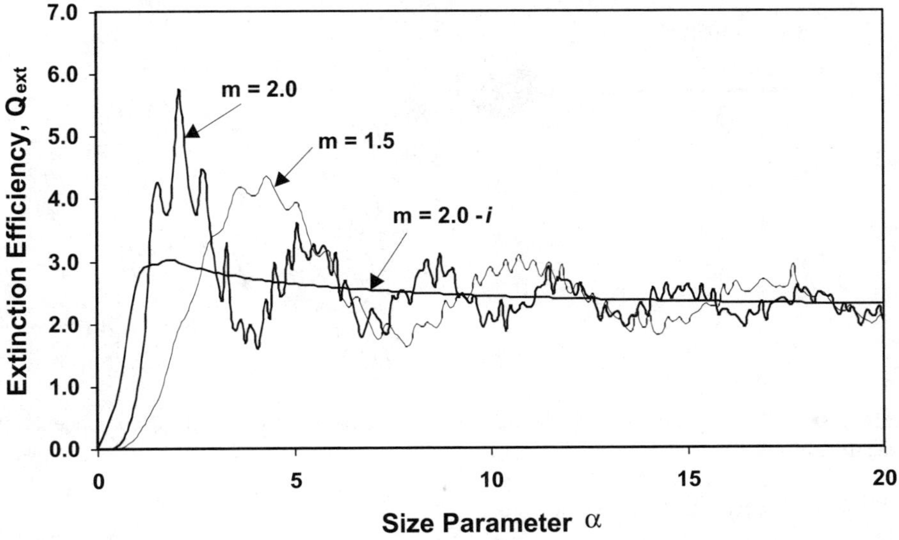

FIGURE 13.6 Extinction efficiency vs. size parameter $\left(\alpha = \frac{\pi d}{\lambda}\right)$.

bends around the particle and is thus removed from the beam when extinction is observed from a long distance away from the particles (distance >> 10 d^2/λ). At distances less than 10 d^2/λ, we observe the more common phenomenon of large everyday objects casting shadows by geometrical blocking. In such cases, of course, Q_{ext} is unity.

For particles between these two extremes (i.e., the particle diameter is of the same order of magnitude as the wavelength of light), the dependence of Q_{ext} on d is very complex and oscillatory. It is calculated using Mie theory, which will be discussed in the following section. Figure 13.6 shows the variation of Q_{ext} with α for several values of particle refractive index. For purely real values of refractive index (i.e., only scattering occurs), the variation is highly oscillatory after rising up sharply in the Rayleigh region and before reaching the asymptotic value of 2. The strong wave interferences between the diffracted and refracted components of scattered light cause these oscillations. For absorbing materials (scattering and absorption occur), the oscillations are damped out because the refracted component is very small.

Using Bouguer's law (Equation 13.10), we can measure the fractional reduction in light intensity as it passes through an aerosol $\left(\frac{I}{I_0}\right)$. If we know the path length of the light beam, we can, in principle, calculate the extinction coefficient, σ_{ext}. However, in many situations, the path length may be short or the aerosol concentration may be low enough that $\frac{I}{I_0}$ may be close to unity. In such cases, it may be difficult to estimate σ_{ext}.

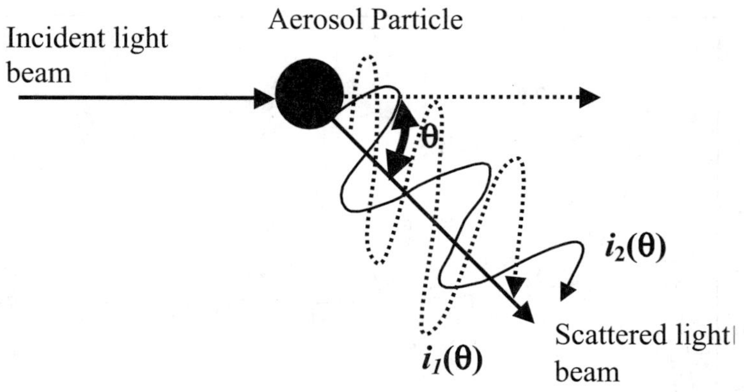

FIGURE 13.7 Diagram showing the angle of scattering and the polarized components of scattered light.

13.6.3 Light Scattering

In the discussion so far, Q_{scat} represents the loss in light intensity in the forward direction as the light beam moves forward through a region containing an aerosol. This energy is scattered in all directions. There is also a significant amount of information about the aerosol that can be gleaned from the amount of light scattered along different directions.

It is useful to establish a frame of reference where the aerosol particle is at the origin. θ is the angle between the direction of the incident light beam and the direction of the scattered beam in the plane formed by the incident and scattered light beams (see Figure 13.7). This is called the angle of scattering and the plane is called the scattering plane. For example, scattering at an angle of $\theta = 0°$ is referred to as forward scattering.

A *scattering intensity coefficient* $q(\theta)$ can be defined as

$$q(\theta) = \frac{\textit{Power scattered at angle } \theta}{\textit{Power geometrically incident on particle}} \tag{13.21}$$

To be precise, $q(\theta)$ is also a function of α and m, so it should be written as $q(\theta, \alpha, m)$. The incident light may or may not be polarized. If it is polarized, then the scattered light is also polarized in the same plane. The incident and scattered light beams can be resolved into two components that are perpendicular to each other — $q_1(\theta)$ is the scattering intensity coefficient for light moving in a plane perpendicular to the scattering plane and $q_2(\theta)$ is the scattering intensity coefficient for light moving parallel to the scattering plane. The scattering intensity coefficients are related to the Mie scattering functions i_1 and i_2 by

$$q_1(\theta) = \frac{i_1(\theta)}{\pi \alpha^2} \tag{13.22}$$

and

$$q_2(\theta) = \frac{i_2(\theta)}{\pi\alpha^2} \tag{13.23}$$

where α is the particle size parameter. For unpolarized light,

$$q(\theta) = \frac{1}{2}\left(q_1(\theta) + q_2(\theta)\right) \tag{13.24}$$

If I_0 is the intensity of an incident beam of perpendicularly polarized light, then the light flux scattered per unit solid angle by a particle of diameter d is given by

$$I_1 = I_0 \frac{\pi d^2}{4} q_1(\theta) = I_0 \frac{\lambda^2}{4\pi^2} i_1(\theta) \tag{13.25}$$

For parallel polarized light, we can write a similar expression:

$$I_2 = I_0 \frac{\pi d^2}{4} q_2(\theta) = I_0 \frac{\lambda^2}{4\pi^2} i_2(\theta) \tag{13.26}$$

For particles that are small compared to the wavelength of light (d < 0.05 µm), we obtain Rayleigh scattering. Here, $q_1(\theta) = \frac{\alpha^4}{\pi}\left[\frac{m^2-1}{m^2+1}\right]^2$, and $q_2(\theta) = \frac{\alpha^4}{\pi}\left[\frac{m^2-1}{m^2+1}\right]^2 \cos^2\theta$. From Equation 13.25 and Equation 13.26, we therefore obtain for incident unpolarized light

$$I = \frac{1}{2}\left(I_1 + I_2\right) = I_0 \frac{\pi^4 d^6}{8\lambda^4}\left[\frac{m^2-1}{m^2+1}\right]^2 \left(1 + \cos^2\theta\right) \tag{13.27}$$

The component I_1 is polarized perpendicular to the scattering plane and I_2 is polarized parallel to the scattering plane. Equation 13.27 shows the dependence of scattering on the fourth power of wavelength. Figure 13.8 shows the relationship between I_1 and I_2 for Rayleigh scattering. $I_1(\theta)$ forms a circle centered at the origin, and $I_2(\theta)$ produces two circles touching each other at the origin. We can see from Figure 13.8 that at 90°, only the perpendicular polarized component of light remains and the parallel polarized component vanishes.

For larger values of α (for particles between 0.1 µm to 10 µm), the Mie theory of light scattering is used to determine the light intensity scattered at different angles

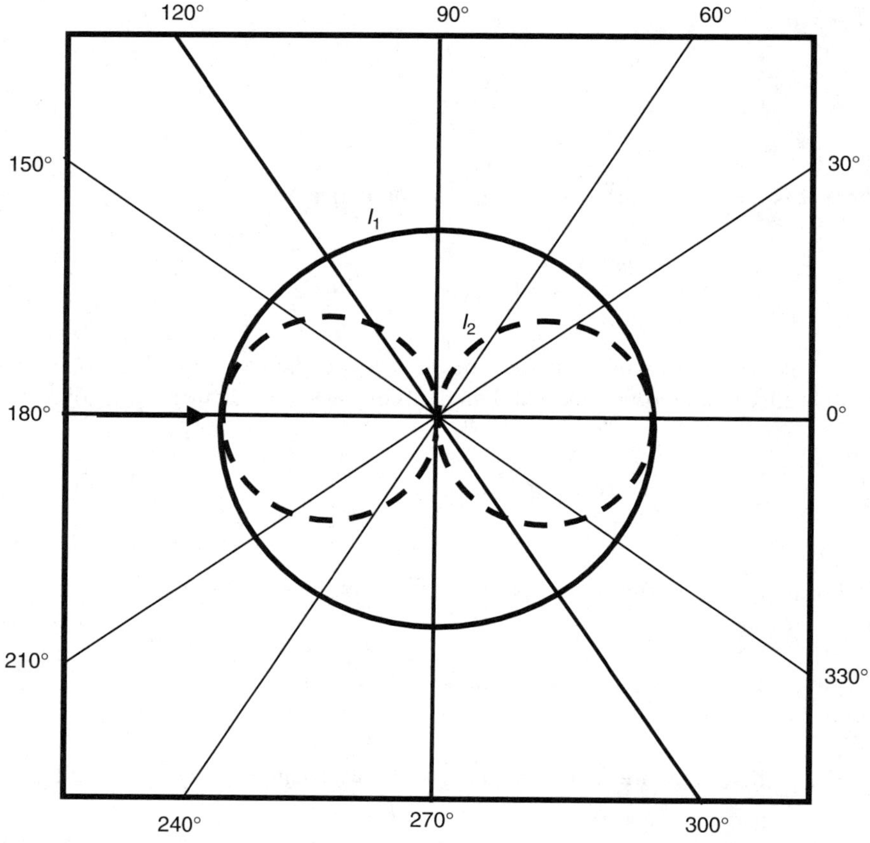

FIGURE 13.8 Polar diagram of angular scattering of perpendicular and parallel polarized light for Rayleigh scattering.

(Kerker, 1969). The equations for Mie theory are complex and the solutions are computationally intensive. Figure 13.9 shows the Mie scattering functions i_1 and i_2 as a function of θ for different values of α.

Several features are worth noting in Figure 13.9. As particle size increases (i.e., as α increases) the light scattered in the forward direction (θ = 0°) increases compared with the light scattered at other angles. For small particles, (e.g., α = 0.5), the light scattered approaches Rayleigh scattering. For large particles, the variation of the Mie scattering functions with scattering angle is quite significant, whereas for small particles, it is much less pronounced.

Figure 13.10 shows the variation of (i_1 + i_2) with the size parameter for three different values of scattering angle (θ = 0°, 90°, and 180°) for particles with refractive index of 1.5 (no absorption). The intensity of scattering in the forward direction increases, whereas backscattering and scattering at 90° decrease in intensity. We can again see how the scattering function becomes increasingly complex and irregularly oscillatory with increasing values of the size parameter. Thus, there are multiple values of particle diameter associated with the same value of scattering intensity.

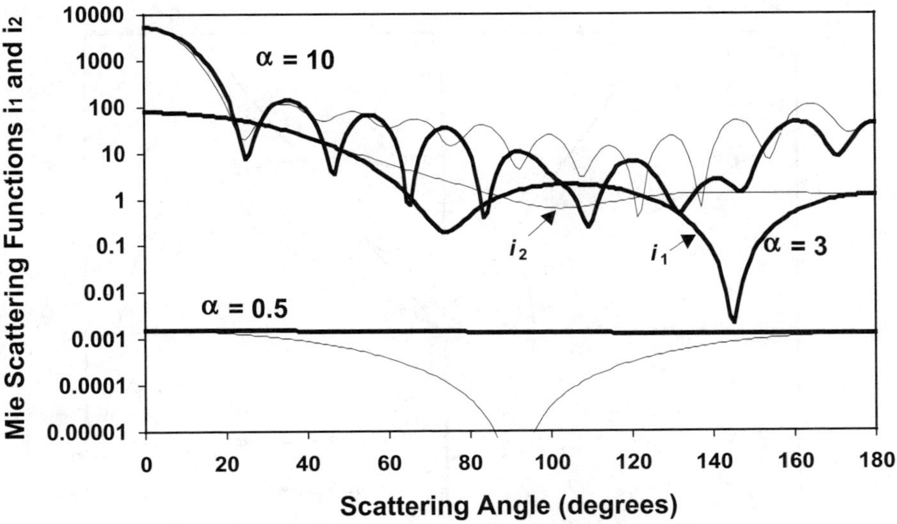

FIGURE 13.9 Mie scattering functions i_1 and i_2 as a function of scattering angle θ for α = 10, 3, and 0.5. The thick lines are i_1 and the thin lines are i_2. The refractive index $m = 1.5 + 0i$, for all three cases.

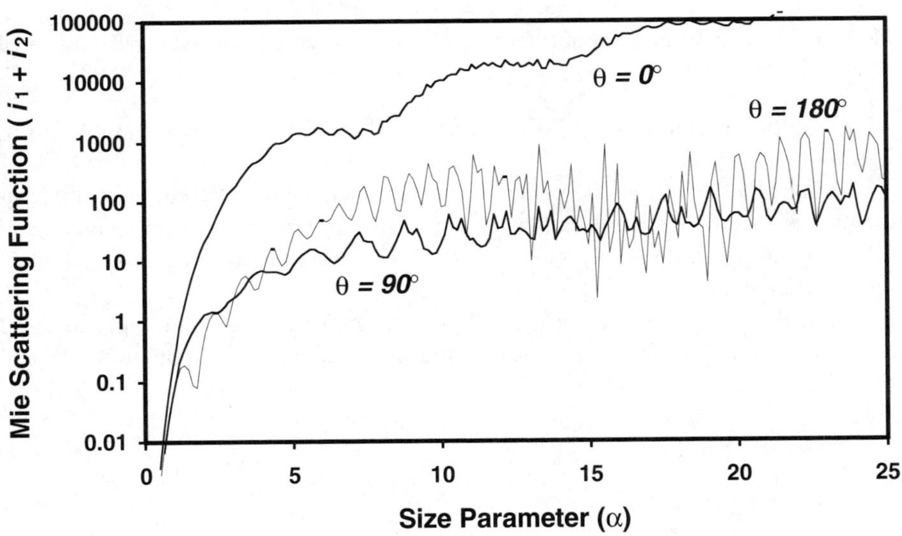

FIGURE 13.10 Mie scattering function $(i_1 + i_2)$ as a function of size parameter for different values of scattering angle.

The oscillations can be smoothed out by accepting light from a range of angles or by using light over a range of wavelengths. Practically, these are achieved by using a large aperture for accepting light over a range of angles and by using white light instead of monochromatic light. The predominance of forward scattering is the most noticeable feature here (see Figure 13.11), and explains why we see more particles

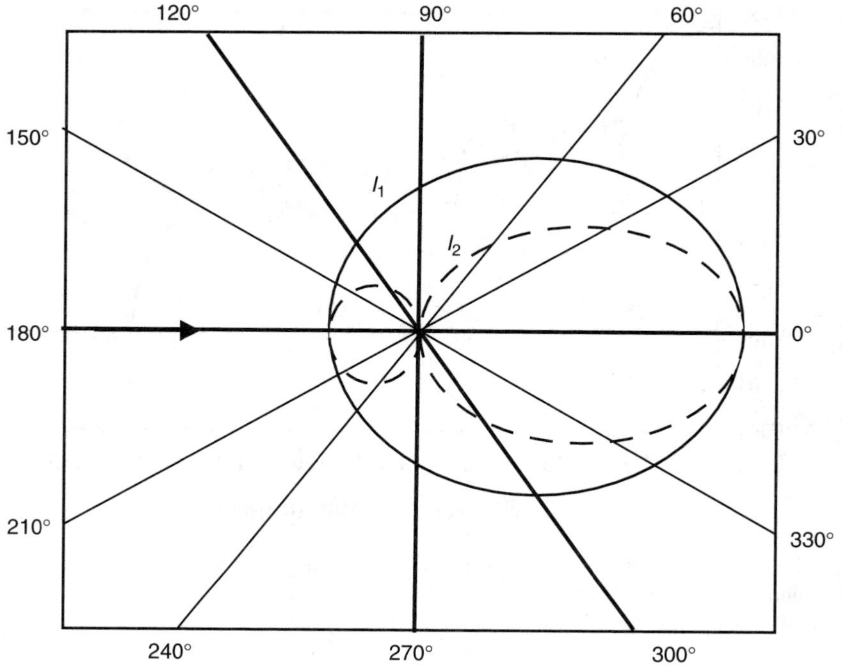

FIGURE 13.11 Polar diagram of angular scattering of perpendicular and parallel polarized light for Mie scattering.

when we look into a beam of light as compared to looking sideways at a beam of light in a dusty room.

Using Mie theory, the theoretical response functions of different optical instruments that employ different scattering angles (or a range of scattering angles) and different wavelengths can be obtained. These response functions are also dependent on the refractive indices of the aerosol particles.

Let $I(\theta, \alpha, m)$ be the intensity of light scattered per unit solid angle in the θ direction where $I = 0.5\ (I_1 + I_2)$ and I_1 and I_2 are defined by Equation 13.25 and Equation 13.26. Thus,

$$I = I_0 \frac{\lambda^2}{4\pi^2} i(\theta, \alpha, m) \tag{13.28}$$

For a given optical instrument with a mean scattering angle θ_0 with a receiving aperture having a solid angle of $\Delta\Omega$, the power collected by the receiving optics due to scattering by a particle of diameter d_p is given by

$$P(\theta_0, d_{p,} \lambda, m, \Delta\Omega) = I_0 \frac{\lambda^2}{4\pi^2} \iint_{\Delta\Omega} i(\theta, \alpha, m) \sin\theta d\theta \tag{13.29}$$

For an ensemble of particles with a size distribution $f(d_p)$ and a number concentration N, the power collected by the detector (the response of the instrument, R) is given by

$$R = N\int_0^\infty f(d_p)P(\theta_0, d_p, \lambda, m, \Delta\Omega)\,dd_p \tag{13.30}$$

For a monodisperse aerosol with all particles having the same refractive index, the response is linearly related to the number of particles, and the instrument can be easily calibrated for this purpose. But in the more general case of a polydisperse aerosol with a nonhomogeneous composition, a given response may arise due to a number of combinations of $f(d_p)$, N, or refractive index.

13.6.4 Light Scattering and Mass Concentration

As we have discussed in previous chapters, most occupational hygiene measurements are desired in terms of mass concentration so that they can be compared with gravimetric standards. Therefore, the measurements made by light scattering instruments need to be related to mass concentrations.

The mass concentration M is related to the number concentration N by

$$M = N\rho_p \int_0^\infty f(d_p)\frac{\pi}{6}d_p^3\,dd_p \tag{13.31}$$

Dividing Equation 13.30 by Equation 13.31, we obtain

$$\frac{R}{M} = \frac{\int_0^\infty f(d_p)P(\theta_0, d_p, \lambda, m)\,dd_p}{\int_0^\infty f(d_p)\frac{\pi}{6}d_p^3\,dd_p}\rho_p \tag{13.32}$$

The response R is linearly related to the mass concentration M only if $P(\theta_0, d_p, \lambda, m)$ is linearly related to particle volume $\frac{\pi}{6}d_p^3$.

We can define a volume scattering function S_v as the amount of light scattered per unit volume (and hence, mass) of the aerosol

$$S_v = \frac{\textit{Power Scattered by Particle}}{\frac{\pi d_p^3}{6}} \tag{13.33}$$

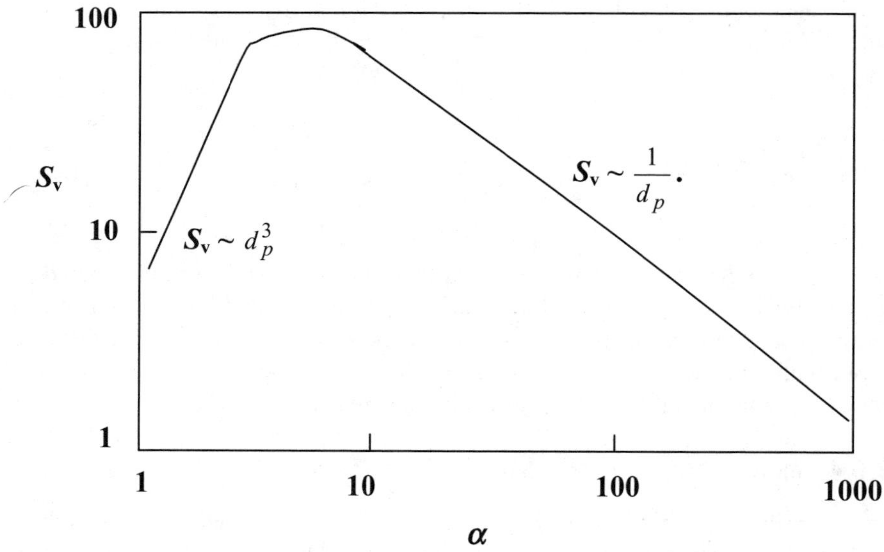

FIGURE 13.12 Relationship between volume scattering function S_v and size parameter α $\left(=\frac{\pi d}{\lambda}\right)$.

From Equation 13.11 or Equation 13.25, we know that the power scattered by a particle is given by

$$Power\ Scattered\ by\ Particle = Q_{ext} \times \frac{\pi d_p^2}{4} \tag{13.34}$$

For large particles (or α), Q_{ext} is a constant (~2), and therefore from Equation 13.33 and Equation 13.34, $S_v \sim \frac{1}{d_p}$. For very small particles in the Rayleigh region, $Q_{ext} \sim d_p^4$, and therefore from Equation 13.33 and Equation 13.34, $S_v \sim d_p^3$. Thus, for very small and very large particles, obtaining mass concentrations from light scattering measurements is not feasible. However, there is a narrow range of particle sizes ($3 < \alpha < 10$) for which S_v is relatively constant, and therefore light scattering is proportional to the mass concentrations, as shown in Figure 13.12. By choosing the wavelength of light carefully, mass concentrations of aerosols that are of relevance to occupational exposures may be obtained.

Such instruments measure the light scattered from particles in the sensing volume (see Figure 13.13), and are quite sensitive even at low concentrations. The measured concentration is independent of the flow rate through the sensing volume. Thus, a range of sampling flow rates can be used.

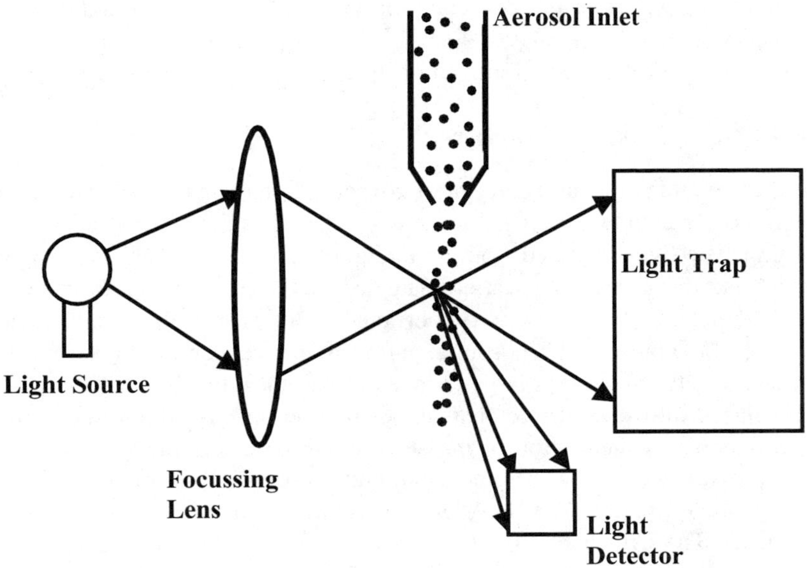

FIGURE 13.13 Schematic diagram for detecting aerosol particle by light scattering.

The DustTrak (TSI Inc., Model 8520) is an instrument of this kind. It measures light scattered at 90° using a solid state silicon photodetector. The laser diode used in the device has a wavelength of 780 nm, which limits the smallest detectable particle to about 0.1 μm. The instrument has an internal pump that continuously draws aerosol through the sensing chamber at 1.7 l/min.

Although such instruments are ideal for measuring the relative concentrations in real time, measuring true gravimetric concentrations is quite cumbersome. For a given particle size, scattered light is directly proportional to the number concentration of particles. Thus, for a given constant aerosol mass concentration, the intensity of scattered light decreases with increasing particle size. If the DustTrak is calibrated using larger particles, e.g., using the respirable fraction of A1 test dust (Arizona Road Dust; MMAD = 4.4 μm), the instrument response to a finer aerosol (e.g., a $PM_{2.5}$ aerosol) will be biased 3 to 5 times higher than the true value, due to the larger number of particles in the finer aerosol for the same mass concentration. Although this can be corrected if one knows the particle size distribution and refractive index of the calibration aerosol and the test aerosol, this is typically not possible in most occupational hygiene or environmental surveys. Then, in order to estimate the true gravimetric concentration in real time, it is necessary to measure a time-weighted average gravimetric concentration independently (e.g., using filter measurements) and then scale the DustTrak measurements according to a calibration factor (Ramachandran et al., 2000, 2003):

$$\text{Calibration Factor} = \frac{\textit{Time - weighted Gravimetric Concentration}}{\textit{Time}\text{ - integrated } \textit{DustTrak Concentration}} \tag{13.35}$$

Another issue is that the concentration measurements of any light scattering instrument increase with relative humidity, due to the increase in particle size associated with condensational growth of hygroscopic components of the aerosol.

13.6.5 Optical Particle Counters

Instead of obtaining the number or mass concentration or an ensemble of particles, optical particle counters are used to detect and size individual particles by light scattering. The light scattered from an individual particle is received by a photodetector placed at a particular scattering angle, and then converted into an electrical pulse. The height of the pulse is proportional to the size of the particle, and the count rate of the pulses is proportional to the number concentration of the aerosol. By measuring the sizes of a large number of particles, the sizes of the particles can be placed into several size channels or bins. From this, the size distribution and the number concentration of the aerosol can be determined. Although such instruments are commonly used in air pollution research, they are not as common in occupational hygiene. A variety of configurations have been used in different instruments. The Climet (Climet Instrument Company, Redlands, CA) is a good example of this type of instrument, which collects scattered light over an angular spread of 15° to 105°. The instrument response increases monotonically with particle size in the range 0.3 to 10 μm. The sample air is surrounded by a sheath of clean air, which allows each particle to be placed accurately in the sensing zone for proper light scattering.

For such instruments, the measurement is dependent on particle composition, i.e., refractive index. The instruments are usually calibrated using polystyrene latex (PSL) spheres and therefore the instrument provides size measurements in PSL-equivalent diameters. However, very low forward scattering angle instruments are not sensitive to particle composition, and several instruments exploit this phenomenon. Because accurate particle sizing depends on the precise placement of the particle in the sensing zone, several types of errors are common in optical particle counters. Coincidence errors occur when more than one particle is present simultaneously in the sensing zone. Grazing errors occur when a particle grazes the sensing zone, causing a signal weaker than that of a similar particle in the center of the zone. The final limitation is that the light scattering equivalent diameter is not related to the aerodynamic diameter, which is more relevant for inhalation exposures.

14 Sampling for Pollutants of Biological Origin

14.1 INTRODUCTION

The sampling methods discussed in the previous chapters typically exploit some physical or chemical property of the pollutant in question, e.g., absorption of infrared radiation by gases or the inertial motion of particles in rapidly turning air streamlines. But for some pollutants of biological origin, these methods, by themselves, may be insufficient. In such instances, the sampling method needs to take into account their biological nature and origin.

Bioaerosols are an important class of such pollutants, and they refer to airborne particles of biological origin. The term includes microorganisms (culturable, non-culturable, and dead) such as bacteria, fungi, and viruses, as well as fragments and particulate metabolic products of biological organisms. These include endotoxins that are components of the cell walls of bacteria and mycotoxins that are fungal metabolic products. More broadly, *biological contaminants* can include gases and vapors of biological origin, microbial growth that can become airborne, and biological constituents shed by animals.

A number of occupational and nonoccupational illnesses are causally linked to exposures to biological contaminants. These range from hypersensitivity (e.g., asthma, allergic bronchopulmonary mycosis [ABPM], and hypersensitivity pneumonitis) to infectious diseases (e.g., the common cold, influenza, and tuberculosis) to inhalation fevers (e.g., humidifier fever). Table 14.1 shows a variety of occupational infectious and hypersensitivity diseases. In order to cause infection, the particle needs to be viable; however, allergenic effects can be caused by nonviable particles as well. Each of these illnesses can be attributed to exposure to a particular biological agent or a group of agents. For example, ABPM is caused by exposures to aspergillosis — a type of fungus; asthma might be caused or exacerbated by exposures to a variety of fungal, arthropodal, avian, and mammalian allergens; the common cold is attributed to rhinoviruses and corona viruses; influenza arises from exposures to the influenza virus; tuberculosis arises from exposures to *Mycobacterium tuberculosis* — a bacterial species; and humidifier fever arises from exposures to endotoxins. In contrast, the so-called *sick building syndrome* is becoming increasingly common and is characterized by nonspecific symptoms such as eye, nose, or throat irritation, headache, and fatigue and cannot be causally linked to a specific biological agent, but is associated with the time spent in a building.

TABLE 14.1
Examples of Airborne Infectious and Hypersensitivity Diseases Associated with Various Occupations

Occupation	Infectious Disease (Pathogen)
Butcher	Anthrax (*Bacillus anthracis*), tularemia (*Francisella tularensis*)
Construction worker	Histoplasmosis (*Histoplasma sp.*)
Farmer	Anthrax (*Bacillus anthracis*), brucellosis (*Brucella abortus*), histoplasmosis (*Histoplasma sp.*), coccidiomycosis (*Coccidioides immitis*)
Meat packer	Brucellosis (*Brucella abortus*), Q fever (*Coxiella burnetti*)
Miner	Tuberculosis (*Mycobacterium tuberculosis*)
Health care worker	Tuberculosis (*Mycobacterium tuberculosis*), rubella (*Togavirus*)
Child care provider	Tuberculosis (*Mycobacterium tuberculosis*), chicken pox (*Herpesvirus*), measles and mumps (*Paramyxovirus*), colds (*coronavirus*), influenza (*Orthomyxovirus*)
Occupation	**Hypersensitivity Disease**
Grain handlers, farmers, agricultural industries	Farmer's lung (hay, grain dust), asthma (grain dust), bagassosis (moldy sugarcane), coffee worker's lung (coffee bean dust)
Veterinarians, animal handlers	Hypersensitivity pneumonitis (animal excreta, furs, feathers), asthma (dander, animal excreta), furrier's lung (animal pelts)
Carpenters, wood industry workers	Asthma (wood dust)
Shellfish processing workers	Asthma (shrimp, prawns, shellfish)

14.2 TYPES OF BIOAEROSOLS

14.2.1 Pollen

Pollen grains are produced by vascular flowering plants, trees, and grasses. They are the main source of allergens in the ambient environment. The most common pollen-caused allergies are due to ragweed (*Ambrosia*), grasses (*Poa*, *Phleum*, and *Lolium*), birch (*Betula*), cedar pollen (*Cryptomeria japonica*), and mugwort (*Artemisia*). Most of the pollen range in size from 10 to 100 μm and can remain airborne over long distances from their sources. They are also resistant to environmental stresses such as temperature extremes and low humidity. The Burkard pollen trap is the most common instrument for collecting pollen. The trap is based on a volumetric method whereby the pollen grains are collected on a film, and microscopically counted and differentiated into species. The measurements are reported in units of number of pollen grains per cubic meter of air.

14.2.2 Fungi

Fungi are unicellular (e.g., yeast) or branched multicellular organisms called hyphae. Fungal spores range in size from 0.5 to 30 μm, and, like pollen, can remain airborne for long distances and are resistant to environmental stresses such as ultraviolet light, extremes of temperature, and low humidity. Most fungi are saprophytic, i.e., they obtain their nutrition from dead organic matter in the presence of adequate humidity. However, some fungal species can invade living tissue and cause infectious diseases. Fungal spores can cause allergic reactions and diseases such as asthma or hypersensitivity pneumonitis. Mycotoxins are toxic chemicals produced by fungi, and examples include those produced by *Aspergillus* (which are carcinogenic) and *Stachybotris* (which cause acute effects such as headaches and dizziness).

In outdoor air, *Cladosporium*, *Alternaria*, *Basidomycetes*, and *Penicillium* are important genera. During the summer and fall, fungal spores are found in large quantities in the ambient environment, with levels up to tens of thousands of spores per cubic meter of air. Spores are collected by volumetric methods whereby they are deposited on culture dishes by impaction. After incubation of the cultures at 20 to 35°C for a minimum of 3 d, the spores are counted as colony-forming units (CFU) per cubic meter of air. The sampling time is short (3 to 5 min), providing information only on a short-term basis. The nonviability of spores is a serious drawback of this method, and microscopic counting yields a much higher number of spores than found in cultivated samples.

14.2.3 Bacteria

Bacteria are unicellular organisms that are found in soils, water, plants, and animals. They occur in a variety of shapes ranging from rod-shaped (e.g., *Lactobacillus*), spherical (*Staphylococcus*), and spiral to filamentous, and their sizes range from 0.5 to 30 μm. A major distinction is made among Gram-negative bacteria, Gram-positive bacteria, and actinomycetes. Gram-positive bacteria (e.g., *Staphylococcus*) have the ability to retain crystal violet dye, whereas Gram-negative bacteria (e.g., *Legionella*) do not. Actinomycetes are soil bacteria (e.g., *Streptomyces*) that produce spores similar to fungal spores. They are found commonly in agricultural settings, office buildings, and residences. Pathogenic bacteria cause a variety of infectious diseases (both contagious and noncontagious) in human beings. Contagious diseases include whooping cough (*Bordetella pertussis*), pneumonic plague (*Yersinia pestis*), tuberculosis (*Mycobacterium tuberculosis*), and nosocomial epidemics (*Staphylococcus aureua*). Noncontagious diseases include legionellosis (*Legionella pneumophila*), anthrax (*Bacillus anthracis*), and respiratory infections (*Pseudomonas aeruginosa*). In indoor settings, the concentration of bacteria in air is determined by the presence of humans and animals, and most of these bacteria are noninfectious. The bacterial concentration in air is determined by methods similar to those used for fungal concentrations, i.e., collection by impaction onto culture plates followed by incubation and counting of colony-forming units. Results are expressed in CFU per cubic meter of air.

A more health-relevant concern in most situations is the presence of bacterial endotoxins. Endotoxins are proinflammatory components of the outer membrane of Gram-negative bacteria and cause inflammation of the airways. In occupational settings, exposure to endotoxins has been related to airway inflammation as well as other symptoms such as fever, chest tightness, airway constriction, edema, and induction of nitric oxide. Similar observations have been made in indoor settings, especially in the context of sick building syndrome.

14.2.4 Viruses

Viruses can reproduce only inside a host cell and cannot grow on nonliving substrates. They consist of either RNA or DNA, and not both, and therefore need the host cell for producing genetic information. Their sizes range from 0.02 to 0.3 μm, and they can be easily transmitted through the air as part of droplet nuclei of respiratory secretions and be inhaled. They can also be transmitted by direct contact or by contact through food and water. Viruses can cause a variety of infectious diseases, e.g., the common cold, influenza, chicken pox, and severe acute respiratory syndrome (SARS).

14.2.5 Other Bioaerosols

In addition to the above microorganisms, bioaerosols also include biological fragments. These include proteins shed, secreted, or excreted by animals, such as dander, saliva, skin, and fur; tannins found in the leaves and stems of woody plants; endotoxins; and proteases, which are enzymes, released into the air in the detergent, pharmaceutical, and food industries.

14.3 BIOAEROSOL EXPOSURE ASSESSMENT STRATEGY

Despite the causal relationship between exposures to specific biological pollutants and health effects, there is insufficient scientific information to establish threshold limit values (TLVs) for these pollutants. For example, the relationship between the actual exposure to airborne microorganisms and the exposure that is measured (e.g., by collecting the microorganisms, culturing them, and then counting the colonies that are formed) is unknown and greatly dependent on the collection and analysis method. Furthermore, human susceptibility to these pollutants varies greatly, and obtaining a reliable dose–response relationship has been very difficult.

Due to the above reasons, there is no standardized exposure assessment strategy for bioaerosols. Each situation is unique in some respect, and the measurement strategy is tailored for each situation. However, the strategy is developed in the context of a *source-pathway-receptor framework*. Figure 14.1 shows the different elements of this framework.

This requires an understanding of:

1. Sources or reservoirs of the biological contaminant in the environment. The source of the contaminant also requires a mode of amplification of the biological contaminant through adequate moisture, temperature, and nutrition for the microorganism.
2. Pathways for dissemination of the biological agent through the environment. The microorganism can be transported by wind, by the HVAC

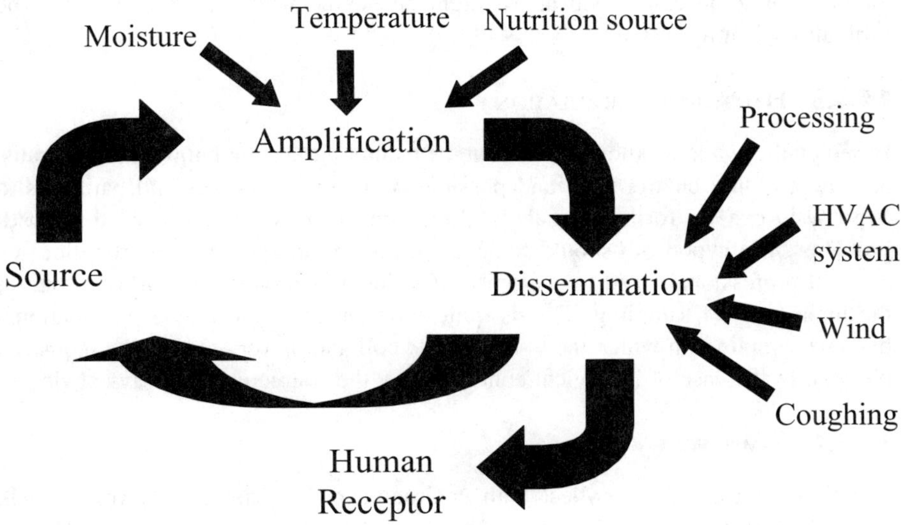

FIGURE 14.1 Schematic diagram of the generation, amplification, and dissemination of biological contaminants in the environment, and human exposure.

system, by various processing activities within an industrial operation, or by human activities such as coughing.

3. Symptoms consistent with exposure to the biological agent exhibited by the human occupants of the environment.

14.3.1 Health Surveys

A good starting point is to gather information regarding the kinds of symptoms being experienced by the inhabitants and the location of the inhabitants within a specific area of the building or buildings, and assess if they are consistent with exposure to biological agents in the building. Some investigations may be conducted to see if a given building is suitable for occupation by a particular susceptible group, e.g., a school building for children, or a home for the elderly. Health surveys of this nature can be helpful in ascertaining the types of environmental samples that need to be collected.

14.3.2 Site Characterization

The next step is the characterization of the workplace or building to see if there are areas that could act as sources or reservoirs of biological agents. These might include areas that have the right combination of dampness, temperature, and nutritional medium, which might promote the growth of microorganisms. Typical areas are outside air intakes, cooling towers, air filters, and heat exchangers such as heating and cooling coils, supply air plenums, supply air diffusers, air-conditioning units, around carpets, humidifiers, plumbing, wet wallboards, and perimeter walls. In most cases, a visual inspection for areas of excess dampness or moisture is sufficient, although in some cases such areas might be behind walls or equipment and be difficult to identify.

14.3.3 Hypothesis Formulation

Based on the available knowledge about the nature of the complaints and symptoms, and the building environment and possible contaminant sources and pathways, a hypothesis can be formulated about the source that is the cause of the health problems. The hypothesis should be developed in consultation with microbiologists, medical professionals, and toxicologists. The identification of the source is one of the main aims of sampling. This is quite different from most other occupational hygiene sampling, in which the source of the pollutant is very clearly the industrial process. In the case of biological contaminants, the source is not always obvious.

14.3.4 Sampling

Sampling should aim to collect both environmental air samples as well as bulk samples from the source. The sampling plan should account for the expected concentrations of the biological agent in bulk and air samples. Enough samples should be collected to quantify the spatial and temporal variability in the concentration levels. The combination of source and air samples should be adequate to test the hypothesis of whether a given source was the cause of elevated bioaerosols of a particular species in an environment.

The information gathered in the previous steps (e.g., the interviews with the inhabitants and the building-site visit) should provide sufficient guidance regarding the places where sampling should be carried out. Indoor levels are typically compared with outdoor levels. Outdoor samples are obtained near the fresh air intake of the building. If there are no indoor sources, then the indoor environment will contain similar microorganisms as the outdoor environment, although with lower bioaerosol concentrations. However, a particular species showing elevated levels is an indication of an indoor source for the microorganism.

Although personal samples are preferable, there is a marked lack of commercially available personal samplers for bioaerosols. Therefore, area samplers placed in the vicinity of the workers or in the location where people spend most of their time is the next best alternative. As in the case of chemical exposure monitoring, it is useful to define similarly exposed groups (SEGs) spanning the full range of exposures from very low to very high, and randomly sample a sufficient number of workers or people in each SEG. Although such a sampling scheme is often useful in estimating the full exposure distribution, in many cases, a much more circumscribed sampling scheme is sufficient. For example, a worst-case sampling scheme targets only the highest exposures or sampling near the source and thus focuses on the tail of the exposure distribution.

Bioaerosol levels vary by several orders of magnitude seasonally as well as diurnally. For example, outdoor fungal spore levels are the highest in late summer. However, in a workplace with an indoor source, fungal levels are likely to be highest during winter. Figure 14.2 shows airborne fungal levels in a school building over

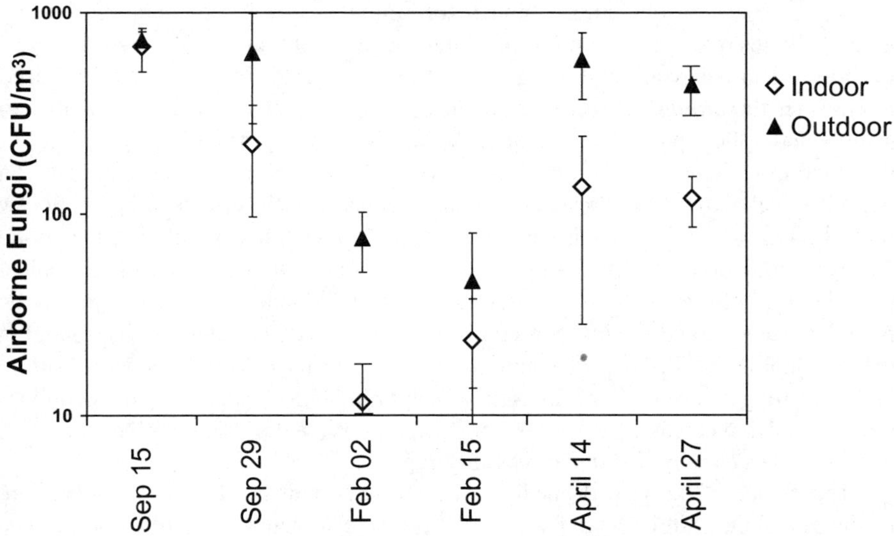

FIGURE 14.2 Airborne fungal levels over time in a school building. The ends of the error bars are the 5th and 95th percentiles of the fungal distributions.

three seasons. We can see that fungal levels can vary by as much as an order of magnitude both within a day and between seasons. We can also see that indoor levels are typically lower than or similar to outdoor levels, indicating the absence of indoor bioaerosol sources.

The issue of the choice of sample averaging time is similar to that for the case of chemical exposures. Ideally, for health effects resulting from chronic exposures, a longer averaging time is preferred (e.g., a full-shift 8-h time-weighted average), whereas for acute health effects, a shorter averaging time is preferable (of the order of several minutes). Such criteria have been established for a few bioaerosols (e.g., wood dust, cotton, and grain dusts), but they do not exist for most bioaerosols, especially viable microorganisms. In addition, many biological contaminants have both chronic and acute effects.

14.3.5 Analyze Data and Test Hypothesis

The sampled data as well as the medical evidence should be analyzed to test the proposed hypothesis. If the data support the hypothesis, further measures can be taken to control the exposures.

14.4 MEASUREMENT METHODS FOR BIOAEROSOLS

Bioaerosols can be either counted under a microscope or cultured in the growth medium on which they are collected. If they are counted, their concentration is expressed in units of particle number per unit volume of air. If they are cultured, their concentration is expressed in units of colony forming units per volume of air (e.g., CFU/m^3).

Many aspects of obtaining a bioaerosol sample are similar to sampling for any aerosol. Issues relating to aspiration efficiency and collection efficiency are identical to those for any aerosol, and are discussed in Chapter 12. However, we also need to consider the *biological recovery efficiency* of the sampler, which is its ability to sample and collect particles without changing the viability or biological activity of the microorganisms. For example, the drying effects of the sample airstream on vegetative cells, the shear stresses on microorganisms, or the effects of high velocity impaction onto a collection surface may affect their viability by causing metabolic and structural damage. Metabolic damage can affect the detection of biological particles by culture methods as well as bioassays that detect components of the particles, such as endotoxins. Structural damage can affect detection by changing the morphology of the particles and thereby potentially causing misidentification. Different fungal species have different susceptibilities to damage during sampling. For example, whereas *Aspergillus* spores can survive for long periods of time, *Stachybotrys chartarum* loses its viability rapidly.

The choice of the growth medium is quite important in this context. Agars are media containing nutrients and water that promote growth of the microorganisms. Whereas malt extract agar is suitable for most saprotrophic and xerophilic fungi, *Stachybotrys chartarum* requires a medium that is not rich in glucose, and hence cellulose agar is preferred. For airborne bacteria, culture media such as blood agars (which by themselves come in various formulations), tryptic soy agar, aerobic plate count agar, and 0.1% (v/v) peptone water are used. The choice of culture medium depends on the bacterial species that are of interest. Agar plates are typically 100 mm in diameter. Thus, it is generally advisable for the hygienist to consult a microbiologist on the choice of the nutrient medium during sampling.

After sampling, the bioaerosol samples are incubated at a specified temperature that is optimal for the growth of the microorganisms of interest. Some species are incubated at 21 to 25°C, whereas others are at 28°C or 35°C.

Three broad categories of sampling methods are in common use for collecting bioaerosols.

14.4.1 Impaction of Bioaerosols onto Agar

The principle of inertial impaction has been described earlier in Chapter 10 and Chapter 12. Several types of impactor designs have been used for bioaerosol sampling. These include *multiorifice, single-stage*, and *cascade impactors*. Instead of collecting the particles on aluminum substrates, they are collected on agar plates (see Figure 14.3). The agar plates are removed after sampling and incubated to recover the culturable bioaerosols. The multiple orifices ensure a uniform distribution of the particles. The Andersen impactors (1 stage with 400 orifices, 2 stages with 200 orifices, and 6 stages with 400 orifices) operate at 28.3 l/min and are commonly used. The 6 stages have cut points of 0.65 μm, 1.1 μm, 2.1 μm, 3.3 μm, 4.7 μm, and 7 μm, respectively. The Surface Air System (SAS) bioaerosol sampler is another commonly used impactor that has a cut point of 2 μm. The Marple personal cascade impactor, described in Chapter 12, operates at 2 l/min and is used for personal sampling. The cascade impactors can provide information on the size distribution of the bioaerosol.

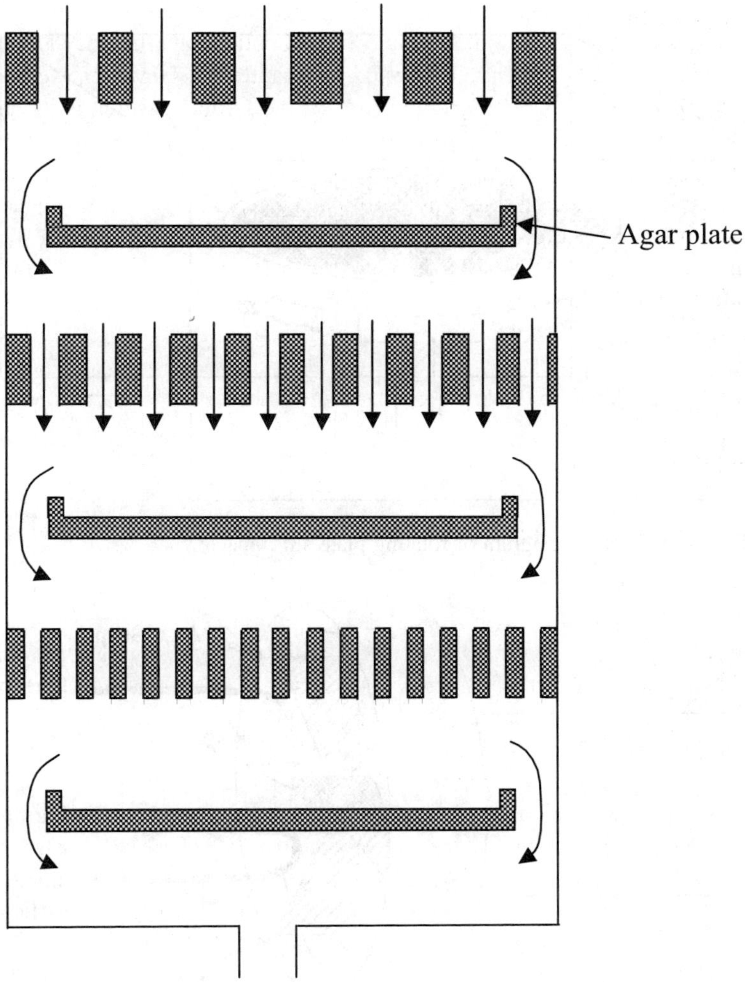

FIGURE 14.3 Multiorifice cascade impactor for bioaerosol sampling.

Slit impactors have a narrow slit through which the bioaerosol is sampled either onto an agar medium for collection and incubation (e.g., the Casella single-slit sampler) or onto a tape strip for microscopic analysis (e.g., various spore and pollen samplers). Typically, the collection medium slowly rotates under the slit so that the sample is spread evenly on the medium without overloading it (see Figure 14.4). Such slit impactors have flow rates ranging from 10 l/min to several hundred lpm and have cut points of 0.5 to 2.0 μm.

Centrifugal samplers such as the RCS biotest sampler also use impaction to collect particles. A rotating impeller is used to sample air at a flow rate of 40 l/min, and the particles are radially impacted onto an agar strip by centrifugal force (see Figure 14.5). The air enters and exits the sampler through the same opening.

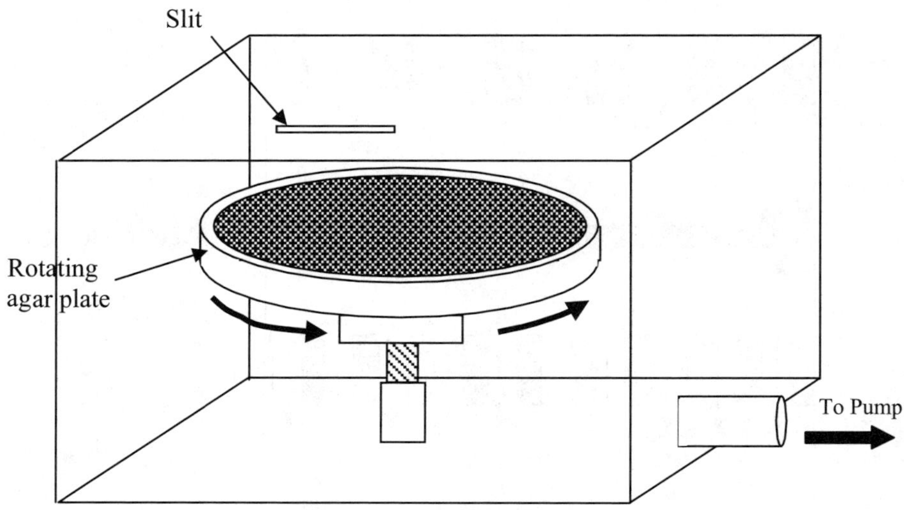

FIGURE 14.4 Schematic diagram of rotating plate slit impactor.

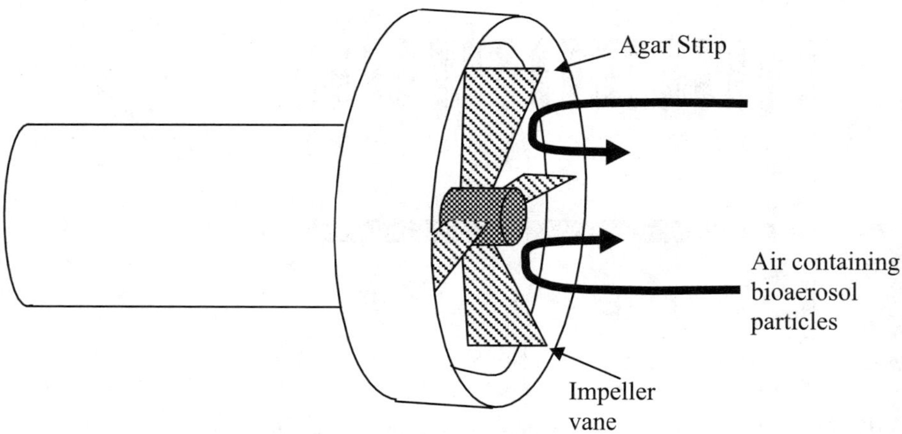

FIGURE 14.5 Schematic diagram of centrifugal impactor.

14.4.2 Impinging of Bioaerosols onto a Liquid

Impingers (described in Chapter 6) also operate using inertial impaction for particle collection. The airstream enters a liquid volume and forms bubbles. The particles larger than about 1 μm impact inside the liquid volume, and the particles are captured in the liquid (see Figure 14.6). Diffusion of smaller particles onto bubble surfaces is also a mechanism for smaller particles. The AGI-4 and the AGI-30 are some of the more commonly used impingers. They operate at a flow rate of 12.5 l/min and have a calculated cut point of 0.31 μm. The distance between the jet exit nozzle and the base of the liquid tube is 4 mm for the AGI-4 and 30 mm for the AGI-30. The midget impinger has a flow rate of 2.83 l/min and a cut point of 0.7 μm. The volume of liquid used is typically 15 to 20 ml.

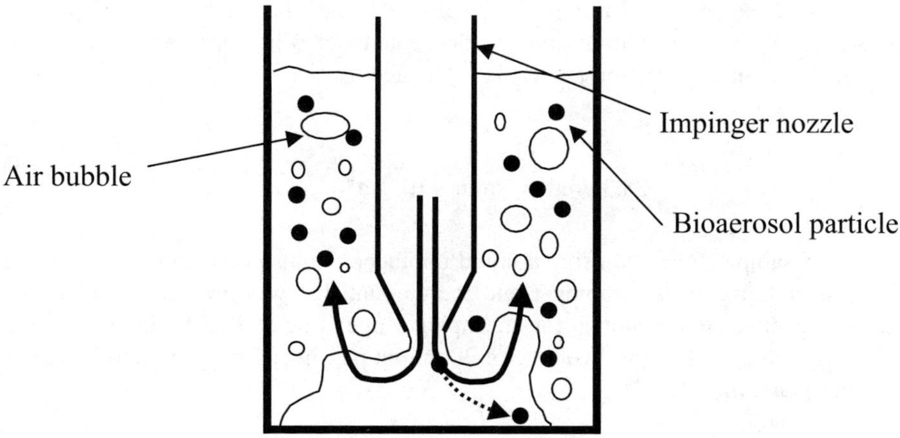

FIGURE 14.6 Bioaerosol collection in an impinger.

Wetted cyclones (also called cyclone scrubbers) have a thin liquid layer that continually washes the inner surface of the tangential inlet cyclone (discussed in Chapter 12). The particles impact on the inner surface and are washed down to the bottom of the cyclone, where they are collected. The volume of liquid used is typically ~20 ml.

As in the case of agars, the choice of the liquid medium depends on the application. Options include sterile water or buffered salt solutions with additives such as amino acids and sugars.

Although impingers are more cumbersome to use than impactors, due to the difficulties of handling the collection liquids, they are preferable in situations of high bioaerosol concentrations. In such situations, impactors can be run for only a very short time period (on the order of a few minutes) before they become overloaded. Impingers can be run for a longer time interval because the liquid can always be diluted by an appropriate factor. Because the sample is collected in a liquid, the propagules break up into individual cells in the water, and thus a more accurate estimate of the bioaerosol concentration is obtained.

14.4.3 Sampling through a Filter

Filter collection of bioaerosol particles is usually performed for the purpose of microscopic examination of the particles. Capillary pore filters and porous membrane filters have been used in this context.

14.5 STATISTICAL ISSUES

14.5.1 Lower Limits of Detection

The lower limits of detection of various bioaerosol sampling instruments can be established by using the detection of 1 CFU as the minimum number that can be detected. If we know the sampling flow rate and the sampling time, the minimum detectable concentration (in units of CFU/m^3) can be calculated. For example, for an Andersen impactor with a sampling flow rate of 28.3 lpm and sampling time of 3 min, the limit of detection (LOD) is calculated as

$$LOD = \frac{1\,\text{CFU}}{28.3\,\text{l/min} \times 3\,\text{min} \times 10^{-3}\,\text{m}^3/\text{l}} \approx 12\,\text{CFU/m}^3 \tag{14.1}$$

For a sample collected using a liquid impinger, we also need to account for the amount of liquid in the impinger and the amount that was used to inoculate the growth medium. For example, for an impinger operating at 12.5 l/min, a sampling time of 30 min, and a liquid volume of 20 ml out of which 1 ml is used to inoculate an agar plate, the LOD is

$$LOD = \frac{1\,\text{CFU/ml} \times 20\,\text{ml}}{12.5\,\text{l/min} \times 30\,\text{min} \times 10^{-3}\,\text{m}^3/\text{l}} \approx 53\,\text{CFU/m}^3 \tag{14.2}$$

14.5.2 Limits of Quantification

As the quantification is carried out by means of counting relatively small numbers of colonies, Poisson statistics are the most appropriate for characterizing the distribution. The coefficient of variation is approximately the reciprocal of the square root of the colony counts. Thus, a count of 1 CFU corresponds to a coefficient of variation of 100%. Therefore, it has been argued that, although using 1 CFU on an agar plate as the minimum number that can be counted is useful for detection of the presence or absence of microorganisms, it leads to unacceptable levels of variability for quantification purposes. Therefore, using 10 CFUs per plate as the minimum number that can be counted has been recommended, which leads to a coefficient of variation of 30%. Others have recommended an even more conservative number of 30 CFUs per plate, which corresponds to a coefficient of variation of 20%. Therefore, the limits of quantification (LOQ) are 10 to 30 times greater than the limits of detection.

14.5.3 Upper Limits of Detection

Ideally, the sampling time interval should be long enough that an adequate quantity (number or mass) of the biological contaminant is collected for analytical quantification, although it should not be so long that the collection medium is overloaded. If the sampling is carried out for a time interval longer than optimum, there is a risk of overloading the collection medium. For example, if too many CFUs are present on an agar plate, the colonies may connect together during incubation and become indistinguishable during counting. Additionally, growth of one fungal species might inhibit the growth of others (i.e., mask them). Recommended levels of surface loading range between 1 and 5 CFU/cm^2 for culturable colonies. For microscopic counting, a surface loading of ~10^4/cm^2 is optimal. If the surface loading density is δ (in CFU/cm^2 or #/cm^2), the collection surface area is A, the sampling time is t, and the sampling flow rate is Q, the maximum concentration (in CFU/m^3 or #/m^3) that can be accurately measured is given by

$$C_{max} = \frac{\delta A}{Q t} \tag{14.3}$$

The above discussion assumes that the CFUs are randomly distributed on the collection surface. However, in the case of collection using multiorifice impactors, the bioaerosol particles deposit underneath the location of each jet orifice. Each such location is called a site. If a colony is formed at such a site, it is referred to as a "positive hole." Because more than one particle may enter through the same orifice and collect on the same spot, the colonies formed by two such particles will be indistinguishable. Thus, CFU may be undercounted. To correct for this potential bias, a positive hole correction factor is applied to the raw CFU counts. Tables for these correction factors are provided in ACGIH (1999). Hinds (1999) provides an expression for this correction factor, which is given by:

$$N_c = N_f \left(\frac{1.075}{1.052 - f} \right)^{0.483} \quad \text{for } f < 0.95 \tag{14.4}$$

where N_f is the number of CFUs or filled sites or positive holes, N_c is the corrected CFUs, and f is the fraction of sites that are filled, i.e., $\dfrac{N_f}{N_{total}}$.

For a 400-hole impactor, we can see a maximum of 400 CFUs. Accounting for the positive hole correction, this implies a total count of ~2628 CFUs. For a sampling flow rate of 28.3 lpm and a sampling time of 3 min, therefore, the maximum concentration that can be measured is

$$C_{max} = \frac{2628 \text{ CFU}}{28.3 \text{ l/min} \times 3 \text{ min} \times 10^{-3} \text{ m}^3/\text{l}} \approx 31{,}000 \text{ CFU/m}^3 \tag{14.5}$$

As we can see, the maximum measurable concentration can be increased by reducing the sampling time. In the above example, if the sampling time is reduced to 1 min, the maximum concentration is increased to ~92,000 CFU/m^3.

Section IV

Exposure Assessment Strategies

15 Variability in Occupational Exposures

15.1 INTRODUCTION

One of the main challenges of occupational exposure assessment is to characterize accurately and efficiently the exposures of large numbers of workers. Because it is frequently not feasible to measure the exposures of all workers due to limited available resources, a common strategy to deal with this problem is to classify the workers who have similar exposures into groups and then sample a limited number of workers from each such group. These groups are called similar exposure groups (SEGs). Within each SEG, the workers have a distribution of exposures that needs to be characterized. This is often referred to as the *exposure profile* of the SEG. The estimation of this exposure distribution requires an understanding of the statistics of sampling and the underlying exposure distribution. A thorough knowledge of exposure variability and its characterization is critical for developing a proper sampling strategy and interpreting the results of sampling.

There are three main categories of variability in measured exposures: (1) *environmental variability* or variation in the levels of exposures in a workplace over time and space and between workers, (2) *sampling and analytical variability* or random errors in the collection and analytical method, and (3) *systematic variation or biases* in worker exposures. In this chapter, we will discuss the characterization of the first two kinds of variability using probability theory because they lend themselves relatively easily to statistical treatment.

However, systematic biases cannot be treated using a statistical approach. Such systematic biases arise from systematic changes in the workplace, e.g., processes, worker activities, or ventilation rates. Such changes can affect the average exposures of workers in the workplace. A sampling strategy that does not account for systematic differences between groups of workers is also likely to underestimate the variability in exposures. For example, consider two groups of workers performing the same jobs and tasks, but during different work shifts. If the ventilation rates are systematically lower during the night shifts and sampling is carried out only during the day shifts, the measured exposure distribution will have a lower average value and variability.

15.2 ENVIRONMENTAL VARIABILITY AND LOGNORMAL DISTRIBUTIONS

Environmental variability refers to the changes in exposure levels from one day to another or from one worker to another. Exposures are affected by the rates of contaminant generation and dilution processes in the workplace. As production rates change with time, contaminant generation rates also change. The processes and operations that occur in a workplace can also vary in complex patterns overlaid with random variations. The airflow patterns are determined by the general ventilation of the work area, which may vary around some mean value. The variations in the mean flow are in addition to the random turbulent eddies as well as molecular diffusion processes that move the contaminant in the workplace. These features cause the work environment to have a spatially and temporally nonhomogeneous distribution of air concentrations. The workers move around in this nonuniform environment, and their activity patterns may also have some variability from day to day. The worker exposures are related to these factors in a multiplicative manner. Irrespective of the distributions of generation rates, ventilation rates, and worker activity patterns, their multiplicative interactions typically lead to exposure distributions that are right-skewed and are described quite well by the *lognormal probability distribution* that we have already discussed in the context of particle size distributions.

This variability can be divided into within-worker and between-worker variability. Within-worker variability refers to the variability of the exposure of an individual worker obtained from repeated measurements over time (assuming that no systematic changes in the work environment have taken place over this time). This arises due to variability in the workplace environment. But there are also variations in the mean exposures between individual workers that arise due to differences in their tasks and work activity patterns. This is referred to as between-worker variability.

If x_i is a sample of N measured exposures obtained from a group of workers, and y_i represents the log-transformed exposure values, then $y_i = \ln(x_i)$. If x_i are distributed lognormally, then y_i are distributed normally. Thus, the log-transformation of the exposure variable allows us to exploit the well-known properties of the normal distribution. Just as a normal distribution is described by its arithmetic mean μ_x and standard deviation σ_x, the lognormal distribution is described by the geometric mean μ_g and geometric standard deviation σ_g. The estimate of the geometric mean, $\hat{\mu}_g$, can be calculated as

$$\log(\hat{\mu}_g) = \frac{\sum_{i=1}^{N} \ln(x_i)}{N} \tag{15.1}$$

and the estimate of the geometric standard deviation, $\hat{\sigma}_g$, is calculated as

$$\log(\hat{\sigma}_g) = \sqrt{\frac{\sum_{i=1}^{N} \left(\ln(x_i) - \ln(\mu_g)\right)^2}{N-1}} = \sqrt{\frac{\sum_{i=1}^{N} \left(\ln(\frac{x_i}{\mu_g})\right)^2}{N-1}} \tag{15.2}$$

Because the variable y_i is distributed normally, we can obtain its mean and standard deviation as $\hat{\mu}_y = \ln(\hat{\mu}_g)$ and standard deviation as $\hat{\sigma}_y = \ln(\hat{\sigma}_g)$. The arithmetic mean is related to the geometric mean and geometric standard deviation by

$$\mu_x = \mu_g \exp\left(\frac{1}{2}\ln^2(\sigma_g)\right) = \exp\left(\mu_y + \frac{1}{2}\sigma_y^2\right) \tag{15.3}$$

It is clear from Equation 15.3 that, because the exponential term is always greater than or equal to 1, μ_x will always be greater than or equal to μ_g. So, the arithmetic mean is always greater than the geometric mean, if σ_g is greater than 1.

The geometric standard deviation is related to the arithmetic mean and standard deviation as follows:

$$\sigma_g = \exp\left(\sqrt{\ln\left(1 + \frac{\sigma_x^2}{\mu_x^2}\right)}\right) \tag{15.4}$$

Here, it should be noted that $\frac{\sigma_x}{\mu_x}$ is the coefficient of variance (CV) of the lognormal variable x.

The lognormal distribution has a form quite analogous to the normal distribution described in Chapter 4.

$$f(x) = \frac{1}{x\ln(\sigma_g)\sqrt{2\pi}}\exp\left(-\frac{\left(\ln(x) - \ln(\mu_g)\right)^2}{2\ln^2(\sigma_g)}\right) \tag{15.5}$$

For a normal distribution, we can calculate the probability that a measurement lies within Z standard deviations (i.e., $Z\sigma_x$) of the true center value μ_x as the area under the curve between $\mu_x \pm Z\sigma_x$. For example, the area under the normal curve between $\mu_x \pm 1.96\sigma_x$ is 0.95. Similarly, for a lognormal distribution the intervals are of the form $\frac{\mu_g}{\sigma_g^Z}$ to $\mu_g \sigma_g^Z$. Thus, 95% of the area under a lognormal curve lies between $\frac{\mu_g}{\sigma_g^{1.96}}$ and $\mu_g \sigma_g^{1.96}$. Figure 15.1 shows a lognormal distribution with a geometric mean of 10 and a geometric standard deviation of 2.3.

Table 15.1 also shows that 68% of the area under a lognormal curve lies between $\frac{\mu_g}{\sigma_g}$ and μ_g/σ_g. Thus, 34% of the area lies between $\frac{\mu_g}{\sigma_g}$ (the 16th percentile) and μ_g (the 50th percentile), whereas the other 34% lies between μ_g and μ_g/σ_g (the 84th

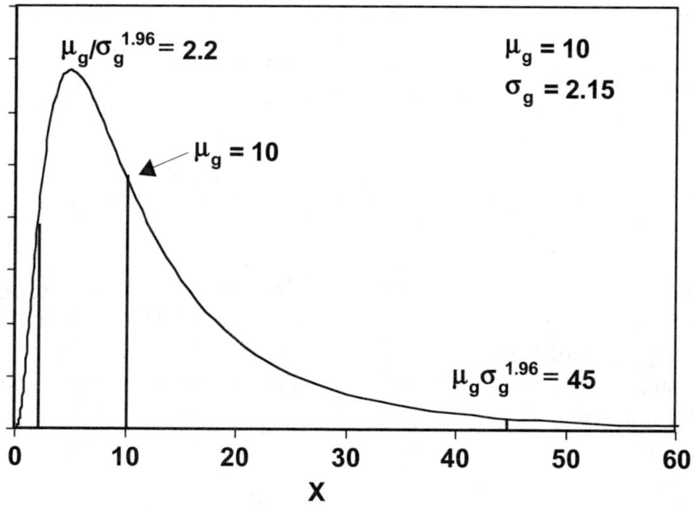

FIGURE 15.1 Lognormal distribution with a geometric mean of 10 and a geometric standard deviation of 2.15.

TABLE 15.1

Fractional Area under the Curve between $\frac{\mu_g}{\sigma_g^Z}$ and $\mu_g \sigma_g^Z$ and is the Probability of a Measurement within *Z* Standard Deviations of the Geometric Mean

Z	Fractional Area under the Curve between $\frac{\mu_g}{\sigma_g^Z}$ and $\mu_g \sigma_g^Z$
1.0	0.684
1.645	0.90
1.96	0.95
2.00	0.954
2.576	0.99
3.0	0.997
3.5	0.9995
4.0	0.9999

percentile). The geometric standard deviation is, therefore, the ratio of the 84th to the 50th percentile (or the 50th to the 16th percentile).

We can illustrate these concepts with a simple numerical example. Table 15.2 shows a data set with 20 measurements of exposure collected for a group of workers. The second column contains the raw measurements, and the third column contains the natural logarithms of the measurements. The average of the log-transformed

TABLE 15.2
Calculations for Estimating Geometric Mean and Geometric Standard Deviation

Measurement Number	Measurement, ppm (x_i)	$y_i = \ln(x_i)$	$(y_i - \bar{y})^2$
1	0.75	–0.287	0.208
2	1.53	0.424	0.065
3	1.61	0.476	0.094
4	0.43	–0.851	1.040
5	3.43	1.231	1.127
6	0.87	–0.136	0.093
7	0.33	–1.095	1.599
8	0.99	–0.010	0.032
9	2.18	0.779	0.371
10	2.41	0.878	0.502
11	1.40	0.336	0.028
12	1.38	0.324	0.024
13	7.43	2.005	3.370
14	3.52	1.258	1.186
15	3.27	1.184	1.029
16	0.56	–0.571	0.549
17	0.64	–0.439	0.370
18	0.51	–0.681	0.723
19	0.74	–0.301	0.222
20	0.32	–1.135	1.701
$N = 20$		$\bar{y} = \frac{\sum y_i}{N}$ $= 0.169$	$s_y = \sqrt{\frac{(y_i - \bar{y})^2}{N-1}}$ $= 0.868$

exposures is 0.169, and the standard deviation of the log-transformed exposures is 0.868. Therefore, the geometric mean is

$$\hat{\mu}_g = \exp(\hat{\mu}_y) = \exp(0.169) = 1.18 \text{ ppm} \tag{15.6}$$

and the geometric standard deviation is

$$\hat{\sigma}_g = \exp(\hat{\sigma}_y) = \exp(0.868) = 2.38 \tag{15.7}$$

Again, as discussed in Chapter 9 for particle size distributions, we can construct a cumulative distribution on log-probability axes. The exposure data are plotted with

TABLE 15.3
Cumulative Distribution of Rank-Ordered Exposure Measurements

Rank Order	Rank-ordered measurements, ppm	Cumulative Percentage, $100 \times \frac{\text{Rank}}{N+1}$
1	0.32	4.8
2	0.33	9.5
3	0.43	14.3
4	0.51	19.0
5	0.56	23.8
6	0.64	28.6
7	0.74	33.3
8	0.75	38.1
9	0.87	42.9
10	0.99	47.6
11	1.38	52.4
12	1.40	57.1
13	1.53	61.9
14	1.61	66.7
15	2.18	71.4
16	2.41	76.2
17	3.27	81.0
18	3.43	85.7
19	3.52	90.5
20	7.43	95.2

the exposure values on the y-axis and cumulative percentage of exposures less than each exposure value on the x-axis. The x-axis uses a probability scale such that it is compressed near the 50% point and expanded near the tails, and the y-axis uses a log scale. Log-probability graphs have the convenient property that the cumulative plot of a lognormal distribution will result in a straight line. First, the exposure data are rank-ordered, i.e., sorted in ascending order. Then, the smallest exposure has a rank order of one, the next smallest has a rank order of two, and so on. The largest value has a rank order equal to N, the number of observations. For each rank-ordered exposure value, a reasonable approximation for the cumulative percentage of exposures less than that exposure value is given by $100 \times \frac{\text{Rank}}{N+1}$. The cumulative distribution is constructed as shown in Table 15.3. The data are then plotted on a log-probability graph as shown in Figure 15.2. Because the data seem to approximately fall on a straight line, we can assume that the data are approximately lognormally distributed.

We can visually fit a straight line to the data. The geometric mean is the median of the lognormal distribution, and hence we can easily read the 50th percentile value

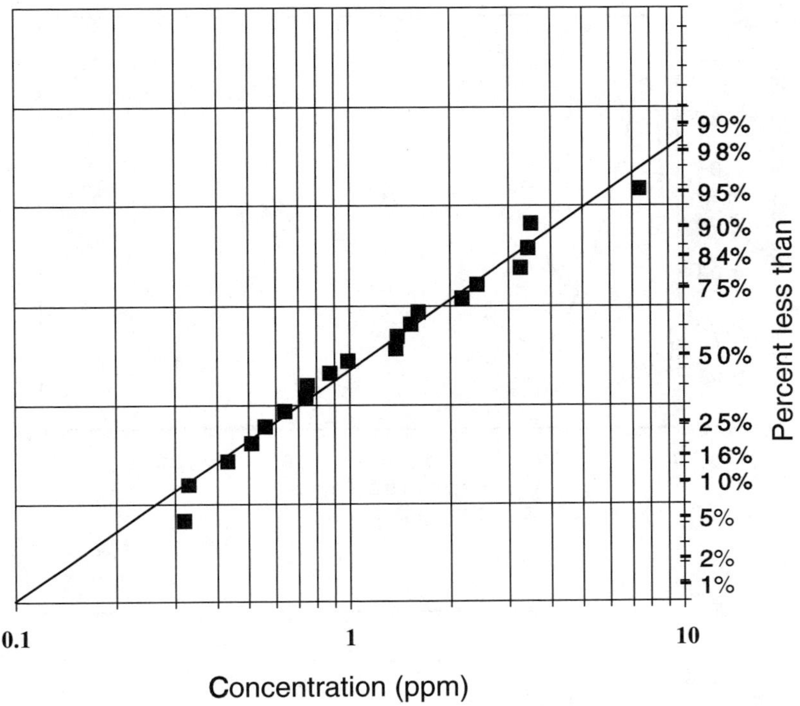

FIGURE 15.2 Log-probability plot of the data shown in Table 15.3.

from the log-probability graph as ~1.2 ppm. The geometric standard deviation is the ratio of the 84th percentile to the 50th percentile, and is approximately equal to 3.1/1.2, i.e., 2.6. These values are reasonably close, although not the same as the more exact values determined by calculations. The discrepancy arises because the straight line was fit to the data on a purely visual basis. We could have adopted more rigorous criteria, such as a least-squares minimization fit.

15.3 SAMPLING AND ANALYTICAL VARIABILITY

Analytical variability arises due to random errors involved in collecting and analyzing samples. These were discussed in detail in Chapter 4. If multiple measurements are made at the same location over the same time interval, then the only source of variability would be the sampling apparatus. This variability can arise, for example, due to variability in the gravimetric determination of filter weights, or due to random fluctuations in pump flow rates. Such measurements will be distributed symmetrically around a mean value and can be described by a normal or Gaussian distribution. Systematic biases can be minimized by following proper calibration and operating procedures. Figure 15.3 shows the relationship between environmental variability and sampling and analytical variability.

Nicas et al. (1991) have obtained useful expressions for the relative magnitudes of analytical and environmental variabilities. If the geometric standard deviation of

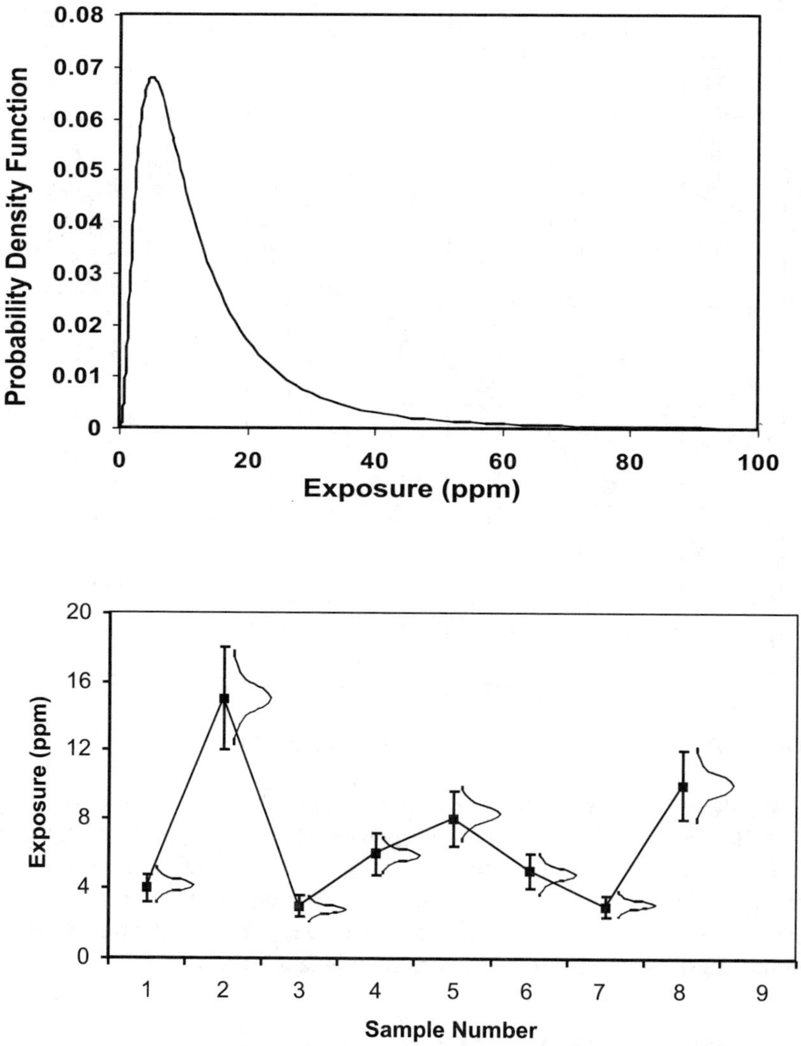

FIGURE 15.3 Environmental and analytical variability. The top figure shows the underlying lognormal distribution for environmental variability. The bottom figure shows a series of samples obtained from this distribution. Each sample has an uncertainty associated with it due to sampling and analytical errors that are distributed normally.

the environmental variability is given by σ_{env} and I is the analytical variability as a fraction of total variability, then I is given by

$$I = 100 \times \frac{\exp[\ln^2(\sigma_{env}) + \ln(1 + CV_{an}^{\;2})] - \exp[\ln^2(\sigma_{env})]}{\exp[\ln^2(\sigma_{env}) + \ln(1 + CV_{an}^{\;2})]} \tag{15.8}$$

where CV_{an} is the coefficient of variation of the analytical method (the coefficient of variation is the ratio of the standard deviation to the arithmetic mean). The first

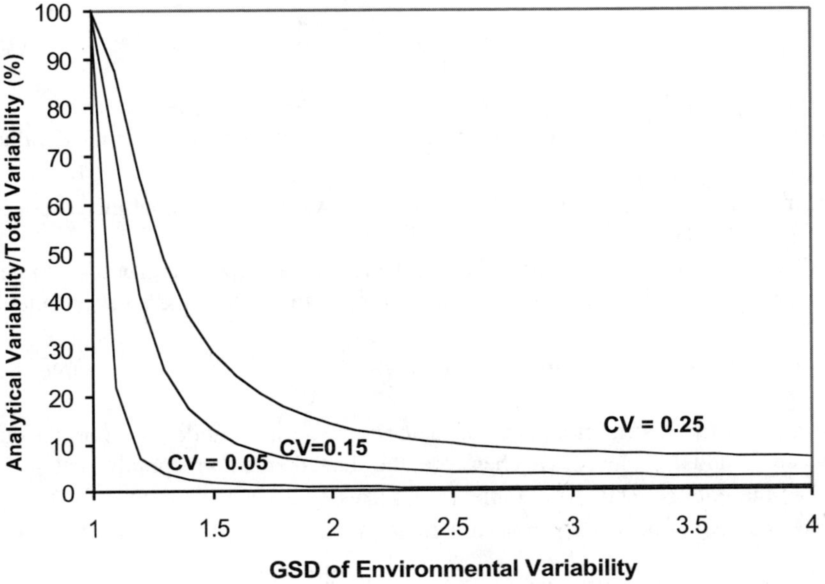

FIGURE 15.4 Analytical variability as a percentage of total variability for relatively low values of coefficient of variance of the analytical method. (Nicas, M., Simmons, B.P., and Spear, R.C., 1991, Environmental versus analytical variability in exposure measurements, *Am. Ind. Hyg. Assoc. J.*, 52: 553–557.)

exponential term in the numerator is the total variability, whereas the second exponential term is just the environmental variability. Equation 15.8 is valid for values of $CV_{an} \leq 0.3$. Figure 15.4 shows the variation of I with σ_{env} for three different values of CV_{an}. It is obvious that for typical levels of environmental variability ($\sigma_{env} \geq 1.5$) and for typical values of CV_{an} ($CV_{an} \leq 0.15$), the value of I is ≤13%. In fact, most *CV*s are less than 0.1, in which case the value of I is less than 6% (Nicas et al., 1991). In addition, Buringh and Lanting (1991) have found that, in many occupational situations, σ_{env} has a value roughly equal to 2.7.

Thus, environmental variability is of much greater importance than sampling and analytical variability for exposure assessment. This implies that, in many instances, it is not cost effective to use a very precise but expensive analytical method when a less precise and less expensive analytical method is available. Using the less precise analytical method may allow us to increase the number of samples we obtain and thus provide a greater overall accuracy and precision in the results. Thus, we will safely ignore analytical variability in the rest of the discussion in this chapter.

15.4 EXCEEDANCE FRACTION

The fact that most occupational exposure measurements can be described by a lognormal distribution allows us to estimate the probability that an exposure measurement exceeds a given value, e.g., an OEL. If the geometric mean of the lognormal exposure distribution is μ_g and its geometric standard deviation is σ_g, then this probability is given by

$$P(x_i > OEL) = P\left[Z > \frac{\ln(OEL) - \ln(\mu_g)}{\ln(\sigma_g)}\right] \quad (15.9)$$

In other words, it is equal to the probability that the standard normal Z-value is greater than $\frac{\ln(OEL) - \ln(\mu_g)}{\ln(\sigma_g)}$. Figure 15.5 shows that this probability is equal to the shaded area under the curve. Thus, if we know the exposure group's geometric mean and the geometric standard deviation along with its OEL, then we can calculate the shaded area corresponding to $Z_{OEL} = \frac{\ln(OEL) - \ln(\mu_g)}{\ln(\sigma_g)}$. From a table of the standard normal distribution, we can determine the area under the normal curve between $-\infty$ and Z_{OEL}, i.e., p_{OEL}. Therefore, the shaded area corresponds to $(1 - p_{OEL})$.

For the data set shown in Table 15.2, let us assume that the OEL = 3.5 ppm. We see that two of the observations are greater than 3.5, i.e., 10% of the observations are greater than the OEL. Therefore, $Z_{OEL} = \frac{\ln(3.5) - \ln(1.18)}{\ln(2.38)} = 1.247$. Then, using a standard normal distribution table, we determine $p_{OEL} = 0.8938$. Therefore, $1 - p_{OEL} = 0.1062$. Thus, the probability for a single exposure exceeding the OEL is 10.62%. Stated differently, 10.62% of the time, we may have an exposure greater

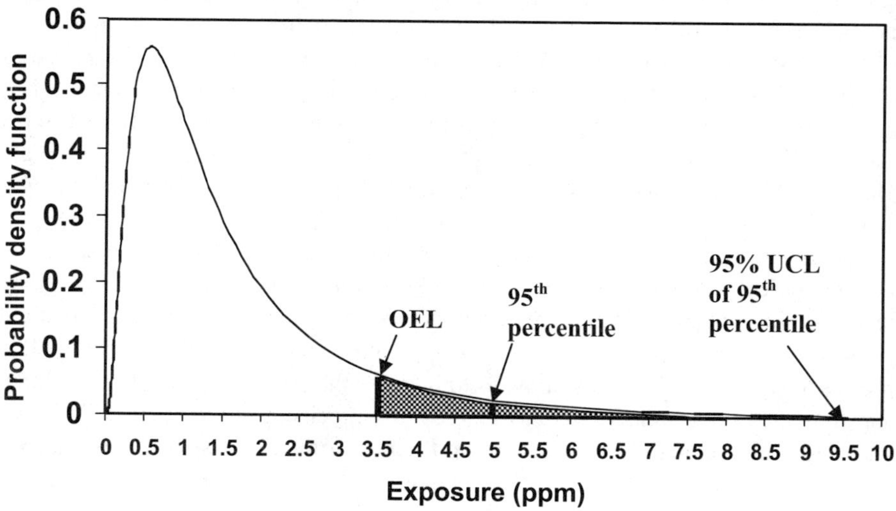

FIGURE 15.5 Probability of an exposure measurement exceeding the OEL (equal to 3.5 in this case) is equal to the shaded area under the lognormal curve. Also shown are the 95th percentile of the exposure distribution and the 95% upper confidence limit for the 95th percentile.

than the OEL. This represents a point estimate of the exceedance fraction, and there is an associated uncertainty in this point estimate.

Hewett and Ganser (1997) have provided a method for estimating 90% confidence intervals around the point estimate. This is based on an established procedure for estimating the confidence intervals around an estimate of a proportion in one tail of the normal Gaussian distribution. Figure 15.6 shows the confidence limits for the exceedance fraction. For a given value of Z_{OEL} calculated for the point estimate of the exceedance fraction and the sample size, Figure 15.6 can be used to determine the confidence intervals. For example, we have calculated the point estimate of the exceedance fraction for the data set in Table 15.2 to be 10.62%. This corresponds to a Z_{OEL} value of 1.247. Using $Z = Z_{OEL}$ for $N = 20$, we can estimate the 95% lower confidence limit (LCL) to be approximately 0.05. Using $Z = -Z_{OEL}$ for $N = 20$, we first obtain the confidence limit as 0.77. Therefore, the 95% upper confidence limit (UCL) is $(1 - 0.77) = 0.23$. Thus, the 90% confidence interval is [0.05, 0.23] or [5%, 23%]. In other words, we are 90% confident that the probability of a single exposure measurement exceeding the OEL lies between 5% and 23%.

There are several benefits in using the procedure described above. First, if the LCL is above a certain level, e.g., 0.05 in the above example, we can conclude with 95% confidence that the true exceedance is greater than 0.05. Conversely, if the UCL is less than a certain amount, say 0.05, then we can conclude with 95% confidence that the true exceedance is less than 0.05. Such conclusions, obtained statistically, are very useful in determining the acceptability of exposure levels in a work environment. Second, as pointed out by Hewett and Ganser (1997), Figure 15.6 can be used to estimate the number of additional measurements needed to lower the UCL below some critical value, e.g., 0.05.

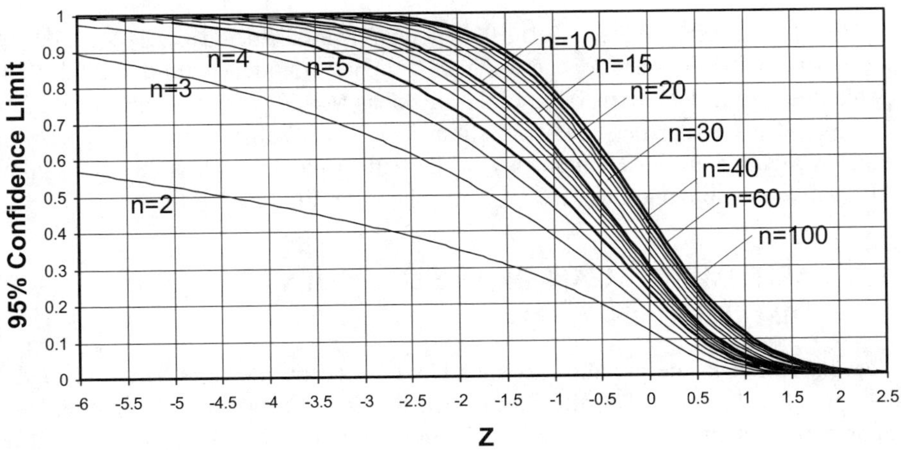

FIGURE 15.6 Confidence limits for the exceedance fraction vs. the Z-value for different sample sizes. (Hewett, P. and Ganser, G.H., 1997, Simple procedures for calculating confidence intervals around the sample mean and exceedance fraction derived from lognormally distributed data. *Appl. Occup. Environ. Hyg.*, 12: 132–142.)

15.5 THE 95TH PERCENTILE

The percentile of a lognormal distribution and the *Z*-value are related by

$$Percentile = \mu_g \left(\sigma_g\right)^{\pm Z} \tag{15.10}$$

Thus, the 95th percentile is given by

$$95th\ \ Percentile = \mu_g \left(\sigma_g\right)^{1.645} \tag{15.11}$$

where $Z = 1.645$ for the cumulative normal distribution. 95% of the exposures in this distribution will be less than this value. However, this is again a point estimate with some associated uncertainty. Therefore, it is again appropriate to estimate confidence limits around this estimate. However, frequently we need to know only the upper confidence limit of this point estimate. For example, we may want to know with a 95% degree of confidence that the 95th percentile is less than a certain value. These are obtained from *K*-factor tables for normal distributions that provide factors $K_{\gamma,\varphi}$ such that the probability is γ that at least a fraction φ of the distribution is less than $\mu_y + K_{\gamma,\varphi,N} \times \sigma_y$ for a sample size of *N*, where μ_y and σ_y are the mean and standard deviation of the normal variate (in this case, it is the log-transformed values of the exposure). Equivalently,

$$Upper\ Confidence\ Level = \mu_g \left(\sigma_g\right)^{K_{\gamma,\varphi,N}} \tag{15.12}$$

For the data set in Table 15.2, the 95th percentile is calculated as $1.18 \times (2.38)^{1.645} = 4.94$ ppm. If we want to know the 95% upper confidence limit for the 95th percentile for the data set in Table 15.2 (which has $N = 20$), then the value of $K_{95,95,20}$ is 2.396. Thus, the upper confidence limit is $1.18 \times (2.38)^{2.396}$, i.e., 9.49 ppm. In other words, we are 95% confident that the 95th percentile is less than 9.49 ppm. The 95th percentile and the 95% UCL are shown in Figure 15.6.

15.6 ARITHMETIC MEAN OF THE LOGNORMAL DISTRIBUTION

The discussion in the previous sections has focused on the right-hand tail of the lognormal distribution, i.e., the exceedance fraction and the 95th percentile. This approach is useful for evaluating the likelihood that the OEL may be exceeded or if the 95th percentile is less than some specified value. It is also useful in evaluating the health risks from chemicals causing acute effects. However, for substances that cause health effects due to chronic exposures, the day-to-day variability is of less importance. For such exposures, the arithmetic mean is the best measure of cumulative exposure over a biologically relevant time period, because the body would have integrated exposures over this time period (Rappaport, 1991). We will also see, in the next section, that this arithmetic mean is independent of the averaging time of the sample.

For a lognormal distribution with a small sample size ($N < 15$), the *sample mean* is an unbiased estimator of the arithmetic mean of the distribution. For larger sample sizes, the maximum likelihood estimate is preferable. As before, it is assumed that x_i is a sample of N measured exposures, and y_i the log-transformed exposure values such that $y_i = \ln(x_i)$. If x_i values are distributed lognormally, then y_i values are also distributed normally. Then, the *maximum likelihood estimate of the arithmetic mean* is given by

$$\hat{\mu}_x(MLE) = \exp\left(\hat{\mu}_y + \frac{1}{2}\left(\frac{N-1}{N}\right)\hat{\sigma}_y^2\right) \tag{15.13}$$

where $\hat{\mu}_y$ is the sample mean of the log-transformed exposures, and $\hat{\sigma}_y$ is the sample standard deviation of the log-transformed exposures. Note that this formula is the same as Equation 15.3 with the crucial difference that $\hat{\mu}_y$ and $\hat{\sigma}_y$ are the sample mean and standard deviation instead of the population mean and standard deviation.

The (1–α) level confidence interval for the arithmetic mean includes the true arithmetic mean 100(1–α)% of the time. The confidence limits (CL) for the maximum likelihood estimate of the arithmetic mean are given by

$$CL_{MLE} = \exp\left(\left(\hat{\mu}_y + \frac{1}{2}\left(\frac{N-1}{N}\right)\hat{\sigma}_y^2\right) \pm t_{\alpha,N-1}\frac{\hat{\sigma}_y\sqrt{N-1}}{N}\right) \tag{15.14}$$

where $t_{\alpha,N-1}$ is the 100α two-tailed percentage point of a Student's t-distribution with (N–1) degrees of freedom. If one-sided intervals are desired, then the two-tailed percentage points of the Student's t-distribution can be replaced with the one-sided percentage points. This confidence interval, however, ignores the sampling variability in $\hat{\sigma}_y$, and thus underestimates the variability.

For the data in Table 15.2, $\hat{\mu}_y$ is equal to 0.169, $\hat{\sigma}_y$ is equal to 0.868, and N is equal to 20. Thus, the maximum likelihood estimate of the mean exposure is equal to 1.695. For a two-tailed 95% confidence interval, $t_{0.05,19} = 2.093$. Therefore, the lower and upper confidence limits are calculated as 1.141 and 2.519, respectively, using Equation 15.14. Thus, we are 95% confident that the maximum likelihood estimate of the mean is between 1.141 and 2.519.

The *minimum variance unbiased estimate* of the arithmetic mean is preferred for small sample sizes or when the sample geometric standard deviation is large. It is given by

$$\hat{\mu}_x(MVUE) = \exp(\hat{\mu}_y)\Psi\left(\frac{\hat{\sigma}_y^2}{2}\right) \tag{15.15}$$

where $\hat{\mu}_y$ is the sample mean of the log-transformed exposures and $\hat{\sigma}_y$ is the sample standard deviation of the log-transformed exposures. The function $\Psi(t)$ is given by

$$\Psi(t) = \left[1 + \frac{(n-1)}{n}t + \frac{(n-1)^3}{n^2(n+1)}\frac{t^2}{2!} + \frac{(n-1)^5}{n^3(n+1)(n+3)}\frac{t^3}{3!} + \frac{(n-1)^7}{n^4(n+1)(n+3)(n+5)}\frac{t^4}{4!}\cdots\right] \tag{15.16}$$

Similarly, a minimum variance unbiased estimate of the variance is obtained as

$$\hat{\sigma}_x(MVUE) = \exp(2\hat{\mu}_y)\left[\Psi(2\hat{\sigma}_y^2) - \Psi\left(\frac{n-2}{n-1}\hat{\sigma}_y^2\right)\right] \tag{15.17}$$

Hewett and Ganser (1997), based on Land's equations, have provided a method for estimating confidence intervals around the point estimate of the arithmetic mean. The 95% confidence intervals around the mean are given by

$$CL_{MVUE} = \exp\left(\left(\hat{\mu}_y + \frac{1}{2}\left(\frac{N-1}{N}\right)\hat{\sigma}_y^2\right) \pm C\frac{\hat{\sigma}_y}{\sqrt{N-1}}\right) \tag{15.18}$$

The C-factor in Equation 15.18 accounts for the variability in the estimate of the mean and the variance of the log-transformed exposures. Figure 15.7 and Figure 15.8 show the dependence of the C-factor on the value of $\hat{\sigma}_y$ and the sample size, N, for calculating 95% confidence intervals.

Again, for the data in Table 15.2, we can estimate the minimum variance unbiased estimate of the arithmetic mean as 1.684 using Equation 15.15 and Equation 15.16. This is slightly lower than the maximum likelihood estimate. From Figure 15.7, we see that for $\hat{\sigma}_y = 0.868$, the C-factor for the LCL is equal to 1.72. From Figure 15.8, we see that, for the same value of $\hat{\sigma}_y$, the C-factor for the UCL is equal to 2.3. Therefore, Equation 15.18 yields the 95% lower and upper confidence limits as 1.231 and 2.732, respectively. Thus, the confidence interval is greater than the confidence interval calculated for the maximum likelihood estimate.

15.7 BETWEEN- AND WITHIN-WORKER VARIABILITY

At the beginning of the chapter, it was stated that the classification of workers into SEGs facilitates the efficient exposure assessment of large numbers of workers. By randomly sampling workers within each SEG, the exposure distribution for each SEG can be estimated.

There are several methods of classifying workers into SEGs. Most commonly, this is done on the basis of an *a priori* understanding of the processes and tasks that each group of workers is engaged in. This approach was first explicated in a landmark

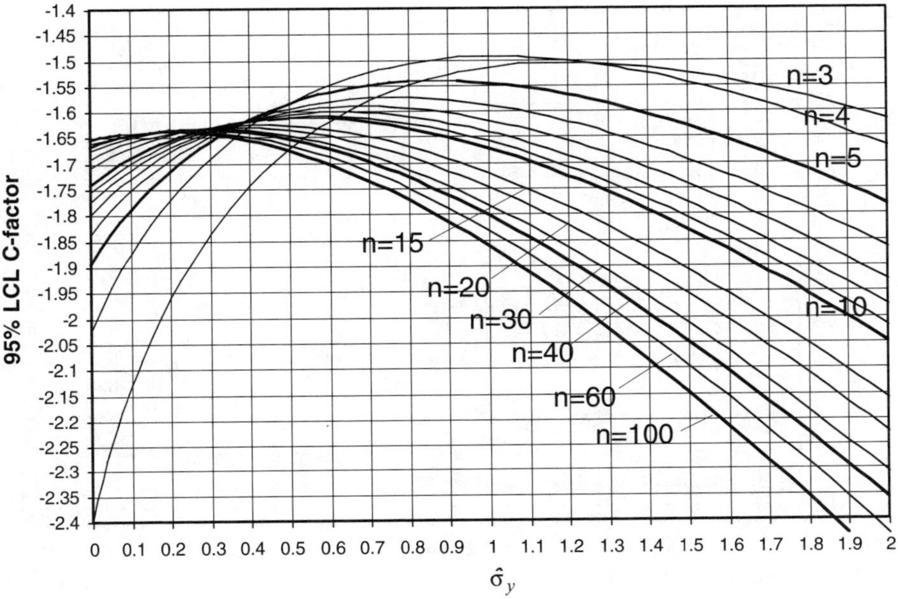

FIGURE 15.7 C-factor for calculating the 95% lower confidence limit (LCL) as a function of the sample standard deviation of the log-transformed exposures and the sample size. (Hewett, P. and Ganser, G.H., 1997, Simple procedures for calculating confidence intervals around the sample mean and exceedance fraction derived from lognormally distributed data. *Appl. Occup. Environ. Hyg.*, 12: 132–142.)

paper by Corn and Esmen (1979), in which workers were prospectively grouped into *exposure zones* on the basis of work similarity (similar profiles of job tasks), similarity of hazardous agents (similar chemicals to which they are exposed), and environmental similarity (ventilation characteristics, processes, etc.). Thus, the classification of the workers is by *a priori* observation alone, and hence this scheme is sometimes called the *observational approach*. The zone is not necessarily a physically defined area of the plant, but refers to a group of workers who share the characteristics mentioned earlier. Corn and Esmen (1979) also made it clear that this classification of workers was a subjective exercise that relied heavily on the professional judgment of the occupational hygienist. After the zones are defined, a certain number of workers are selected in each zone for sampling. However, the zones should not be changed on the basis of measurement data. A critical assumption in such a classification is that the workers within each such zone have similar exposure distributions, i.e., each worker's exposure profile is very similar to every other worker in that zone. If this condition is satisfied, then the only effective measures for reducing exposures are those that affect each worker in the group, i.e., ventilation controls and process changes. However, verification that this condition is indeed satisfied requires multiple measurements on every sampled worker in an SEG so that the exposure distribution of each worker can be individually determined and compared with the exposure distributions of other workers. Such exhaustive measurements are rarely possible due to constraints of time and money.

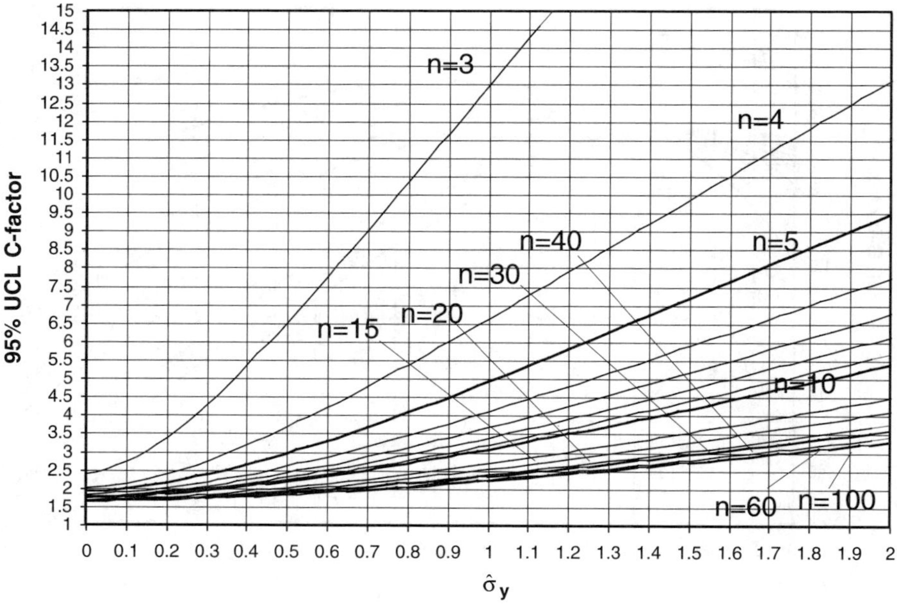

FIGURE 15.8 C-factor for calculating the 95% upper confidence limit (UCL) as a function of the sample standard deviation of the log-transformed exposures and the sample size. (Hewett, P. and Ganser, G.H., 1997, Simple procedures for calculating confidence intervals around the sample mean and exceedance fraction derived from lognormally distributed data. *Appl. Occup. Environ. Hyg.*, 12: 132–142.)

A one-way random-effects model can be used to parse out the between-worker and within-worker components of variability (Kromhout et al., 1993; Rappaport et al., 1993). Let there be k workers who have been selected for sampling from within an SEG. For the ith worker, there are n_i measurements. Thus, the total number of measurements made for this SEG is given by $N = \sum_{i=1}^{k} n_i$. Let y_{ij} be the log-transformed exposure of the ith worker on the jth day. It can expressed as

$$y_{ij} = \mu + b_i + w_{ij} \quad (15.19)$$

where b_i is the random deviation of the ith worker's mean exposure (μ_i) from the mean exposure of the group (μ), and w_{ij} is the random deviation of the exposure of the ith worker around that worker's mean exposure μ_i. Thus, b_i refers to between-worker variability, and it is normally distributed with a mean of zero and a standard deviation of σ_B. Likewise, w_{ij} refers to the within-worker variability, and it is normally distributed with a mean of zero and a standard deviation of σ_W. The two components of variability are independent, and the total variance, σ_T^2, is given as $\sigma_W^2 + \sigma_B^2 = \sigma_T^2$.

The estimate of σ_W^2 obtained by the analysis of variance (ANOVA) is given by

$$\hat{\sigma}_W^2 = MSW = \frac{\sum_{i=1}^{k}\sum_{j=1}^{n_i}\left(y_{ij} - \bar{y}_i\right)^2}{(N-k)} \tag{15.20}$$

where *MSW* is the mean square within error obtained from the ANOVA table, and $\bar{y}_i$ is the mean log-transformed exposure for the *i*th worker, i.e., $\bar{y}_i = \left(\sum_{j=1}^{n_i} y_{ij}\right) / n_i$.

The estimate of σ_B^2 is given by

$$\hat{\sigma}_B^2 = \frac{MSB - MSW}{n_0} \tag{15.21}$$

where *MSB* is the mean square between error obtained from the ANOVA table, given by $MSB = \left(\sum_{i=1}^{k} n_i \left(\bar{y}_i - \bar{y}\right)^2\right) / (k-1)$. Here, $\bar{y}$ is the mean of the log-transformed exposure for all workers, i.e., $\bar{y} = \left(\sum_{i=1}^{k}\sum_{j=1}^{n_i} y_{ij}\right) / N$. In Equation 15.21, n_0 is equal to $\left(N - \sum_{i=1}^{k} \frac{n_i^2}{N}\right) / (k-1)$.

An *F*-statistic is computed using *MSW* and *MSB* as $F_{k-1,N-k} = \frac{MSB}{MSW}$, in which *k*–1 is the degree of freedom associated with the mean square between term, and *N*–*k* is the degrees of freedom associated with the mean square within term. This *F*-statistic is compared with the critical *F*-value for a given level of confidence (which is obtained from an *F*-distribution, found in most statistical texts). However, most statistical software packages automatically carry out the *F*-test during ANOVA calculations. If the *F*-value is greater than the critical *F*-value, then we can conclude that the between-worker variability is significant, i.e., the workers in the SEG have significantly different means.

From the above, we can estimate the parameters of the within- and between-worker exposure distributions. From Equation 15.3, the exposure distribution of the *i*th worker has a mean value that is given by $\mu_{x,i} = \exp\left(\mu_i + \frac{1}{2}\sigma_w^2\right)$. The between-worker distribution (i.e., the distribution of the means of individual workers, μ_i) has a mean of μ and variance σ_B^2. Also, $\ln(\mu_{x,i})$ is normally distributed with a mean of $\exp\left(\mu + \frac{1}{2}\sigma_w^2\right)$ and variance σ_B^2. The geometric standard deviation of within-worker variability is given by $\exp(\hat{\sigma}_W)$, and the geometric standard deviation of between-worker variability is given by $\exp(\hat{\sigma}_B)$, in which $\hat{\sigma}_W$ and $\hat{\sigma}_B$ are given by Equation 15.20 and Equation 15.21, respectively.

Using the above framework, Kromhout et al. (1993) and Rappaport et al. (1993) challenged the assumption of the observational approach of Corn and Esmen (1979). They analyzed a large number (183) of such worker groups obtained from 45 different studies reported in the literature, with a minimum of two personal measurements per worker in each group. Whereas some of the workers were assigned to their groups by the hygienists of the individual studies, the rest were classified by Kromhout et al. (1993) and Rappaport et al. (1993) on the basis of their job titles at a given location. The ANOVA model described above was used to determine the between-worker and within-worker components of variance in each worker group. It was found that roughly 80% of the groups had workers who were not similarly exposed. The variation between workers in an SEG (as expressed by ${}_B\hat{R}_{95}$, the ratio of the 97.5th percentile to the 2.5th percentile) varied between 1 and 2000. Thus, the approach can sometimes lead to excessively high variability within an SEG, so that some workers at the tail of the distribution may face much higher health risks. In other words, some of the workers' exposures may be misclassified.

If the within-worker variability is the dominant source of variability, then the exposure is being driven by process variables and ventilation, which affect all workers to approximately the same extent. However, if individual workers have exposures that are significantly different, then the differences most likely arise due to differences in individual tasks and work practices, and not due to differences in the environment. An observational classification approach may not be able to detect these differences, and thus could cause misclassification.

In view of these findings, Rappaport proposed a retrospective classification scheme (Rappaport, 1991) in which the entire population of workers is randomly sampled and subsequently divided into groups such that ${}_B\hat{R}_{95}$ for each group does not exceed 2 (i.e., $GSD_B < 1.2$). Such groups are called *monomorphic groups*. Others have suggested a more lenient criterion, e.g., the Health and Safety Executive (HSE) of the U.K. prefers that ${}_B\hat{R}_{95}$ for each group not exceed 4 (i.e., $GSD_B < 1.4$). It is clear that this approach requires multiple measurements of the sampled workers' exposures to estimate the between- and within-worker components of variance. Because the classification of workers is done after sampling, this approach is commonly referred to as the *sampling approach* to classification.

Consider the data set shown at the top of Table 15.4, which shows the exposures of six workers who were each randomly sampled five times. The exposures are log-transformed and a one-way ANOVA is carried out. Below that is shown the mean and the variance of the log-transformed exposures for each worker. We suspect that something is amiss because the averages of the first four workers are similar, but

TABLE 15.4
Sample Exposure Data Set (in ppm) of Six Workers being Sampled on Five Days

Sample ID	Worker 1	Worker 2	Worker 3	Worker 4	Worker 5	Worker 6
1	1.36	2.14	2.85	2.32	4.56	6.78
2	3.67	1.54	2.51	2.87	2.36	1.80
3	1.29	4.13	3.34	1.80	6.54	3.56
4	2.41	1.62	1.40	2.53	4.98	2.24
5	2.35	2.07	2.82	1.82	7.08	15.52

Groups	Count	Sum	Average	Variance
Worker 1	5	3.6018	0.7204	0.1900
Worker 2	5	3.8182	0.7636	0.1543
Worker 3	5	4.5501	0.9100	0.1128
Worker 4	5	4.0072	0.8014	0.0422
Worker 5	5	7.8171	1.5634	0.1884
Worker 6	5	7.3176	1.4635	0.7695

Source of Variation	SS	df	MS	F	*p*-value	*F*-critical
Between groups	3.528128	5	0.70563	2.90555	0.03444	2.62065
Within groups	5.828509	24	0.24285	—	—	—
Total	9.356638	29	—	—	—	—

the averages of the fifth and sixth workers are quite different. The ANOVA output table is shown at the bottom of Table 15.4. We see that the p-value is less than 0.05, and the F-value calculated is greater than the critical F-value for the 0.05 level of significance. Hence, the between-worker variability is significant.

We can calculate the within-worker variance as $\hat{\sigma}_W^2 = MSW = 0.24285$. The between-worker variance is obtained from Equation 15.20 and is equal to $\hat{\sigma}_B^2 = 0.092554$. The total variability is $\hat{\sigma}_T^2 = \hat{\sigma}_W^2 + \hat{\sigma}_B^2 = 0.33541$. Thus, $\frac{\hat{\sigma}_B^2}{\hat{\sigma}_T^2}$ is equal to 0.2759, or roughly 27% of the variability in the exposures is due to differences between workers.

The within-worker geometric standard deviation is given by $\exp(\hat{\sigma}_W) = 1.63$, and the geometric standard deviation of between-worker variability is given by $\exp(\hat{\sigma}_B) = 1.35$.

The situation can be seen graphically in Figure 15.9, in which the cumulative exposure distributions of the individual workers are shown. We can see that Workers 1, 2, 3, and 4 have roughly similar means, whereas Workers 5 and 6 form a distinctly different population. This confirms our suspicion aroused from the calculation of the means of the log-exposures of the individual workers in Table 15.4. Figure 15.9 also shows the cumulative distribution of all the measurements taken together. It is clear that the overall distribution masks the underlying differences between workers

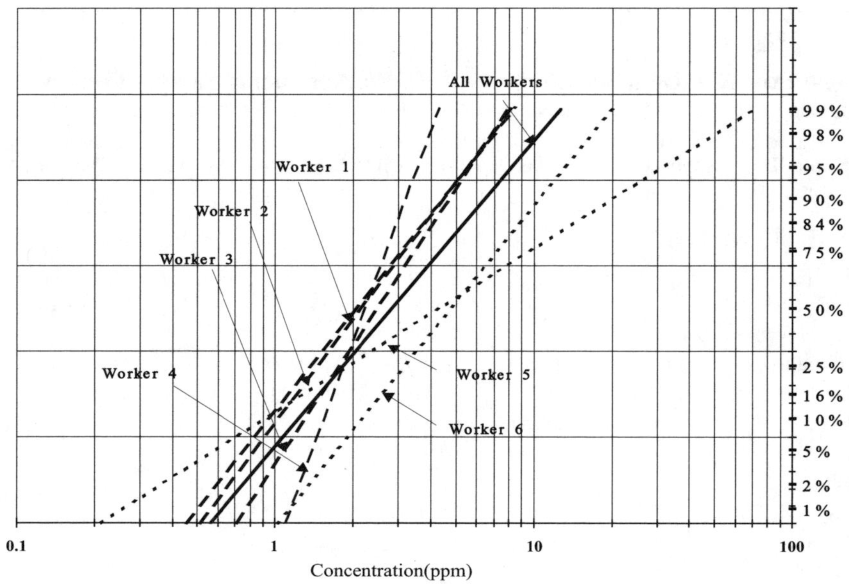

FIGURE 15.9 Cumulative exposure distributions of the six workers' data shown in Table 15.4.

within an SEG. Clearly, Workers 5 and 6 have been misclassified and should not belong to the same SEG as the other four workers. One point to note is that the model assumes that the within-worker geometric standard deviation is the same for all workers and is calculated using Equation 15.20. However, if we plot the exposure data for each of the workers, as shown in Figure 15.9 in which a straight line is fit to the data, then the slopes of the individual lines are slightly different from each other. The model, on the other hand, calculates an average within-worker geometric standard deviation using the data of all the workers.

15.8 AVERAGING TIME AND EXPOSURE DISTRIBUTIONS

As discussed in Chapter 1, the concentration of the air pollutant in the breathing zone of the worker is a reasonably good approximation of the concentration to which the worker is exposed. If $C(t)$ is the instantaneous concentration of a given pollutant in the breathing zone that a worker is exposed to over a time interval T, then the exposure over this time interval is defined as

$$x(T) = \frac{1}{T}\int_{t=0}^{T} C(t)\,\mathrm{d}t \tag{15.22}$$

Here, T is also known as the averaging time. The averaging time can be as short as a few seconds, which is typical of most direct reading instruments operating in near real time. It can also be of the order of several hours, e.g., the standard 8-h time-weighted average exposure. The distribution of $x(T)$ is what we have been studying so far in this chapter. However, we also need to consider the effect of the averaging time on the exposure distribution and the relationship between distributions with different averaging times. For example, consider a worker who is wearing both a direct reading instrument that measures concentrations over very short time intervals, as well as an integrating sampler, such as a passive badge that provides 8-h TWA concentrations. Let the two averaging times be denoted by T_{short} and T_{long}, where $T_{long} = nT_{short}$. What is the relationship between the mean and variance of the short-term and long-term measurements?

Spear et al. (1986) showed mathematically that the mean value of the distribution is independent of the averaging time, and hence the short-term and long-term measurements have the same mean. In other words, $\mu_{x(T_{short})} = \mu_{x(T_{long})}$. This result is intuitively obvious for just one long interval. For example, an 8-h interval comprises thirty-two 15-min intervals, and the 8-h TWA is equal to the average of the thirty-two 15-min averages. Spear et al. (1986) generalized this result and showed that if there is a distribution of 8-h TWAs and a distribution of 15-min intervals that comprise the 8-h intervals, then the means of both these distributions are the same.

The relationship between the variances of the two distributions is a bit more tricky. If the values of the 15-min averages were truly randomly distributed, then because each 8-h TWA is the average of thirty-two 15-min averages, we can say that

$$\sigma_{x(T_{long})} = \frac{\sigma_{x(T_{short})}}{\sqrt{n}} \tag{15.23}$$

where n is the number of short-term intervals within each long-term interval. This is the same as the relationship seen in Chapter 4 between the standard deviation of individual measurements and the standard deviation of the mean. Thus, the standard deviation decreases as the averaging time increases. From Equation 15.4, this implies that the geometric standard deviation also decreases as the averaging time increases. However, from Equation 15.3, we see that the geometric mean increases as the averaging time increases.

Equation 15.23 is valid only if, as mentioned earlier, the short-term exposures are random. However, this may not always be the case. The value of an exposure at time t_n is likely to be influenced by its values at t_{n1}, t_{n2}, etc. This is immediately obvious from a graph of the output of a real-time instrument measuring concentration at a fixed location. Concentrations at successive time intervals are not at all random; they are related to concentrations at preceding time intervals. Let us assume that concentrations separated by one time interval are correlated, concentrations separated by two time intervals are correlated, and so on. In the general case for concentrations separated by k time intervals, we can define a quantity $r(k)$ as

$$r(k) = \frac{E\left[\left(x_i - \mu_x\right)\left(x_{i+k} - \mu_x\right)\right]}{\sigma^2_{x\left(T_{\text{short}}\right)}} \tag{15.24}$$

where $E(.)$ refers to the expected value of the parameter within parentheses. The function $r(k)$ is referred to as the *autocorrelation function*, and denotes the fractional contribution of the covariance of values of exposures separated by different time lags. If the x_is are uncorrelated, then the numerator in Equation 15.24 will be equal to zero. However, in the general case, the concentration x_i may be related not just to the concentrations x_{i+1} and x_{i-1}, but to concentrations x_{i+k} and x_{ik}.

In this case, Equation 15.23 is modified to

$$\sigma^2_{x\left(T_{\text{long}}\right)} = \frac{\sigma^2_{x\left(T_{\text{short}}\right)}}{n}\left[1 + \left(\frac{2}{n}\right)\sum_{k=1}^{n-1}(n-k)\,r(k)\right] \tag{15.25}$$

When $r(k)$ is zero, i.e., the sequential values are uncorrelated, then Equation 15.25 reduces to Equation 15.23. When $r(k)$ is equal to unity for all values of k, we obtain

$$\sigma^2_{x\left(T_{\text{long}}\right)} = \sigma^2_{x\left(T_{\text{short}}\right)} \tag{15.26}$$

In other words, the variances are equal. Because the means are also equal, the short-term and long-term exposure distributions are identical. For all other values of $r(k)$ between 0 and 1, the variance of the long-term distribution is less than the variance of the short-term distribution by an amount that depends on the autocorrelation function. However, there is very little evidence that significant autocorrelation exists in occupational exposures. Thus, an easy way to improve the precision of exposure assessment is to use long averaging times during measurements.

16 Occupational Exposure Assessment Strategies

16.1 INTRODUCTION

The design of an exposure assessment strategy should be driven by the reason for obtaining samples, i.e., the question that needs to be answered or decision that needs to be made using the data. In Chapter 1, several reasons for carrying out sampling for air contaminants were discussed. The most common reason is routine monitoring of worker exposures to chemicals in a workplace and comparison of these exposures with occupational exposure limits (OELs). This can be carried out by occupational hygienists employed by the company to make decisions about restricting workplace exposures to acceptable levels, or by regulatory enforcement agencies to determine if worker exposures meet legal standards. Another important reason might be to determine a relationship between exposure and the health outcome in an occupational epidemiology study, which, in turn, might lead to the establishment of new standards. Although other special reasons might exist, they usually fall under the umbrella of the two reasons cited above. The sampling strategy includes the collection, statistical analysis, and interpretation of exposure data relative to an OEL. Several factors need to be considered in designing exposure assessment strategies. Exposure variability, which has been discussed at length in Chapter 15, is one of the most important factors. Exposures vary between workers, and over time, shift, and location. The sampling strategy should be effective in capturing this variability. At the same time, the strategy must be feasible and efficient in that it should not require an inordinately large number of samples. Occupational hygienists usually operate with limited resources that preclude large sample sizes. The dual requirements of effectiveness (i.e., the ability to provide correct exposure decisions) and efficiency (i.e., the need to minimize the number of measurements) have led to vigorous debate on the optimal sampling strategies. This debate also has implications regarding the "correct" interpretation of OELs. The following sections will address these issues of effectiveness and efficiency.

16.2 SAMPLE COLLECTION

There is broad consensus within the occupational hygiene community that *personal samples* obtained from the breathing zone of the worker are the most representative of the worker's exposure, in that the concentration measured by the personal sampler is close to the concentration of the pollutant being inhaled by the worker. *Area samples* obtained from samplers at fixed locations in the workplace are not well correlated with personal measurements. In most situations, personal samplers measure higher concentrations than static area samplers.

It is also critical to know the *exposure metric* that has relevance to the biological effect of interest. Although this seems like a fairly obvious point, it has often proved difficult to achieve in practice. For the measurement of aerosols, the choice of inhalable, thoracic or respirable fractions depends on the disease that we are interested in. Traditional exposure assessment of diesel exhaust aerosol has been based on the mass concentration metric. However, this may not accurately reflect the full complexity of the exposure. Recent studies have suggested that particle number and surface area concentrations may be more health-relevant indices than mass concentration, although the issue is far from settled. The choice of exposure metric also affects the classification of workers into similar exposure groups (SEGs). In a study of exposures to diesel exhaust aerosol, three concentration exposures — mass, surface area, and number — of bus drivers, parking garage attendants, and mechanics were measured. The three groups did not differ statistically significantly in terms of their mass exposures to elemental carbon. Thus, if the mass metric were used, workers from all three categories would occupy the same SEG. Surface area concentrations indicated that the garage mechanics had an exposure distribution distinctly different from those of bus drivers and ramp attendants (who had exposure distributions very similar to each other). Therefore, garage mechanics would be in a different SEG from the other two categories of workers. The ramp booth attendants had much lower number concentration exposures than garage mechanics, and thus they would be in different SEGs. Thus, we see that depending on the exposure metric chosen, the three occupational groups have similar or different exposures.

The selection of the optimal *sampling period* (the length of time over which the sample should be obtained) should be based on the toxicokinetics of the pollutant in the human body (Rappaport, 1991). For chronic toxicants, health effects are related to the body burden accumulated over long periods of time, typically of the order of several years or decades. The rates of elimination or repair are also very slow. Thus, transient spikes in exposures over a time period of a work shift or less will not affect the body burden significantly. In other words, there is a body damping of such transient exposure spikes. When the elimination half life of a toxicant ($T_{1/2}$) is between 10 and 100 h, the transient spikes within a shift (<8 h) are effectively damped. Day-to-day variability is unimportant for toxicants that have a $T_{1/2}$ greater than 40 h (Rappaport, 1991). The above is true only if we assume that the kinetics of accumulation and removal of the toxicant are first-order linear processes. For such chronic toxicants, the biological effects, and therefore the risk of disease, will be related to the arithmetic mean exposure and time, which determine body burden. An important implication of this is that fewer measurements — but with long sampling times (longer than single-shift averages) — are sufficient when the objective is the assessment of the risk of disease, e.g., in an epidemiological study. However, if the objective is the assessment of compliance with an OEL, such long-term averages are not useful because most OELs were not established with long-term averages in mind.

Nonlinear kinetics can result if there is damage resulting from short periods of high exposure. The biological time constants are less than the time period of a single shift. For such cases of acute toxicity, the exposure variability is transmitted to the tissue with high fidelity, and there is little body damping. In such a scenario, short-term exposure variability is important, and the existence of a number of short-term exposure limits (STELs) is a reflection of this fact. Such periods of very high exposures may be rare, but their consequences might be severe. There is evidence that some acute respiratory responses are precursors of chronic physiological changes (Wegman et al., 1992). Acute irritant events may cause severe discomfort that might lead to increased risk of accidents. It is essential to characterize three features of peak exposures: duration, magnitude, and frequency. A single brief "excursion" may be important for the study of an acute effect, but irrelevant for studying a chronic effect. For example, a brief 10-fold increase in ammonia exposure for 10 min may be a relevant peak in the study of acute irritation. But a similar excursion of a brief duration in silica levels will be irrelevant in increasing the risk of silicosis. The minimum height (magnitude) of the peak required for eliciting a specific physiological response requires knowledge of the threshold below which no detectable response occurs. For each potential threshold, only exposures exceeding that level should be defined as relevant peaks and evaluated against acute responses. The timing of the peak exposure (which is related to its frequency), combined with knowledge of the latency period of the biological effect, determines the appropriate time to examine the onset of the effect. The pharmacodynamics, thresholds, and latency periods of acute irritants are poorly understood. The above issues of duration, magnitude, and frequency illustrate the difficulty in relating acute exposure events with symptoms. Continuous sampling methods are invaluable in this context. Whereas such methods use mostly static area samplers that monitor the general environment, notable exceptions include, for example, the use of personal monitors to monitor both acute and chronic exposures to hydrogen sulfide in the pulp and paper industry.

16.3 OCCUPATIONAL EXPOSURE LIMITS

It is useful at this point to discuss occupational exposure limits (OELs), their evolution and interpretation, and the implications of differing interpretations of sampling strategies. The most influential OELs are the threshold limit values (TLVs) that are issued by the American Conference of Governmental Industrial Hygienists (ACGIH), a voluntary organization with members from federal, state, and local bodies as well as industry and academia. These TLVs have been published annually by ACGIH since 1946 and have had a profound influence on occupational standards internationally.

The TLVs and other OELs assume that for every substance, there exists a concentration below which no adverse health effects occur, no matter how frequent the exposure. For chemical carcinogens in which there may not be a threshold or dose at which zero risk would be expected, a risk threshold (e.g., 1 in 1,000 or 10,000 workers) is used for setting the OEL. For example, in the early 1980s, the background workplace mortality risk was estimated to be around 1 in 1,000, and this theoretical cancer risk was used in setting some OELs for carcinogens. Currently, the ACGIH TLVs are set on the basis of available occupational epidemiologic studies and animal toxicology tests.

The current preferred interpretation of the TLVs is in the preamble of the TLV booklet, (ACGIH, 2004) which says:

> Threshold Limit Values (TLVs) refer to airborne concentrations of substances and represent conditions under which it is believed that nearly all workers may be repeatedly exposed day after day without adverse health effects. Because of wide variation in individual susceptibility, however, a small percentage of workers may experience discomfort from some substances at concentrations at or below the threshold limit; a smaller percentage may be affected more seriously by aggravation of a preexisting condition or by development of an occupational illness .... Individuals may also be hypersusceptible or otherwise responsive to some industrial chemicals because of genetic factors, age, personal habits, medication, or previous exposures. Such workers may not be adequately protected from adverse health effects from certain chemicals at concentrations at or below the threshold limits ....

Although the TLV committee of the ACGIH has also claimed that the TLVs are set to protect the health of workers without regard to economic or technical feasibility, this has been challenged in several studies. Some studies have remarked that, whereas the TLVs showed poor correlation with the incidence of adverse effects, they were strongly correlated with prevailing achievable levels of exposure in industry (Roach and Rappaport, 1990). Thus, they should be seen as levels that have been achieved, and not as thresholds. Other studies have pointed to the undue influence of corporate representatives on the TLV committee in the setting of the TLVs (Castleman and Ziem, 1988). Since these critical studies appeared, the operational philosophy, the procedures, and the composition of the TLV committee have changed to reflect greater sensitivity to the criticisms leveled against it.

The ACGIH TLVs, although not legal standards by themselves, have driven the legally enforceable standards of the Occupational Safety and Health Administration (OSHA). The OSHA exposure limit standards are called permissible exposure limits, or PELs. Hansson (1998) found in an analysis of occupational standards in Germany (the maximum workplace concentrations or the MAK values) that these values were also not purely health-based. By comparison, Swedish OELs were the lowest and most protective. In all these instances, the OELs are not assumed to protect all the workers, but most of the workers.

There have been conflicting interpretations of the OELs for chronic diseases. Rappaport (1991) has argued that the OELs represent long-term limits of time-weighted averages. This interpretation flows from the wording of the TLV-TWA, as the "... time-weighted average concentration for a normal 8-h workday and 40-h workweek ...."

Rappaport (1991) argued that, because OSHA equates risk with cumulative exposure and also considers economic and technical feasibility, and because the mean exposure is the best predictor for individual risk, the OSHA PELs should also be interpreted as the average exposure received by a worker or SEG over a 45-year period. In other words, the conventional TWA OEL should be interpreted as upper limits to the long-term average (LTA) exposure experienced by each worker. In such a case, the sampling strategy would focus on determining the probability that an arbitrary worker in an SEG experiences an LTA greater than the OEL.

However, OSHA has not accepted this interpretation and maintains that the PELs are levels that should never be exceeded for any shift-long measurements. However, this is an impossible requirement because workers' exposures form a distribution in which the PEL is but one point. The exposures will exceed the PEL frequently in some workplaces and rarely in others. Based on estimates of the parameters of the exposure distribution, it is possible to calculate the frequency with which the PEL is exceeded in a given workplace. However, OSHA defines a workplace to be in compliance only if all measured exposures are less than the PEL. Even if a single measurement exceeds the PEL, the workplace is declared to be out of compliance. For chemicals with specific standards such as benzene, lead, or cadmium, engineering and administrative controls are required to bring exposures to acceptable levels. This interpretation is further complicated by the fact that the OSHA sampling strategy calls for very few measurements, a point we will discuss later.

Hewett (2001) has argued that the TWA OELs issued by ACGIH, OSHA, and National Institute for Occupational Safety and Health (NIOSH) are concentrations averaged across each single shift, which should not be exceeded. In this case, the sampling strategy focuses on determining the probability that an arbitrary worker in an SEG experiences a shift-long exposure that exceeds the OEL, and a statistic such as the 95th percentile is compared with the OEL. If the exceedance fraction is low (<5%), then the worker exposure is nominally controlled. These different interpretations of OELs lead to different sampling strategies, which will be discussed later in this chapter.

16.4 CLASSIFICATION OF WORKERS INTO SIMILARLY EXPOSED GROUPS

Because the time and resources needed for assessing the exposure of every worker in the workplace can be prohibitive, the standard approach has been to classify workers into SEGs and then randomly sample a subset of workers within each SEG. A critical assumption in such a classification is that the workers within each SEG have similar exposure distributions, i.e., each worker's exposure profile is very similar to every other worker's. Rappaport (1991) has proposed a more precise definition of such a monomorphic group as one in which 95% of the individual mean exposures lie within a factor of 2, i.e., in which the ratio of the 97.5th percentile to the 2.5th percentile (${}_{B}\hat{R}_{95}$) is less than or equal to 2. This corresponds to the between-worker geometric standard deviation, GSD_B, less than 1.2. There are several methods of classifying workers into SEGs.

16.4.1 The Observational Approach

This approach was described in Chapter 15 and requires an understanding of the processes and tasks that each group of workers is engaged in. The approach, first proposed by Corn and Esmen (1979), has now become an important element of the standard approaches adopted by American Industrial Hygiene Association (AIHA) and Comité Européen De Normalisation (CEN) (Mulhausen and Damiano, 1998; CEN, 1995). Workers are prospectively assigned to groups, or exposure zones, on the basis of work similarity (similar profiles of job tasks), similarity of hazardous agents (similar chemicals to which they are exposed), and environmental similarity (ventilation characteristics, processes, etc.). The occupational hygienist needs to collect basic information about the workplace and processes, the workers and the jobs and tasks being performed, the chemicals in use, and the various mechanisms to control and limit exposures. Exposure predictions developed using physical or chemical exposure modeling techniques can also be used. Thus, the SEGs are established by observations of process, job, task, and environmental agent. This information gathering might involve tours of the facility, interviews of the workers, managers, and process engineers, as well as reviews of existing documentation regarding the operating procedures, production records, engineering controls, and previous environmental sampling records (Mulhausen and Damiano, 1998). A key feature of the observational approach is that exposure monitoring data are not needed. Thus, it is a subjective exercise that relies on the professional judgment of the occupational hygienist. Therefore, it is likely that two occupational hygienists may arrive at different SEG classifications. Corn and Esmen (1979) also cautioned that the exposure zones should not be changed *post facto* on the basis of the measurement data.

Rappaport (1991) pointed out that if the value of ${}_B\hat{R}_{95}$ is less than 2 (i.e., $GSD_B < 1.2$), then the variability in exposure is primarily due to within-worker variability and driven by process, job, task, and control variables. These are precisely the variables that are characterized during the observational phase of the exposure assessment, and, therefore, the observational approach would work well for such situations. However, if individual workers have exposures that are significantly different, i.e., the value of ${}_B\hat{R}_{95}$ is greater than 2 (i.e., $GSD_B > 1.2$), then differences in individual work practices in performing the jobs and tasks are driving exposure variability. In other words, the between-worker variability is driving overall exposure variability. Rappaport et al. (1993) showed that characteristics used to establish SEGs by the observational approach are only marginally related to the between-worker component of variability. At this point, observational schemes can only be improved by ever-finer classifications based on observations of minute differences between the tasks performed by individual workers. An observational classification approach may not be able to detect these differences. Thus, workers in two different SEGs may have overlapping exposure distributions, which in turn cause misclassification of exposures.

16.4.2 The Sampling Approach

To overcome the shortcomings of the observational approach, Rappaport (1991) proposed a classification scheme where the entire population of workers is randomly sampled and subsequently divided into monomorphic groups as defined earlier. This approach requires multiple measurements of exposures of every sampled worker in an SEG to estimate the between- and within-worker components of variance. The determination of these components of exposure variability was described in Chapter

15. The occupational hygienist does not spend any time in observations of the workplace to classify the workers. Because the classification of workers is done on the basis of sampling alone, this approach is commonly referred to as the sampling approach to classification.

Rappaport et al. (1995) proposed a hybrid scheme that uses a very crude observational approach (e.g., one based solely on job title and the primary building where the job is carried out) followed by a more thorough sampling plan. It was claimed that this might be an optimal approach. For each observational group thus defined, a minimum of 10 workers are sampled at least twice (for a total of at least 20 measurements). For each observational group, the random effects analysis of variance (ANOVA) model is fit to the log-transformed exposure data, and the standardized parameters of this model are determined as described in Chapter 15. If the model fit is acceptable, then the observational group is deemed to be a monomorphic group. For observational groups with less than ten workers, all the workers would need to be sampled. Because the total number of workers in this case would be less than 20, Rappaport et al. (1995) suggested combining several small groups that still share a common factor (e.g., department or building) but not the same job title. It was recognized that this might also increase between-worker variability. It was also recognized that whereas 20 measurements might be sufficient when the group mean exposures is less than 20% of the OEL, more measurements might be needed when the mean is higher. The large sample sizes were justified on the basis of the large exposure variabilities.

Such approaches do not depend on the subjective professional judgments of the hygienists. They are based solely on measurements and are thus more objective. However, many measurements are required from each worker in the SEG, and this may not always be feasible due to constraints of time and money. Mulhausen and Damiano (1998) argue that the whole point of classifying workers into SEGs is to minimize the number of measurements that need to be obtained, and the sampling approach undermines that rationale.

16.4.3 A Hybrid Approach

The standard approach proposed by AIHA (Mulhausen and Damiano, 1998) combines the observational and sampling approaches for defining SEGs. Unlike the approach of Rappaport et al. (1995), which is also a hybrid of sorts, this method still retains the primacy of the observational approach. Although the observational approach has the advantage of efficiency (fewer number of measurements), it could in some situations be ineffective, i.e., it does not classify workers in the correct groups. However, the risks of such potential misclassification vary from one SEG to the next. The occupational hygienist should be able to identify the SEGs for which the potential for misclassification are significant. The workers in these SEGs, referred to as *critical SEGs*, would be monitored more thoroughly for obtaining estimates of within- and between-worker variability. Several rules of thumb were proposed to identify these critical SEGs. SEGs with exposure profiles above the OEL would not be sampled, as resources would be better spent in controlling those exposures. Similarly, SEGs with exposures below 10% of the OEL could also be excluded from sampling. Sampling is recommended for all SEGs that have exposure profiles above 10% of the OEL. For SEGs that have exposure profiles even closer to the OEL (e.g., between 50% and 100% of the OEL), multiple measurements for each sampled worker might be needed to further refine the exposure profiles using the ANOVA model described in Chapter 15. However, no clear-cut rule is presented for when such additional monitoring and analysis is needed; instead, the decision is left to the professional judgment of the occupational hygienist.

16.5 SAMPLE SIZE REQUIREMENTS — STRATEGIES FOR DECISION MAKING

16.5.1 AIHA Strategy

In day-to-day occupational hygiene practice, the determination of exposure is a vital part of the assessment of compliance with either regulatory or voluntary standards, i.e., making a decision about rating an exposure group profile as either acceptable or unacceptable (Mulhausen and Damiano, 1998). An acceptable exposure group is one where the true group 95th percentile exposure (for a reasonably homogeneous group) is less than the single-shift limit, or OEL_{TWA}. An unacceptable exposure group is one where the true 95th percentile exceeds the limit. This dichotomous rating scheme can be subdivided into four categories: three representing acceptable exposure profiles and one representing unacceptable exposure profiles. An exposure profile may be considered acceptable if the occupational hygienist determines that exposures are highly controlled, well-controlled, or (nominally) controlled. An exposure profile is unacceptable if exposures are poorly controlled.

Table 16.1 lists each of these categories along with statistical description for each control zone recommended by the AIHA. It follows from the statistical description of the highly controlled rating category that any combination of true group geometric mean (G) and group geometric standard deviation (D) which results in a 95th percentile that is less than or equal to 10% of the limit can be considered a highly controlled exposure profile. Similar reasoning applies to the other control zones.

Because almost all employers provide only limited resources for exposure assessment and control, the AIHA recommends that occupational hygienists prioritize their SEGs using methods described earlier (Mulhausen and Damiano, 1998). The occupational hygienist assigns an initial "exposure rating" of 1, 2, 3, or 4 as in Table 16.1. SEGs that merit a high initial exposure rating (e.g., nominally controlled or uncontrolled), or that involve high-toxicity substances or low certainty in the initial exposure rating should be placed at the top of the priority list for quantitative studies. SEGs at the opposite end should be lower in the priority list. In reality, those SEGs that receive low exposure ratings are rarely evaluated using more objective techniques. Corporate occupational hygienists often state that, due to resource limitations, they do not quantitatively sample more than 90% of their processes, but instead rely upon the initial ratings. In these cases, the initial exposure ratings become the final exposure ratings.

TABLE 16.1
AIHA Exposure Category Rating Scheme

AIHA Exposure Rating	Proposed Control Zone Description	Qualitative Description	AIHA Recommended Statistical Interpretation
1	Highly controlled (HC)	Exposures infrequently exceed 10% of the limit	$X_{0.95} \leq 0.10\ OEL$
2	Well controlled (WC)	Exposures infrequently exceed 50% of the limit and rarely exceed the limit	$0.10\ OEL < X_{0.95} \leq 0.5\ OEL$
3	(Nominally) controlled (NC)	Exposures infrequently exceed the limit	$0.5\ OEL < X_{0.95} \leq OEL$
4	Poorly controlled (PC)	Exposures frequently exceed the limit	$OEL < X_{0.95}$

The AIHA strategy requires randomly selecting 6 to 10 workers in an SEG and collecting one measurement from each worker (Mulhausen and Damiano, 1998). The basis for this recommendation was a finding that having fewer than six measurements led to a lot of uncertainty. The 95th percentile of the exposure profile, as well as its upper confidence limit (UCL), is estimated. If the 95th percentile is less than the OEL, then the exposure profile is deemed acceptable, although reassessment is recommended. If the 95th percentile is greater than the OEL, then further investigation or control measures (or both) are required. If the UCL is less than the OEL, then the exposure is acceptable with some estimated degree of confidence. The Health and Safety Executive (HSE) in the U.K. recommends a similar strategy of 5 to 10 measurements per SEG (Gardiner, 1995). The CEN (1995) strategy also shares important elements with the AIHA strategy. Indeed, many corporations have developed similar schemes, often referring to the AIHA scheme as their model.

16.5.2 OSHA Strategy

As mentioned earlier, OSHA defines a workplace to be in compliance only if all measured exposures are less than the PEL. Even if a single measurement exceeds the PEL, the workplace is declared to be out of compliance, and engineering and administrative controls are required to bring exposures to acceptable levels, especially for chemical-specific standards. Employers are encouraged to select the maximum-risk employees for monitoring. Thus, the strategy involves a simple comparison of each measurement with the PEL. At the same time, the OSHA sampling strategy calls for very few measurements. Only some of the PELs specify minimum numbers of measurements to be obtained, and OSHA relies partly on voluntary compliance on the part of employers. Rappaport (1984) showed that, for any level of exceedance, the probability of noncompliance increases with the number of measurements. Let f_{PEL} be the exceedance, i.e., the probability that an exposure x is greater than the PEL, i.e., P(x > PEL), and n be the total number of measurements. The probabilities of compliance and noncompliance are given by

$$P(c) = \left(1 - f_{\mathrm{PEL}}\right)^{n} \tag{16.1}$$

$$P(\bar{c}) = \left\{1 - \left(1 - f_{\mathrm{PEL}}\right)^{n}\right\} \tag{16.2}$$

Figure 16.1 shows how the probability of noncompliance varies with the exceedance fraction and sample size. As sample size increases, the probability of noncompliance increases. For even small values of the exceedance fraction, noncompliance is highly likely, even for modest sample sizes. Thus, the OSHA strategy sets up a perverse incentive for employers to obtain as few measurements as possible, preferably none at all.

The OSHA strategy compares each measurement with the PEL and assumes that the measurement is in compliance if the upper confidence level of the measurement (defined only in terms of the sampling and analytical error) is below the PEL. Likewise, the measurement is out of compliance if the lower confidence limit of the measurement is above the PEL. If the confidence limits encompass the PEL, then there is a potential for overexposure. Thus, another serious criticism of the OSHA strategy is that the role of the sampling and analytical error is enhanced, even though it is a minor contributor to the overall variability, as discussed in Chapter 15.

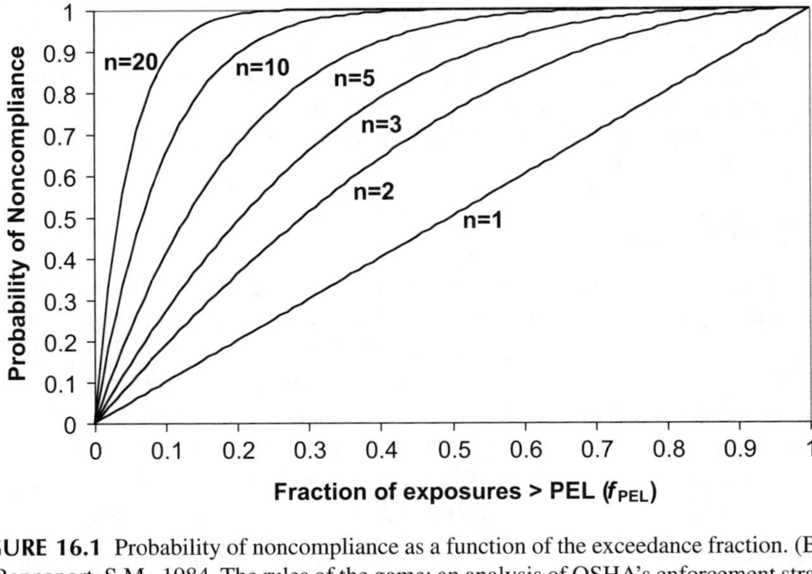

FIGURE 16.1 Probability of noncompliance as a function of the exceedance fraction. (Based on Rappaport, S.M., 1984, The rules of the game: an analysis of OSHA's enforcement strategy, *Am. J. Ind. Med.*, 6: 291–303.)

16.5.3 Effectiveness and Efficiency of Strategies for Decision Making

Thus, regulatory compliance compels occupational hygienists to design sampling strategies aimed at satisfying the minimum requirements. However, such minimalist strategies are often incapable of reliably detecting poorly controlled exposures (Tuggle, 1981; OSHA, 2001). In general, any strategy that requires only a small number of measurements may lead to an incorrect decision that the entire distribution of exposures for a group of workers is acceptable. The fewer the number of measurements, the less is our confidence in the estimate of exposure variability. Estimates of the upper tail of the distribution (e.g., the 95th percentile or the exceedance fraction) are even less certain. Ideally, routine exposure assessment in occupational settings should be carried out for the purpose of risk management, and, in this sense, it has been compared to quality control (Hewett, 2001). In other words, meeting exposure assessment and control objectives should be the focus of an exposure assessment program that aims to minimize health risk. The sampling strategy for a baseline exposure assessment should be designed so that there is a high probability of detecting a clearly unacceptable group exposure profile.

The goal of an employer's exposure management program should be to minimize the number of workers whose upper percentile exposures are greater than the OEL. Thus, for a typical exposure limit, an appropriate measure of compliance would be the probability that a randomly selected worker's 95th percentile exposure is greater than the OEL. However, there are no published exposure assessment strategies that directly estimate this probability.

Hewett (2003), using computer simulations, analyzed the effectiveness (the ability to achieve a specific objective) and efficiency (the number of measurements or resources required of the strategy) of several common exposure assessment strategies such as the OSHA 6b strategy (Leidel et al., 1977; the OSHA Z-table strategy (OSHA, 2002), the AIHA SEG strategy (Mulhausen and Damiano, 1998), and the CEN strategy (CEN, 1995). Although the two OSHA strategies were found to be highly efficient, (i.e., a decision can be reached in 1 to 2 measurements), they are not very effective (i.e., they do not have sufficient power to reliably detect poorly controlled group exposure profiles). The probability of detecting clearly unacceptable exposure profiles or power is around 42%. In this context, a poorly controlled group exposure profile was defined as one in which the exceedance fraction was 25%. At least six measurements are required to achieve a power of at least 90%.

Hewett (2003) found that the AIHA SEG strategy with six measurements is effective at detecting poorly controlled exposure profiles. For 10 measurements, the AIHA strategy has a very high power (>99%) to detect clearly unacceptable exposure profiles (which were defined to have an exceedance fraction of 25%).

16.5.4 Comparing the Mean with an OEL

Rappaport (1984) argued that the OSHA PELs were set by assuming that the risk of chronic disease was directly proportional to the cumulative exposure (mean exposure multiplied by the time over which the exposure occurred), and therefore to the exposure mean. At the same time, compliance is defined in terms of the probability of a single measurement exceeding the PEL. Thus, many exposure distributions having the same probability of noncompliance could have very different means, and therefore very different risks. Rappaport (1984) argued that, therefore, it makes more sense to estimate the long-term mean exposures for an SEG, because they are more directly related to the risk of chronic disease. Additionally, because the estimate of the mean becomes more precise with more measurements, there would be an incentive to increase the number of measurements. This would be in contrast to the existing strategy that seemed to penalize obtaining more measurements by increasing the odds of being out of compliance.

One consequence of this line of thinking was to view the PELs as long-term average (LTA) exposure limits and not simply as the limit for an 8-h TWA. The mean of the exposure distribution was tested against the PEL that was interpreted as an LTA-OEL (Lyles et al., 1997). This interpretation has been controversial, and has generated a lively debate in the literature (Hewett, 1998a; Rappaport et al., 1998a; Hewett, 1998b; Rappaport et al., 1998b; Hewett, 2001).

The second concern regarding testing the mean of a distribution against an OEL is the relatively large number of measurements required for the purpose. Rappaport (1994) showed that the sample size required for testing the hypothesis that the mean is less than the OEL is given by

$$n = \frac{\left(z_{(1-\alpha)} + z_{(1-\beta)}\right)^2 \left(\sigma^2 + 0.5\sigma^4\right)}{\left[1 - \left(\mu_x / OEL\right)\right]^2} \tag{16.3}$$

where α is the level of significance, $(1-\beta)$ is the power required, σ is the standard deviation of the log-transformed exposures, μ_x is the mean exposure and the two z terms are the values from the standard normal distribution associated with probabilities $(1-\alpha)$ and $(1-\beta)$, respectively. Table 16.2 shows the required sample sizes

TABLE 16.2
Sample Size Requirements for Testing if the Mean Exposure Is Less than the OEL for $\alpha = 0.05$ and $(1-\beta) = 0.90$

	Sample Size				
μ_x/OEL	$\sigma_g = 1.5$	$\sigma_g = 2.0$	$\sigma_g = 2.5$	$\sigma_g = 3.0$	$\sigma_g = 3.5$
0.10	2	6	13	21	30
0.25	3	10	19	30	43
0.50	7	21	41	67	96
0.75	25	82	164	266	384

Source: Rappaport, S.M. (1994), Interpreting levels of exposure to chemical agents, in *Patty's Industrial Hygiene and Toxicology*, 3rd ed., Vol. 3, Part A, Harris, R.L., Cralley, L.J., and Cralley, L.V. Eds., John Wiley & Sons, New York.

for various values of the mean and geometric standard deviation. When the GSD of the distribution is less than or equal to 2, and the mean exposure is 25% or less of the OEL, the number of measurements required is ~10. However, for larger GSDs, and when the mean exposure approaches the OEL, the number of measurements required for testing the mean is very large (several hundred samples).

As described earlier, Rappaport et al. (1995) also proposed a scheme that uses a very crude observational approach followed by a more thorough sampling plan. For each observational group, a minimum of 10 workers should be sampled at least twice (for a total of at least 20 measurements). Again, this would work well in classifying exposures as acceptable only if the group mean exposure is less than 20% of the OEL. Sample sizes would need to dramatically increase if the mean exposures are higher and approach the OEL.

Rappaport (1994) has argued that, even though this approach leads to higher sample sizes, the method is more scientifically defensible than the other approaches. In view of the fact that sampling and analytical errors are minor contributors to the total exposure variability, there is a need to develop inexpensive and less precise monitoring techniques so that large sample sizes become economically feasible. When, in some situations, the sample numbers are daunting, it would also provide appropriate incentives for the employer to install mechanisms to control exposures.

In contrast, Hewett (2001) has argued that approaches involving testing or estimating the mean are more appropriate for epidemiological studies than for compliance monitoring. In epidemiological studies, accurate estimates of cumulative or long-term exposures are required to develop an exposure–response relationship. Compliance-driven monitoring is more akin to risk management than risk assessment. The OEL is used to determine if current exposures are being effectively managed. Conceptually, if the worst-case exposures are below the TWA OEL, then the long-term average exposure will be much less than the TWA OEL. Thus, compliance-driven monitoring is thought to be more protective. However, it must be emphasized that this debate is far from settled.

16.5.5 Estimating the Mean

If our goal is to estimate the mean of the distribution, then we can use our knowledge of normal statistics to achieve this. If we know the exposure distribution parameters (e.g., the geometric mean and GSD) *a priori*, then the calculation of the number of samples required to estimate the mean within a certain amount of error and with a certain degree of confidence is straightforward (Hewett, 1995). The approximate number of samples, n, is given by

$$n = \left(\frac{t\,CV}{E} \right)^2 \tag{16.4}$$

Here, CV is the coefficient of variation, defined as the ratio of the standard deviation to the mean and expressed as a percent value, where the standard deviation and the mean are given by their minimum variance unbiased estimates obtained from Equation 15.17 and Equation 15.15. E is the desired amount of the percent error in the estimate of the mean and t is the t-distribution value for the required degree of confidence for a (1–α) confidence level and (n–1) degrees of freedom.

If the parameter of interest is the geometric mean instead of the arithmetic mean, then the required sample size is

$$n = \left(\frac{t \ln(GSD)}{\frac{1}{2} \ln\left(\frac{1+E}{1-E}\right)} \right)^2 \tag{16.5}$$

Equation 16.5 specifies the sample size required to estimate the geometric mean (GM) within plus or minus a certain amount of fractional error with a certain degree of confidence.

Equation 16.4 and Equation 16.5 require some knowledge of the exposure distribution parameters. These need to be obtained from pilot studies or measurements made in other similar situations. Hewett (1995) showed that the sample size could be quite large when the estimated GSD is large. One way to reduce the sample size is to reduce the required accuracy (i.e., E is increased); another is to reduce the degree of confidence (1–α) required in the estimate.

16.6 EXPOSURE MEASUREMENT ERROR AND ITS IMPLICATIONS FOR EPIDEMIOLOGY

The previous subsections have dealt with various exposure assessment strategies from the perspective of compliance monitoring. These strategies can lead to varying amounts of misclassification error, i.e., a worker is placed in an SEG incorrectly. Because the data collected using such strategies is often also used for epidemiological purposes, it is useful to consider the effect of these exposure misclassification errors on the relationship between exposure and health response. The exposure–response relationship is typically obtained as a standard linear Gaussian regression model. For example, we might have a regression of the response y (e.g., log mortality or a morbidity measure such as change in FEV-1 over some time period) on the exposure x:

$$y = \alpha_x + \beta_x x + \varepsilon \tag{16.6}$$

where α and β are regression coefficients to be estimated, and ε is the measurement error. The error is random and independent of the covariate x. We can assume that ε is normally distributed with variance σ_ε^2. The true exposure x is normally distributed with variance σ_x^2. The coefficient β is the expected change in mortality (or morbidity) per unit change in the true exposure and can be estimated using ordinary least squares regression.

Let us assume that we do not know the true exposure level x, and instead only have some approximation z. If we regress the response y on z, we will obtain new negression coefficients and a different error term,

$$y = \alpha_z + \beta_z z + \varepsilon^* \tag{16.7}$$

What is the relationship between $\hat{\beta}_x$ and $\hat{\beta}_z$? To answer this question, we need to understand the relationship between the true and measured exposures, i.e., between x and z. The relationship is of two basic types.

16.6.1 Classical Error Model

The first type of relationship is called the *classical error model*. Here, we assume that z is an imperfect measure of x, i.e., the average value of z within each x stratum is equal to x, or $E(z \mid x) = x$. The measurement error z–x is uncorrelated with x. One example of this is the relationship between a measurement made using an instrument and the true value of the parameter, which we discussed in Chapter 4. Thus, when the true concentration is x, an unbiased instrument will measure x on average, even though individual measurements z can be different from x. In the context of worker exposures, the within-worker component of variability obtained by repeatedly sampling an individual worker can be considered to follow the classical error model. It is assumed that the repeat measurements on a worker vary about a true value.

Under the classical error model, the regression coefficient $\hat{\beta}_z$ is a biased estimate of β_x. In a simple linear regression with one variable of exposure, $\hat{\beta}_z$ is expected to be smaller than β_x. In other words, it is attenuated.

$$\beta_z = R\beta_x \tag{16.8}$$

where R is a attenuation factor between 0 and 1, and is given by

$$R = \frac{\sigma_x^2}{\sigma_x^2 + \sigma_\varepsilon^2} \tag{16.9}$$

The denominator is the variance of the observed measurements and can be written as σ_z^2. R can also be expressed as $\frac{\sigma_z^2 - \sigma_\varepsilon^2}{\sigma_z^2}$, and is a measure of the reliability of z as a measure of x. Equation 16.9 can be rewritten as

$$R = \frac{1}{1 + \frac{\sigma_\varepsilon^2}{\sigma_x^2}} = \frac{1}{1+\lambda} \tag{16.10}$$

where λ is the variance ratio. The variance ratio of the average of k repeat measurements is equal to the variance ratio for the separate measurements divided by k. So, the expression for R is given by

$$R = \frac{1}{1 + \lambda / k} \tag{16.11}$$

The value of R can be used to assess the magnitude of bias in regression. The components of the variance ratio can be obtained from an analysis of variance, where σ_ε^2 is the within-worker or "error" variance and σ_x^2 is the between-worker or "true" variance. From Equation 16.11, we can see that if the error variance is large, then repetition of exposure measurements for each subject is a method for reducing the bias in regression. In fact, Equation 16.11 can be used to determine the number of repeat measurements needed to reduce the bias in the regression coefficient to a multiplication factor of at least R. Thus, if λ equals 0.5 and we can tolerate an R equal to 0.8, then k equals 2. Brunekreef et al. (1987) argue that, because it is usually not possible to have estimates of the variance ratios before an epidemiological study is conducted, there is a need to conduct a pilot study to obtain estimates of the variance ratios in the exposure variables before the main study is conducted. The above discussion is valid only for cases where there is only one exposure variable. In the multivariate case, the analysis is much more complex. Interested readers can find further discussion in Cochran (1968), Brunekreef et al. (1987), Zeger et al. (2000), and Heederik and Attfield (2000).

16.6.2 Berkson Error Model

The second type of measurement error is called *Berkson error*. In this error model, we assume that the average value of the true exposure within each stratum of measured value z is equal to z, or $E(x \mid z) = z$. This model is useful when z is a measured value (e.g., exposure) that is shared by a group of individuals whose individual exposures x might vary. For example, when z is the mean true exposure for an SEG ($z = \bar{x}$) and its value is assigned to all workers in that SEG, then the difference between the assigned and true (but unobserved) values of individual exposure is defined as Berkson error.

In the case of Berkson error, if we regress y on z according to Equation 16.7, then the estimate of the regression coefficient $\hat{\beta}_z$ is an unbiased estimate of β_x. Having z rather than x does not lead to bias in the regression coefficient. But the exposure measurement error increases the variance of the regression coefficient. This is because having a surrogate z instead of the actual exposure x does not provide as much information about the coefficient β_x (Armstrong, 1990). Direct estimation of Berkson error depends on the availability of data providing the true exposure of each individual. Levin et al. (2000) have used sophisticated statistical methods such as bootstrapping to estimate this type of error in occupational exposure studies.

However, in practice, z itself is an approximation of the true mean exposure $\bar{x}$ of the workers in that SEG. The difference ($\bar{x}$–z) will often follow the classical error model. Thus, most regressions based on this type of exposure estimation will have both Berkson and classical types of measurement error.

It is now interesting to consider the situation when area measurements are used to approximate the personal exposures of workers in an SEG. The difference between x and z now comprises several components of error. If the true personal exposure of a worker is x_i, then it can be expressed as

$$x_i = z + (x_i - \bar{x}) + (\bar{x} - z^*) + (z^* - z) \quad (16.12)$$

where $(x_i - \bar{x})$ is the error due to having aggregated rather than individual data. $(\bar{x} - z^*)$ is the difference between the average personal exposure and the true area measurement value, and $(z^* - z)$ is the difference between the true and measured area measurement. The term $(x_i - \bar{x})$ is Berkson error, where having aggregate instead of individual data does not bias the regression coefficient. The second term $(\bar{x} - z^*)$ is a source of bias. The last term $(z^* - z)$ is the classical error in the area measurement instrument.

Heederik and Attfield (2000) compared several exposure assessment strategies in a study of the relationship between dust exposure and the change in lung function over an 11-year time period. The data set included 1,172 miners with 36,824 concurrently measured personal dust samples obtained from the 1969 to 1981 U.S. National Study of Coal Workers' Pneumoconiosis. The long-term average exposure for each miner was calculated in several different ways. The first method used all the measurements available per worker, as well as random samples of these measurements (leading to sample sizes of 3, 6, 9, and 12 measurements per worker). The second method created job exposure matrices (JEMs). The exposure categories of these JEMs were made by aggregating workers having job titles with similar exposures. The exposure measurements were merged with individual work histories to calculate average exposures. Finally, the JEM was modified by adding a time variable and a variable for the mine where the measurement was obtained. Several other types of JEMs were also studied.

Table 16.3 shows the effect of sample size on the regression coefficient. As fewer measurements were used per worker, the regression coefficient (the slope of the lung function change on dust exposure) became smaller. The slope of the exposure–response relationship based on three measurements was roughly a third of that found when all measurements were used (which corresponds to an average of 31 measurements per worker, 36,824/1,172). This was a significant amount of attenuation. An analysis of variance showed that within-worker variability was three times greater than between-worker variability, i.e., the variance ratio was three. The influence of this error variance on the true variance can be reduced to insignificance

TABLE 16.3
Regression Analysis of the Relationship between 11-Year Individual Mean Exposure to Respirable Coal Dust and Change in Lung Function (FEV-1) over the Same Time Period for 1105 Workers after Adjusting for Age, Height, and Smoking — National Study of Coal Workers' Pneumoconiosis, 1969 to 1981

Samples per Worker	FEV-1, Coefficient (ml/mg/m^3)	Standard Error (ml/mg/m^3)
All samples	−4.5	1.5
15	−3.8	1.4
12	−3.6	1.4
9	−3.2	1.3
6	−2.5	1.3
3	−1.8	1.1

Source: Heederik, D. and Attfield, M. (2000), Characterization of dust exposure for the study of chronic occupational lung disease: a comparison of different exposure assessment strategies, *Am. J. Epidemiol.*, 151: 982–990.

when all 31 measurements are used. This finding is consistent with our earlier discussion of classical errors.

Table 16.4 compares the slopes of the exposure–response relationship found using the various exposure assessment strategies. The slopes are not statistically significantly different from each other, even though the slope is greatest when estimated by a JEM using a combination of six exposure categories and coal mine as a main effect. In other words, the confidence intervals of all these estimates overlap. However, the standard errors for the regression coefficients are the smallest when the individual measurements are used. The standard errors for the regression coefficients become greater when JEMs are used, and sometimes cause the regression coefficient to become statistically insignificant. This is related to between-worker variability and is due to Berkson-type errors.

Thus, we can see the trade-offs in the different exposure assessment strategies. Although the individual exposure assessment strategy requires a large number of measurements, it leads to the smallest standard error. Various grouping strategies require fewer measurements and lead to unbiased slope estimates with larger standard errors.

The success of a grouping strategy depends on the within-group variability (i.e., how homogeneous the SEG is), the between-group variability (i.e., how different the groups are), the standard error of the mean exposure for each group (i.e., the precision), and the number of exposure measurements available per worker. The grouping is optimal when each SEG is as homogeneous as possible, the greatest contrast exists between SEGs, and there are enough measurements

TABLE 16.4
Regression Analysis of the Relationship between 11-year Individual Mean Exposure to Respirable Coal Dust and Change in Lung Function (FEV-1) over the Same Time Period for 1105 Workers after Adjusting for Age, Height, and Smoking for Different Exposure Assessment Strategies — National Study of Coal Workers' Pneumoconiosis, 1969 to 1981

Exposure Assessment Strategy	FEV-1, Coefficient ($ml/mg/m^3$)	Standard Error ($ml/mg/m^3$)
Individual	–4.4	1.6
6 categories	–2.2	3.2
6 categories + time (10 strata)	–3.2	3.4
6 categories + time (4 strata)	–2.0	3.1
6 categories + coalmine	–5.9	2.4

Source: Heederik, D. and Attfield, M. (2000), Characterization of dust exposure for the study of chronic occupational lung disease: a comparison of different exposure assessment strategies, *Am. J. Epidemiol.*, 151: 982–990.

available to estimate the mean exposure with the greatest precision. These criteria may, at times, be at odds with each other. For example, the requirements for homogeneity may require the formation of larger numbers of SEGs with fewer workers in each of them. This reduces the number of measurements per SEG and, therefore, the precision of the exposure estimates. The above discussion illustrates the need for pilot studies to be performed prior to a large epidemiological study to quantify estimates of bias and precision. There is also a need to analyze the data, using multiple exposure assessment strategies to evaluate their effect on the exposure–response relationships.

17 Exposure Modeling

17.1 ROLE OF MODELING IN EXPOSURE ASSESSMENT

Although exposure monitoring has been the most common method of evaluating worker exposures, it is not necessarily the optimal method, or even a feasible method, in many instances. Exposure estimates will be most accurate when high-quality measured data are available in sufficient quantities over relevant time periods. However, such data may not always be available. For instance, in many epidemiological studies, there is a need for exposure estimates of workers in processes that no longer exist. Sometimes, one may want to estimate exposures for a new process that is still in its planning stages to evaluate the adequacy of the proposed engineering controls or respirator selection. Another reason might be to prioritize monitoring efforts so that resources, which are limited, are spent on monitoring the workers at maximum risk. Thus, model outputs can act as a guide for monitoring efforts. In all these scenarios, there is a need to estimate exposures without actually carrying out monitoring. Exposure modeling is a tool that provides such estimates. In more general situations, there may be some available monitoring data, but they may be incomplete or of poor quality. In such cases, a judicious combination of monitoring data and exposure model outputs may provide better exposure estimates than any one source of information by itself.

An exposure model describes how various workplace parameters affect exposures. More precisely, in this context, the exposure model is a set of equations that predicts the airborne concentration of contaminants at different times and at different positions in the workplace. Typically, models include a source (or contaminant generation) term and allow for the transport and fate of the contaminant through space and over time to predict concentrations. The workers who move through the contaminated environment are exposed to the contaminant in proportion to the amount of time they spend in different spatial locations.

The workplace parameters that affect exposures are called *determinants of exposure*. Some determinants increase exposures (e.g., the throughput rate in a production facility), others decrease exposures (e.g., the local exhaust ventilation), and yet others might either increase or decrease exposures. Whereas some of the exposure determinants are intuitively obvious, others are more subtle in their effects. A number of studies over the last several decades have identified these determinants of exposure (Burstyn and Teschke, 1999). Unfortunately, the measurement of exposure determinants has not received the same level of attention as the measurement of exposures, with the result that exposure modeling is still a relatively new field. Our understanding of exposure mechanisms is still somewhat crude, and many available models have been invalidated. However, it is being increasingly recognized that, in most occupational situations where actual exposure monitoring data are relatively sparse and exposure variability is large, mathematical modeling may provide a more accurate exposure estimate (Nicas and Jayjock, 2002). This provides a rationale for allocating more resources for development and validation of exposure models. This, in turn, may encourage the increased use of modeling for purposes such as assessing compliance, designing appropriate exposure controls, and making retrospective exposure assessments for epidemiological purposes.

The models described in the next section differ in their levels of sophistication. Each level increases the cost (in terms of the amount of information needed as inputs to the models), but yields more accurate estimates. The exposure models discussed in this chapter provide only a starting point or an introduction to the modeling perspective. Whereas some of the models start from basic physical principles and are therefore causal models, others are more empirical and thus are merely predictive models.

The first tier comprises the saturation vapor pressure model, which provides the most conservative exposure estimates and is the least onerous in terms of data required to use the model. Clearly, this model is only applicable to gas and vapor exposures. The next tier comprises the well-mixed room model with ventilation. This model generally provides lower estimates of exposure than the saturation vapor pressure model because it takes into account the ventilation through the workplace. At the same time, it ignores the effect of proximity to the source. At the third tier, the near-field far-field model is more sophisticated because it attempts to capture the effect of source proximity on exposure. However, it comes at the cost of making measurements of the interzonal flow rate. A number of other models, such as the eddy diffusion model, are also available, but these are increasingly resource intensive. At the end of the spectrum, there are models based on computational fluid dynamics and mass transfer, as well as probabilistic Markov chain Monte Carlo analysis, all of which require substantial computing resources. These are beyond the scope of this chapter. Frequently, the use of modeling in occupational settings does not extend to anything more sophisticated than that discussed in this chapter.

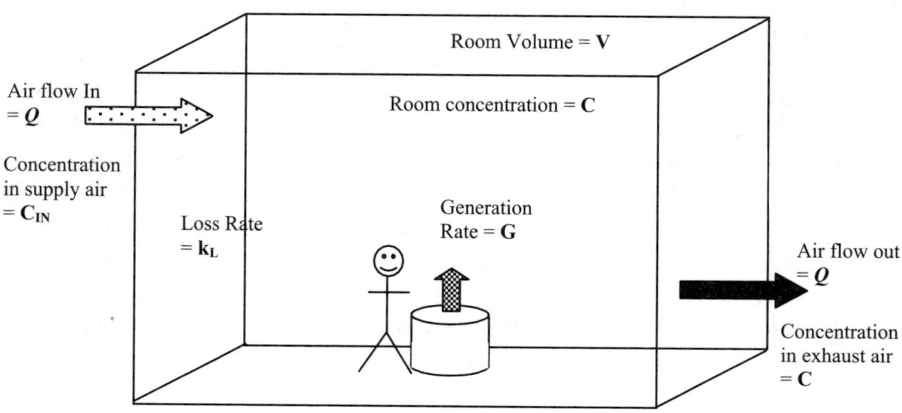

FIGURE 17.1 Diagram of well-mixed room model.

17.2 SATURATION VAPOR PRESSURE MODEL

To start with, let us consider a situation in which we do not have any information about the dimensions of the workplace, the airflow through the workplace, the amount of the chemical being used, or the activities of the workers. The only information available is about the chemical itself. The ideal gas law and the saturation vapor pressure of the chemical can be used to predict the saturation concentration of the chemical in air.

So, if the partial pressure of a chemical equals its saturation vapor pressure value, the saturation concentration of the chemical in air is:

$$C_{sat}\text{ (in ppm)} = \frac{P_v\text{ in mm Hg}}{760\text{ mm Hg}} \times 10^6 \tag{17.1}$$

This is the same as Equation 2.14. In essence, this equation makes the worst-case assumption that the partial pressure of the chemical in air will equal its vapor pressure value. This is equivalent to saying that the airborne concentration of the chemical is the same as its saturation concentration in air.

This worst-case assumption requires that (1) the chemical is continually exposed to room air, (2) there is no room ventilation, or $Q = 0$ m³/min the air flow rate, (3) the room and liquid temperatures are constant, (4) there is sufficient time to reach equilibrium, (5) there is a sufficient mass of chemical in the room such that the liquid (or solid) chemical remains at equilibrium, and (6) the ideal gas law holds.

Consider a situation in which a worker is exposed to a chemical with a saturation vapor pressure of 10 mm Hg (at 20°C). If there is no further information about the situation, we can estimate the exposure in the worst-case scenario. From Equation 17.1, $C_{sat}\text{ (in ppm)} = \frac{10\text{ mm Hg}}{760\text{ mm Hg}} \times 10^6 = 13{,}158\text{ ppm}$. If a container with this chemical is left open in a nonventilated storage cabinet, and an employee opens the cabinet, then the estimated concentration would be a good estimate of the exposure of the employee in the first few breaths (i.e., peak exposure). If the ceiling limit for this chemical is 300 ppm, then we see that the estimated acute exposure is ~40-fold higher. On the other hand, if a chemical had a saturation vapor pressure of 0.1 mm Hg, then the saturation concentration would be 131 ppm. If the TWA OEL for this chemical was 300 ppm, then we may safely conclude that the OEL will not be exceeded, even in the worst case. By providing an upper-bound estimate of the exposure, the model facilitates decision-making about whether further concern is warranted or not, which could lead to additional modeling or monitoring.

17.3 THE WELL-MIXED ROOM MODEL

This model is more sophisticated than the saturation vapor pressure model, in that it incorporates information about the flow rate of air through the workroom and the generation rate of contaminant within the room, among other factors. This well-known model assumes that the air in the room is completely well mixed, so that the concentration at any point in the room is the same at any point in time. In other words, there is no spatial variability within the room. The contaminant is dispersed instantaneously throughout the volume of the room. Although clearly a physically unrealistic assumption, it leads to a certain simplification of the mathematical solution. The cost of this simplification is that the model underestimates the exposures of workers near the contaminant source. However, the model is reasonable for situations where the workers are not very close to the source, and the process is a continuous one that has reached a quasi-steady state (i.e., there are no large variations in the process variables over time). There are several variations on the basic theme, and so it is instructive to delve into the details of this model.

17.3.1 Constant Emission Rate

Let us consider a room of volume V (e.g., in m^3) through which the ventilation airflow rate is a constant equal to Q (e.g., in units of m^3/min) as shown in Figure 17.1. The air entering the room (at a flow rate of Q) has a contaminant concentration of C_{in} (e.g., in units of mg/m^3). There is also a contaminant source within the room that is generating the airborne contaminant at a constant rate of G (e.g., in units of mg/min). This may be a reasonable assumption when we are interested in chronic health effects, and short-term variations in the generation rate (and hence the exposure) are not important. Thus, the air entering the room, as well as the in-room source, increase the amount of contaminant in the room.

Air may enter a room via mechanically driven supply air systems (e.g., diffusers in ceilings and walls) and via infiltration through open windows and doors and cracks around windows and doors. Air may exit a room via mechanically driven exhaust air systems (e.g., exhaust registers, local exhaust hoods) and via exfiltration through open windows and doors, and cracks around windows and doors. We assume a balance in the volumetric rate (m^3/min) of air entering a room Q_{in} and leaving the same room Q_{out}. Therefore, we drop the subscripts and simply refer to Q as the supply or exhaust air rate of the room.

The airflow Q will also remove some of the contaminant from the room. In addition, there might be other routes by which the contaminant may be removed. In the case of gases and vapors, these might include adsorption onto room surfaces (e.g., walls, wall and floor coverings, etc.) or chemical reactions, or both. In the case of aerosols of a given size, this might include gravitational settling, diffusion onto walls, thermophoresis, and condensation and evaporation, to name just a few mechanisms. All these loss mechanisms can be combined into one term, i.e., a loss rate coefficient k_L (e.g., in units of per minute), i.e., the fractional mass of contaminant in the room removed per minute. Thus, the airflow rate as well as various loss mechanisms decrease the amount of contaminant in the room.

The principle of mass conservation can be used to develop an expression for the contaminant concentration in the room. A mass balance equation for the contaminant in room air can be written by considering all the contaminant mass entering room air and leaving it in an infinitesimal interval t to $t + dt$. The change in contaminant mass in this interval is the mass gain minus the mass loss.

$$\text{Change in Mass in } dt = \text{Mass Gain in } dt\text{–Mass Loss in } dt \tag{17.2}$$

The change in mass in the interval t to $t + dt$ must equal the product of the room volume V (m^3) and the infinitesimal change in the contaminant concentration in room air, denoted by dC (mg/m^3), during this interval. Thus, the mass balance is as follows:

$$V \cdot \mathrm{d}C = \mathrm{G} \cdot dt + C_{\mathrm{IN}} \cdot Q \cdot dt - C(t) \cdot Q \cdot dt - \mathrm{k_L} \cdot C(t) \cdot V \cdot dt \tag{17.3}$$

The first two terms on the right-hand side represent mass gain terms due to the contaminant source within the room and the contaminant being brought into the room by the incoming airflow. The third and fourth terms are mass loss terms due to contaminant being removed from the room by the airflow and other loss mechanisms. After dividing both sides of Equation 17.3 by V and dt, and with some algebraic rearrangement of the terms, we obtain

$$\frac{\mathrm{d}C}{\mathrm{d}t} + \left(\frac{Q + k_{\mathrm{L}}\, V}{V}\right) C(t) = \frac{G + C_{\mathrm{IN}}\, Q}{V} \tag{17.4}$$

This is a first-order ordinary differential equation. Let us assume that at time $t = 0$, the concentration in the room is $C(0)$. Then, the solution to Equation 17.4 is given by

$$C(t) = \frac{G + C_{\mathrm{IN}}\, Q}{Q + k_{\mathrm{L}}\, V}\left(1 - \exp\left(-\frac{Q + k_{\mathrm{L}}\, V}{V} t\right)\right) + C(0)\exp\left(-\frac{Q + k_{\mathrm{L}}\, V}{V} t\right) \tag{17.5}$$

Equation 17.5 is the general solution to the differential equation and represents the concentration in the well-mixed room as a function of time. Typically, it is also assumed that the contaminant concentration in the incoming flow is zero, and that the loss term denoted by k_{L} is zero. Equation 17.5 then reduces to

$$C(t) = \frac{G}{Q}\left(1 - \exp\left(-\frac{Q}{V} t\right)\right) + C(0)\exp\left(-\frac{Q}{V} t\right) \tag{17.6}$$

The steady-state concentration (i.e., the concentration after infinite time has passed) is given by setting $t = \infty$ in Equation 17.5 and Equation 17.6. We obtain

$$C_{\text{steady state}} = \frac{G + C_{\mathrm{IN}}\, Q}{Q + k_{\mathrm{L}}\, V} \tag{17.7}$$

from Equation 17.5, or

$$C_{\text{steady state}} = \frac{G}{Q} \quad (17.8)$$

from Equation 17.6.

Figure 17.2 shows how concentration varies with time in a workplace modeled as a well-mixed room for four different scenarios. The generation rate is 105 mg/min, the room volume is 240 m^3, and the flow rate is 15 m^3/min. All other parameters are set to zero, as in Equation 17.6. The steady-state concentration is given by Equation 17.7 and is equal to 7 mg/m^3. This is the baseline scenario or Scenario 1 in Figure 17.2.

In Scenario 2, the initial concentration in the room is 10 mg/m^3 and other conditions are the same as those in Scenario 1. Even though the concentration profile starts differently, the steady-state concentration is the same as that in Scenario 1. Thus, the initial state of the system does not affect the steady state.

In Scenario 3, the supply air has a contaminant concentration of 5 mg/m^3, and other conditions are the same as those in Scenario 1. From Equation 17.7, we know that this will affect the steady-state concentration. The steady-state concentration is equal to 12 mg/m^3, which is just the sum of the steady-state concentration predicted for Scenario 1 and the 5 mg/m^3 in the supply air. In Scenario 4, the loss rate constant is equal to 0.1 min^1 and other conditions are the same as those in Scenario 1. This

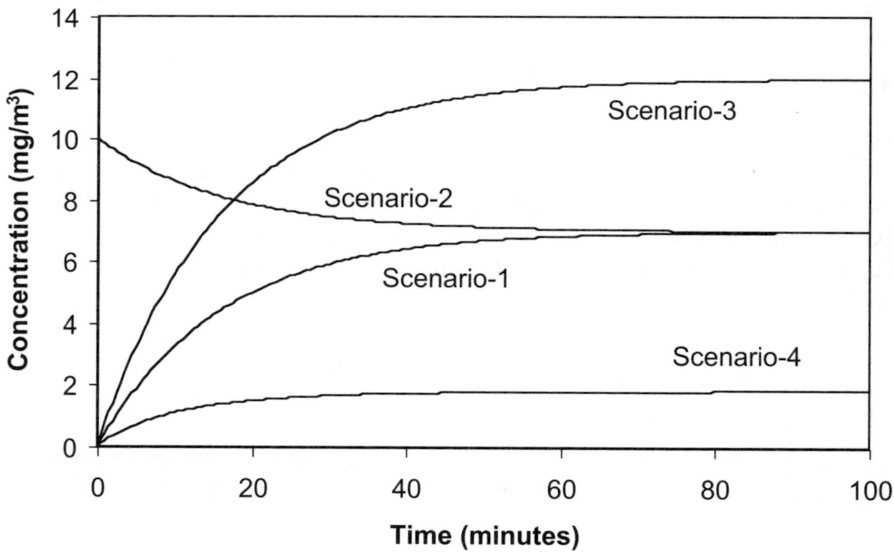

FIGURE 17.2 Predictions of the well-mixed room model for four scenarios. In all four scenarios, G = 105 mg/min, V = 240 m^3, and Q = 15 m^3/min. Scenario 1 corresponds to $k_L = C_{IN} = C(0) = 0$. Scenario 2 corresponds to $C(0)$ = 10 mg/m^3, $k_L = C_{IN} = 0$. Scenario 3 corresponds to C_{IN} = 5 mg/m^3, $k_L = C(0) = 0$. Scenario 4 corresponds to k_L = 0.1 min^1, $C_{IN} = C(0) = 0$.

loss rate is very high (and, admittedly, has been chosen quite arbitrarily for this example) and causes a significant reduction in the steady-state concentration. The steady-state concentration for this scenario is 2.69 mg/m^3.

Equation 17.6 can be used to consider the scenario in which the generation rate is zero and there is an initial nonzero concentration in the room. In this case, Equation 17.6 will only have the second term and will reduce to an exponential decay curve.

$$C(t) = C(0)\exp\left(-\frac{Q}{V}t\right) \tag{17.9}$$

This represents the well-known purging equation. The exponent, Q/V, is termed as the nominal number of air changes per unit time. Typically, the units are air changes per hour (ACH). When $\ln[C(t)]$ is plotted against time, a straight line is obtained with a slope of $-Q/V$.

Equation 17.8 can be easily modified for the case of aerosol exposures. If, for example, the only loss mechanism is aerosol deposition due to gravitational settling, then the steady-state concentration is given by

$$C_{\text{steady state}} = \frac{G}{Q + v_{\text{TS}} A} \tag{17.10}$$

where v_{TS} is the terminal settling velocity of the aerosol particles and A the horizontal cross-sectional area of the workroom (i.e., floor area).

17.3.2 Exponentially Decreasing Contaminant Emission Rate

A variation on the well-mixed room model described earlier is the generation rate not remaining constant, but exponentially decreasing. This is a reasonable model for the generation rate of vapor from a small spill or an off-gassing of residual fumigants such as ethylene oxide and methyl bromide. As the chemical in the spill evaporates, the liquid cools. In turn, the tendency of the chemical to evaporate decreases. Further, as the chemical evaporates, the pool size shrinks. Consequently, the surface area from which the chemical can evaporate decreases. The generation rate at any point in time is assumed to be proportional to the amount of liquid left in the spill, and the amount of liquid left in the spill decreases exponentially.

$$m = m_0 \exp(-\alpha t) \tag{17.11}$$

where m is the amount of liquid in the spill and α the emission rate constant (e.g., in units of per minute). The generation rate is given by

$$G = \alpha m = \alpha m_0 \exp(-\alpha t) \tag{17.12}$$

When the liquid has completely evaporated, the generation rate becomes zero — a fact that is intuitively clear and is also captured by Equation 17.12. A mass balance equation can be set up as before. Assuming that the supply air is contaminant-free and that there are no loss mechanisms other than ventilation,

$$V \cdot dC = \alpha m_0 \exp(-\alpha t) \cdot dt - C(t) \cdot Q \cdot dt \tag{17.13}$$

The solution to this differential equation (assuming that the initial concentration $C(0) = 0$) is given by

$$C(t) = \frac{\alpha m_0}{\alpha V - Q}\left[\exp\left(-\frac{Q}{V}t\right) - \exp(-\alpha t)\right] \tag{17.14}$$

From Equation 17.14, it is clear that the steady-state concentration from a spill is zero. The concentration increases from zero to a maximum and then exponentially decays to zero. The time at which the concentration reaches a peak can be obtained by differentiating Equation 17.14 and setting the first derivative equal to zero.

$$t_{\text{peak}} = \frac{V \ln\left(\frac{\alpha V}{Q}\right)}{\alpha V - Q} \tag{17.15}$$

Again, assuming a spill of 10 g (10,000 mg), and an evaporation rate of $0.15/\text{min}^{-1}$ for the same room and airflow rate as before, we can plot the concentration profile in the room. Figure 17.3 shows this plot.

17.4 THE NEAR-FIELD FAR-FIELD MODEL

Although the well-mixed room model is adequate in many situations, it underestimates the exposure of workers who are close to the contaminant source. To account for this deficiency, a slightly more complicated two-compartment model can be used (Nicas, 1996; Nicas, 2000). Conceptually, it is a small step from a one-compartment to a two-compartment model. The region very near and around the source is modeled as one well-mixed box, the so-called near-field, and the rest of the room is another well-mixed box that completely encloses the near-field box. This box is called the far-field, and there is some amount of air exchange between the two boxes. Figure 17.4 shows the two zones schematically.

The supply and exhaust flow rates are the same and equal to Q (e.g., in units of m^3/min). The airflow rate between the two zones is β (in units of m^3/min). Whereas the determination of Q is straightforward, the determination of β is not so. It is dependent, to some extent, on the dimensions of the near-field zone. One approach that has been proposed is to determine it as the product of the random airspeed (v)

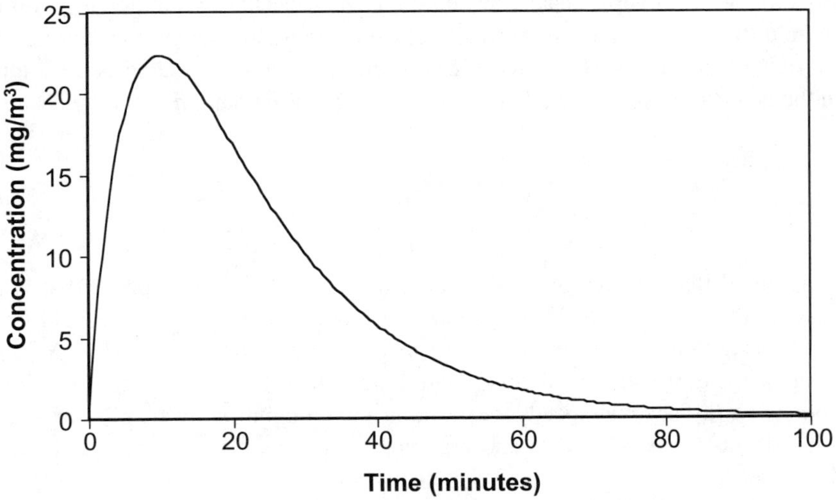

FIGURE 17.3 Air concentration profile for a well-mixed room with a small spill with evaporation. Q = 15 m^3/min, V = 240 m^3, m_0 = 10,000 mg, α = 0.15 min^1.

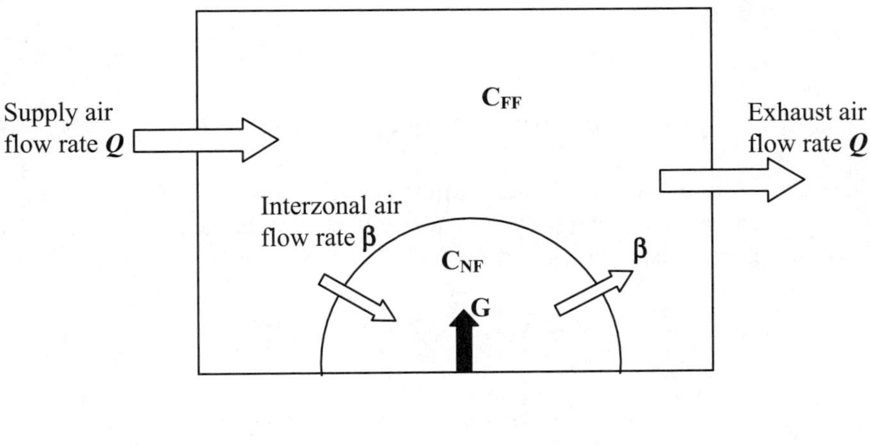

FIGURE 17.4 The near-field and far-field zones.

at the boundary of the near-field and one half of the free surface area (SA) of the near-field.

$$\beta = \frac{1}{2} SA \times v \tag{17.16}$$

The factor of 1/2 arises because the flow rate of β occurs by air flowing into the near-field through one half of the free surface area and air flowing out through the other half of the free surface area. Thus, if the contaminant source is on a table, then the near-field can be modeled as a hemisphere of diameter *d* around the source,

$$\beta = \frac{1}{2}\left(\frac{1}{2}\pi d^2\right) \times v \tag{17.17}$$

It is assumed that air cannot flow through the base of the hemisphere that is the surface of the table. However, the model does not depend on the near-field being modeled as a hemisphere (or any other shape for that matter).

An estimate of v can be obtained with a nondirectional anemometer. In a study of indoor workplaces, airspeeds were found to be lognormally distributed with a median of 3.6 m/min (12 fpm) and a geometric standard deviation of 2 (Baldwin and Maynard, 1998).

For the sake of simplicity, it is assumed that the initial concentration in both zones is equal to zero, the supply air is free of contaminant, and the only removal mechanism for the contaminant is by ventilation. The mass balance equations for the near-field and far-field zones are, respectively,

$$V_{NF}\cdot dC_{NF} = [G\cdot dt + \beta\cdot C_{FF}\cdot dt] - \beta\cdot C_{NF}\cdot dt \tag{17.18}$$

$$V_{FF}\cdot dC_{FF} = \beta\cdot C_{NF}\cdot dt - [\beta\cdot C_{FF}\cdot dt + Q\cdot C_{FF}\cdot dt] \tag{17.19}$$

where the subscripts NF and FF refer to the near- and far-fields. This gives a pair of coupled differential equations that can be solved to yield the near-field and far-field concentrations as a function of time. The solutions are of the form

$$C_{NF} = \alpha_1 \times \exp(\lambda_1 t) + \alpha_2 \times \exp(\lambda_2 t) \tag{17.20}$$

$$C_{FF} = \alpha_3 \times \exp(\lambda_1 t) + \alpha_4 \times \exp(\lambda_2 t) \tag{17.21}$$

where the parameters λ_1, λ_2, α_1, α_2, α_3, and α_4 are functions of V_{NF}, V_{FF}, Q, and β. The full solutions and a more detailed exposition of the model are presented in Nicas (2000). In this chapter, we shall only consider the steady-state concentrations in the two zones that are given by

$$C_{NF,SS} = \frac{G}{Q} + \frac{G}{\beta} \tag{17.22}$$

$$C_{FF,SS} = \frac{G}{Q} \tag{17.23}$$

Thus, the near-field steady-state concentration is greater than the far-field steady-state concentration. It is clear that if $\beta \leq Q$, then $C_{NF,SS} \geq 2\ C_{FF,SS}$. In general, Q increases relative to β as the room size increases. In turn, the model predicts relatively higher exposure intensity near the emission source compared with the well-mixed room model. Therefore, using the well-mixed room model leads to a more substantial underestimate of exposure near the source as the room size (and Q) increases. Although the two-zone model improves this situation, it comes at the cost of requiring knowledge of the interzonal flow rate.

Consider the same room as in the previous examples, where the generation rate is 105 mg/min, the room volume is 240 m^3, and the flow rate is 15 m^3/min. But let us assume that the contaminant source is on a table, and the worker is at an arm's length from the source (i.e., the radius of the hemisphere is ~0.8 m). Thus, the volume of the near-field zone is $V_{NF} = \frac{2}{3} \cdot \pi \cdot r^3 = 1.1 m^3$. The room volume is equal to the volume of the far-field. Strictly speaking, we need to subtract the near-field volume from the room volume to obtain the far-field volume. However, the near-field volume is so small compared with the room volume that we can ignore this correction. It is assumed that the random air velocity is 3.6 m/min, which is the median airspeed in workplaces as estimated by Baldwin and Maynard (1998). The value of β is calculated using Equation 17.16 to be ~7.25 m^3/min.

Figure 17.5 shows the concentration profile for the near- and far-fields for this scenario. The far-field steady-state concentration (7 mg/m^3) is the same as that in Figure 17.3 for the one-box well-mixed room scenario. The near-field steady-state concentration is ~21.5 mg/m^3, roughly three times greater than the far-field concentration.

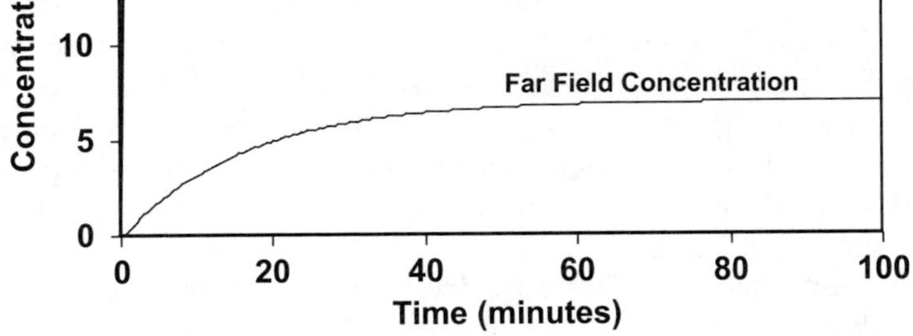

FIGURE 17.5 Predictions of the near-field far-field model for G = 105 mg/min, V_{FF} = 240 m^3, Q = 15 m^3/min, V_{NF} = 1.1 m^3, β = 7.25 m^3/min.

17.5 EMPIRICAL EXPOSURE MODELS

Whereas the models described above are derived from fundamental physical principles (albeit with simplifying assumptions), there is another class of models that is purely empirical. These models use descriptive information about the jobs and processes in a structured fashion to estimate relative exposures.

One example of this type of model is the EASE (Estimation and Assessment of Substance Exposure) model developed by the Health and Safety Executive in the U.K. (EASE, 1997). The EASE model was developed for modeling exposures across a wide range of scenarios encountered in the workplace. Although the model considers both inhalation and dermal exposures, the discussion here is limited to inhalation exposures. The model focuses on exposures resulting from normal use of substances in the workplace and does not deal with spills, loss of containment, or breakdown of normally reliable control mechanisms. For each category of substances (e.g., gases and vapors, and dusts, which are further divided into fibrous and nonfibrous categories), logical criteria have been developed to classify exposures into a limited number of categories. An expert system has been developed that analyzes each exposure scenario and provides an exposure range.

For example, for gases and vapors, the types of exposures possible are based on: (1) *volatility* of the chemical, (2) *use patterns*, and (3) *patterns of control.* Volatility, or the tendency to become airborne, has six levels: (1) gas, (2) liquid or solid, high vapor pressure, (3) liquid or solid, medium vapor pressure, (4) liquid or solid, low vapor pressure, (5) liquid or solid, very low vapor pressure, and (6) aerosol. Each of these levels is further divided into logic trees to determine the tendency of the chemical to become airborne. The use pattern has four levels: (1) closed system, (2) within a matrix, (3) nondispersive, and (4) widely dispersive. The pattern of control has six levels: (1) full containment, (2) local exhaust ventilation, (3) segregation, (4) direct handling with dilution ventilation, and (5) direct handling. The combinations of these three criteria lead to 120 possible exposure scenarios. For dusts, in addition to the three criteria described above, the model also considers the particle size distribution and the type of dust (fibrous or nonfibrous) in estimating exposures.

For each of the exposure scenarios, the model predicts an exposure range as the output. For example, in the case of vapors, the lowest exposure range is 0 to 0.1 ppm and the highest is greater than 1000 ppm. The ranges were obtained from the U.K. National Exposure Database, which contains exposure-monitoring data from a wide variety of industries and industrial processes. Although the data were obtained for a variety of reasons (e.g., compliance, exposure control) and thus might be biased, the expert system accounts for these biases in assigning exposure ranges. The EASE model is still in the process of being validated by users in several countries.

Cherrie and Schneider (1999) have developed a model of the exposure process based on characterizing emission from sources in the workplace, the dispersal of the contaminant in the work environment, and the interaction of the workers with the dispersed contaminant. The active emission from the source comprises the intrinsic emission of the contaminant, the method of handling, and the efficiency of any local controls, e.g., local exhaust ventilation. Intrinsic emission, ε_i, is the potential of the substance to become airborne, and depends on the physical characteristics of the contaminant such as the vapor pressure for gases and vapors or particle size distribution for aerosols. The handling method determines the amount of energy being supplied to the substance, h. For example, the height from which a dust is being dropped will be a factor in the amount of dust becoming airborne. Similarly, the amounts of dust generated by sawing a log of wood and by stacking wooden logs are different. Local exhaust ventilation reduces the exposure according to its efficiency, η_{lev}. Thus, the active emission is expressed as

$$\varepsilon_a = \varepsilon_i \cdot h \cdot (1 - \eta_{lev}) \tag{17.24}$$

In addition, fugitive sources may cause passive emissions, ε_p. These might be due to sources that are not controlled by local exhaust ventilation. The model also accounts for the fraction of time that the source is actively emitting t_a, and the efficiency of personal protective equipment, η_{ppe}. Thus, the exposure from a source close to the worker is given by C_{NF}, where

$$C_{NF} = \left(\varepsilon_i \cdot h \cdot (1 - \eta_{lev}).t_a + \varepsilon_p\right).(1 - \eta_{ppe}) \tag{17.25}$$

The contribution of sources that are far away from the worker is affected by general exhaust ventilation in the workplace. This contribution is expressed in a manner very similar to Equation 17.25 as follows:

$$C_{FF} = \left(\varepsilon_{i,FF} \cdot h_{FF} \cdot (1 - \eta_{lev,FF}).t_{a,FF} + \varepsilon_p\right).(1 - \eta_{ppe}) \cdot d_{gv} \tag{17.26}$$

where the subscript FF refers to the far-field, and the term d_{gv} refers to the dilution effect caused by general exhaust ventilation.

If a worker performs a number of tasks during a work shift, each of which can be modeled according to Equation 17.25 and Equation 17.26, then the exposure of the worker is given by

$$E = \sum_{j=1}^{n} \left(C_{NF,j} + C_{FF,j}\right) \cdot \Delta_j \tag{17.27}$$

where the subscript j refers to the jth task, and Δ_j is the fraction of time in a workshift spent in the jth task.

Numerical values for each of the parameters of the model need to be provided. Because these are typically unavailable, subjective judgments are used to arrive at the values of these parameters. For example, a logarithmic scale can be chosen for each of the input parameters. Cherrie and Schneider (1999) provide guidance for selecting parameter values (see Table 17.1). The values in Table 17.1 are nondimen-

TABLE 17.1
Example of Assigning Numerical Values to Input Parameters for the Empirical Exposure Model of Equation 17.27

Parameter Values	Description	Meaning
Intrinsic emission, ε_i		
10	Very high	Very dusty
3	High	Dusty material
1	Moderate	Some dust produced
0.3	Low	Little dust produced
0.1	Very low	Very little dust produced
0	None	Contaminant is contained
Handling, *h*		
10	Very high	High-energy crushing
3	High	Breaking, dropping 0.5 to 2 meters
1	Moderate	Dropping less than 0.5 meters
0.3	Low	Lifting, stacking
0.1	Very low	Careful lifting
0	None	No handling or processing
Local Exhaust, (1 η_{lev})		
1	None	No local controls
0.3	Some controls	Local ventilation installed
0.1	Effective controls	Well-designed and maintained LEV

Source: Cherrie, J.W. and Schneider, T. (1999), Validation of a new method for structured subjective assessment of past concentrations, *Ann. Occup. Hyg.*, 43: 235–245.

sional, and hence the exposure estimate will also be nondimensional. Thus, the model output will be a relative exposure. If actual monitoring data exist on specific tasks or jobs, then they can be used to convert the nondimensional exposures into actual exposure values by appropriate scaling.

17.6 MONTE CARLO SIMULATION ANALYSIS IN MODELING

The discussion of the various models in this chapter has tacitly assumed that the input parameters are known precisely. Thus, if there is a given set of input parameters, then there is one value of the output for the model. However, complete and precise knowledge of the values of the input parameters (or anything else, for that matter) is impossible. The exposure determinants (the input parameters) are known with some degree of uncertainty. Therefore, selecting one value for each of the input parameters is not advisable. It is better to find a way to represent the uncertainty in the input parameters and consider how this uncertainty leads to uncertainty in the model output. Monte Carlo sampling analysis is a powerful technique for propagating the uncertainties in the model inputs to determine the uncertainties in the model outputs. It can provide insights into the relative importance to the model conclusions of the various assumptions and uncertainties in the model inputs. It can help in deciding whether it is worthwhile to gather more information to reduce uncertainty. It also helps avoid disputes over the best value chosen for point estimates, because the full range of possible results is considered.

The conceptual basis for error propagation can be illustrated using a simple example of a model where the input and output parameters are discrete variables. Let y be a function of x_1 and x_2.

$$y = x_1 + x_2 \tag{17.28}$$

Both x_1 and x_2 can each take only one of three possible values. But these values have different probabilities associated with them. Thus, x_1 can only take the values of 0.3, 1.0, and 1.7 with probabilities of 0.2, 0.6, and 0.2, respectively. The probabilities add up to 1.0. Similarly, x_2 can only take the values of 0.5, 1.0, and 1.5 with probabilities of 0.33, 0.34, and 0.33, respectively, adding up to 1.0. To investigate the possible interactions between the effects of all the inputs at various levels, one has to look at all possible combinations of input values. This is done by constructing a *probability tree* as shown in Figure 17.6. The uncertainty in the inputs can be expressed as a discrete probability distribution. There will be probabilities attached to each branch of the probability tree. Thus, y can take nine possible values. The probability of each value is obtained by the product of the probabilities of the two input variables. Thus, y can take a value of 0.8 only if $x_1 = 0.3$ ($p = 0.2$) and $x_2 = 0.5$ ($p = 0.33$). Thus, the probability associated with $y = 0.8$, P, is 0.2×0.33, i.e., 0.066. The probabilities of all the possible values that y can take also add up to 1.0. Figure 17.6 shows the values of the input variables and their associated probabilities.

Thus, Figure 17.6 shows how the uncertainty in the two input parameters gets reflected in the uncertainty in the model output. Although the example is illustrative, it does show the limitation of using such an approach when the input variables are continuous or when there are more than two variables that can make more than three values each. In such cases, the probability tree will have an infinite number of nodes and branches.

One way out of this quandary is to select a moderate-sized, random sample of scenarios for evaluation. This is called Monte Carlo sampling. Each scenario is generated by selecting a branch at a node according to its assigned probability. The branch values are generated from the underlying continuous probability distribution. The accuracy of Monte Carlo sampling can be improved by increasing the sample size.

Jayjock (1997) has identified two sources of uncertainties in the determinants of worker exposure. The first source is the natural variability of these parameters, and the second is the lack of knowledge about the parameters. The first kind of uncertainty can be described by sampling statistics, which has been discussed in earlier chapters. This uncertainty can be expressed using normal or lognormal distributions (for most occupational measurements). The second kind of uncertainty

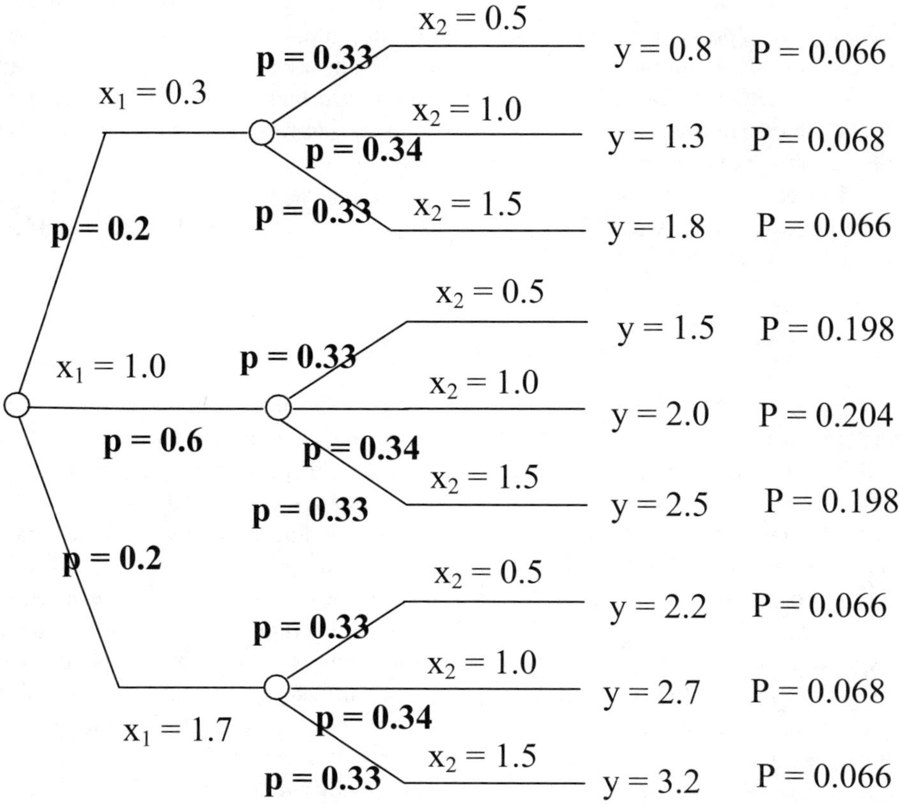

FIGURE 17.6 Propagation of uncertainty through a model with two discrete variables as input parameters.

represents a more fundamental ignorance about the parameter, and is usually the dominant kind of uncertainty. A variety of other distributional shapes can be used to represent this uncertainty. Uniform distributions (where every value between an upper and lower limit is equiprobable) and triangular distributions (with a minimum, maximum, and modal value) are examples of distributions used to represent such uncertainties. Figure 17.7 shows the shapes of these commonly used distributions.

If there are some available measurements for an input parameter, e.g., the ventilation flow rate through a work area, then one can estimate the mean and standard deviation of these measurements and represent the distribution of the parameter using a normal or lognormal distribution. The measurements obtained are assumed to be from an underlying distribution of airflow rates. If, however, there is very little or no information regarding a parameter, then the probability distribution is a reflection of the subjective state of uncertainty or lack of knowledge on the part of the assessor. For example, if one were asked to estimate the airflow rate (air changes per hour) through a room in the absence of any measurements, then an "expert" can estimate it to be between 5 and 9 air changes per hour, with each value being equally likely. But there is no population of airflow measurements from which

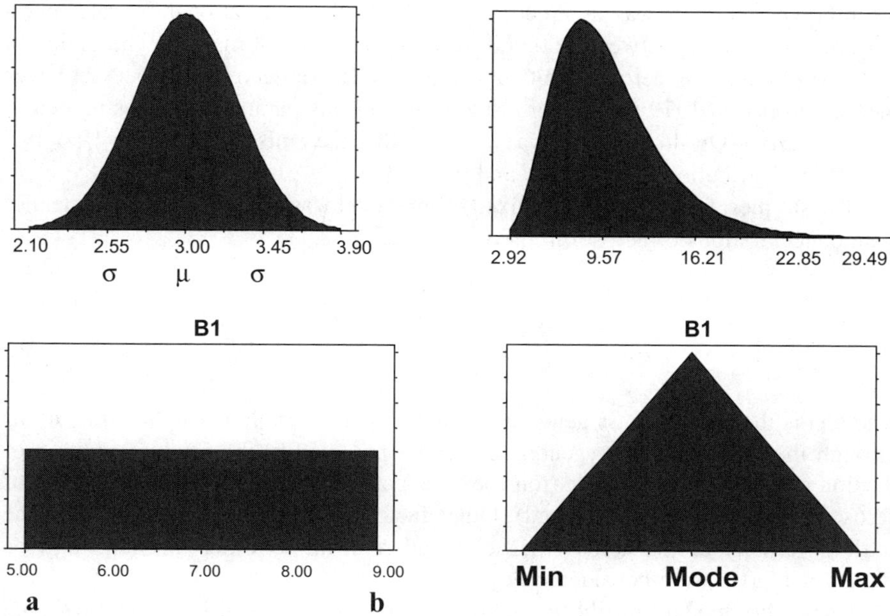

FIGURE 17.7 Examples of probability distributions commonly used in exposure modeling. Clockwise from top left: normal, lognormal, triangular, and uniform distributions.

samples have been obtained. The estimate is subjective and can differ from person to person.

Thus, each input parameter is represented as a probability distribution. A large number of independent sets (say, 100,000) of input parameters are obtained by sampling randomly from their respective probability distributions. For each set of input parameters, a model output is predicted using the model. Thus, 100,000 values of the output are obtained, which can be plotted as a probability distribution (e.g., a histogram). This represents the uncertainty in the model output.

The following example, from Ramachandran (2001), relating to the reconstruction of historical exposures to airborne nickel aerosol in a smelter, illustrates the use of Monte Carlo sampling in exposure modeling. Little data exist that characterize exposures that occurred several decades ago (1960 to 1978). However, modeling using process information can be utilized to reconstruct air concentrations and exposures. Such process information is sometimes available, even though air-monitoring data may not be available. This includes data on production rates, ventilation, and emission factors. Although these data were not available on an annual basis, it seemed reasonable to use the few measurements that were available from some years to make reasonable assumptions about the values of these parameters for the other years. For the year of interest, 1965, the nominal production of Bessemer matte, an intermediate product in the manufacture of nickel, was 330,800 tons. This is a measurement that is, in fact, available on an annual basis from company records. Although no ventilation rate information was available for 1965, there was one ventilation survey carried out in 1970 that estimated a net flow rate of 160,000

m^3/min. Therefore, it was assumed that in 1965, the ventilation flow rate had a uniform distribution between 100,000 m^3/min and 200,000 m^3/min. The emission factor (kilograms of aerosol emitted per ton of Bessemer matte processed) was measured once in 1979 in a rather crude way, and this parameter was estimated to be 0.19 kg/ton. On this basis, it was assumed that the emission factor in 1965 had a uniform distribution between 0.1 and 0.3 kg/ton.

The simplest form of the well-mixed room model was used for predicting steady-state concentrations of aerosol in the workplace.

$$C_{\text{steady state}} = \frac{G}{Q} = \frac{PR \times EF}{Q} \tag{17.29}$$

where G is the aerosol mass generation rate and Q is the volumetric flow rate of air through the workplace. The generation rate is modeled as the product of the production rate of Bessemer matte (tons per year) and the emission factor (kilogram of aerosol per ton of matte produced). Other factors, such as the contribution of the settling velocity of the aerosol particles and removal by other mechanisms (see Equation 17.10), were considered negligible.

Using this model and the probability distributions described above, a Monte Carlo simulation was carried out. By randomly sampling from their probability distributions, 100,000 sets of the three input parameters (PR, EF, and Q) were obtained. For each set of input parameters, the steady-state concentration was calculated using the model. The histogram of these 100,000 output values represented the variability or uncertainty in the estimate of the steady-state concentration of aerosol in the nickel smelter in 1965. Figure 17.8 shows this process.

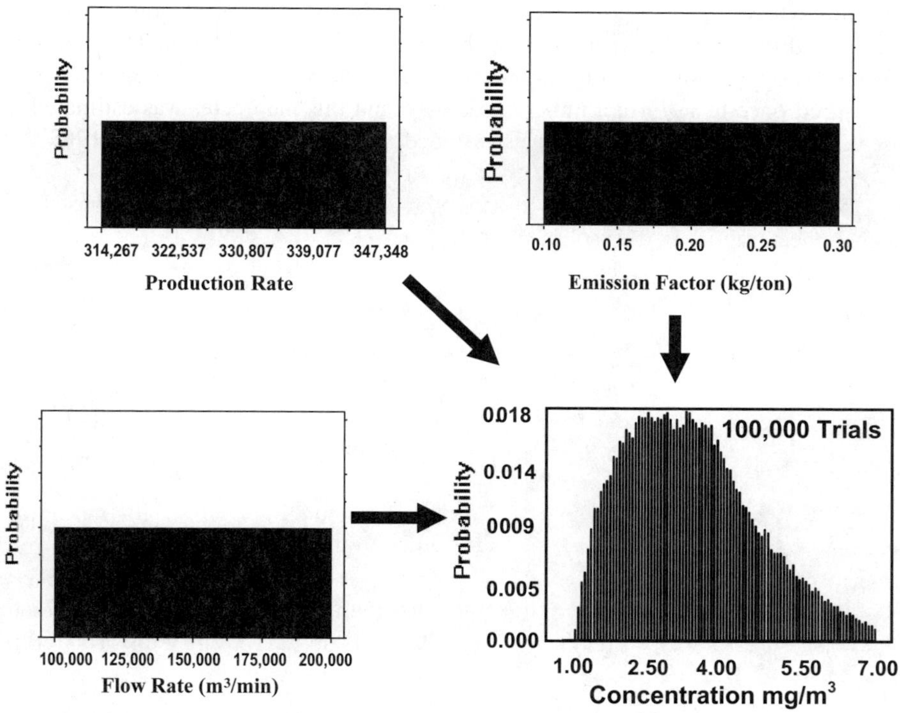

FIGURE 17.8 Monte Carlo sampling from the probability distributions for the ventilation rate, production rate, and emission factor to estimate the probability distribution of the steady state aerosol concentration in a nickel smelter. (From Ramachandran, G., 2001, Retrospective exposure assessment using Bayesian methods, *Ann. Occup. Hyg.,* 45(8): 651–667.)

18 Reconstructing Historical Exposures

18.1 INTRODUCTION

There are many documented cases (e.g., asbestos, silica, and radon daughters) of a causal relationship between the health risk for disease and long-term exposure to airborne environmental contaminants. The biologically effective dose in such instances is related to the temporal history of an individual's exposure, the kinetics of uptake and clearance of the inhaled material, and some measure of the harmfulness or potency of the contaminant. All of these are time-dependent quantities, and the integrated dose at time t since the start of the exposure may be expressed in a general form as

$$\text{Dose} = \int_0^T f\{E(t), R(t), G(t)\}\mathrm{d}t \tag{18.1}$$

Here, $E(t)$ is the exposure history derived from measurements of exposure concentration. $R(t)$ is a function describing the retention of the inhaled contaminant in the body. For example, retention in the lung tissue is well-documented in lung deposition models (ICRP, 1994) and toxicological data. Finally, $G(t)$ describes the time-dependent potency of the contaminant to cause harm to the tissue (Vincent et al., 1988; Vincent and Donaldson, 1990). For example, in the case of radioactive particulate matter, the potency to cause harm is related to the ionizing radiation of a well-defined type that derives from radioactive decay. Most exposure-based epidemiology assumes that cumulative exposure, i.e., $\int_0^T E(t)dt$, is a good measure of dose. It is important to realize that this is an approximation that is only valid when $R(t)$ and $G(t)$ are unity. Unlike simpler models that calculate dose as the cumulative exposure in which each exposure is equally weighted, the model in Equation 18.1 gives greater weight to the effect of earlier exposures through the parameter $G(t)$. Thus, it is reasonable to expect that the deposited particles that stay a long time in the lung from earlier exposures have a greater impact on the health outcome than particles deposited more recently. In this manner, exposure histories can be used in conjunction with pharmacokinetic and pharmacodynamic models to obtain better estimates of biologically relevant doses to organs or tissues.

The above model underscores the importance of having exposure data expressed as a function of time. Although long-term prospective epidemiological studies can be very useful in determining the relationship between exposure and disease, this is not a luxury that can often be afforded by industries and standards-setting bodies, which have to act on information available currently. Therefore, to establish robust quantitative dose–response relationships for epidemiological purposes, it is vital to reconstruct past exposures of individuals or populations as functions of time over the periods of interest.

The above model underscores the importance of the toxicokinetics of the pollutant in the human body (Rappaport, 1991). For chronic toxicants, health effects are related to the body burden accumulated over long periods of time, typically of the order of several years or even decades. Transient spikes in exposures over a time period of a shift or less are not significant contributors to the overall body burden. For such chronic toxicants, the biological effects, and therefore the risk of disease, will be related to the arithmetic mean exposure and time that determine body burden. Most of the rest of this chapter is devoted to the problem of estimating exposure as a function of time, $E(t)$. In the last few sections, the problem of estimating the functions $R(t)$ and $G(t)$ will be addressed.

18.2 EXPOSURE RECONSTRUCTION

18.2.1 The Exposure Data Matrix

Because the goal of retrospective exposure assessment is to develop estimates of dose for use in epidemiological studies, it is clear that the estimation of exposure histories (i.e., exposure as a function of time) of various job classes is critical. These job exposure histories are then combined with worker employment histories to obtain exposure histories for individual workers. Figure 18.1 shows how exposure histories are used within an epidemiological study to estimate a dose–response relationship.

The *exposure data matrix* shown in the top left of Figure 18.1 is a simple way of organizing exposure data that allows describing, analyzing, estimating, and linking exposure data to workers more explicitly (Seixas and Checkoway, 1995). The exposure data matrix shown in Figure 18.1 is quite simple and has only two dimensions — job title and time. However, the matrix can have many dimensions such as plant, type of process or machine, and availability of exposure controls. In instances where the exposures to multiple chemicals need to be accounted for, a separate dimension for each chemical of interest might be included. Other information, such as production and ventilation records, modeling estimates, and subjective judgments of exposures made by plant occupational hygienists, can also be included as separate dimensions. Ideally, one would prefer highly specific dimensions with all pieces of information included, so that the exposure estimates are as precise and free of bias as possible.

18.2.2 Measurement Errors in Exposures

There is a paucity of historical exposure data for many occupational air contaminants — with exceptions such as those in the coal mining industry (Hurley et al., 1982, 1987) — which is compounded by the long latency periods associated with the

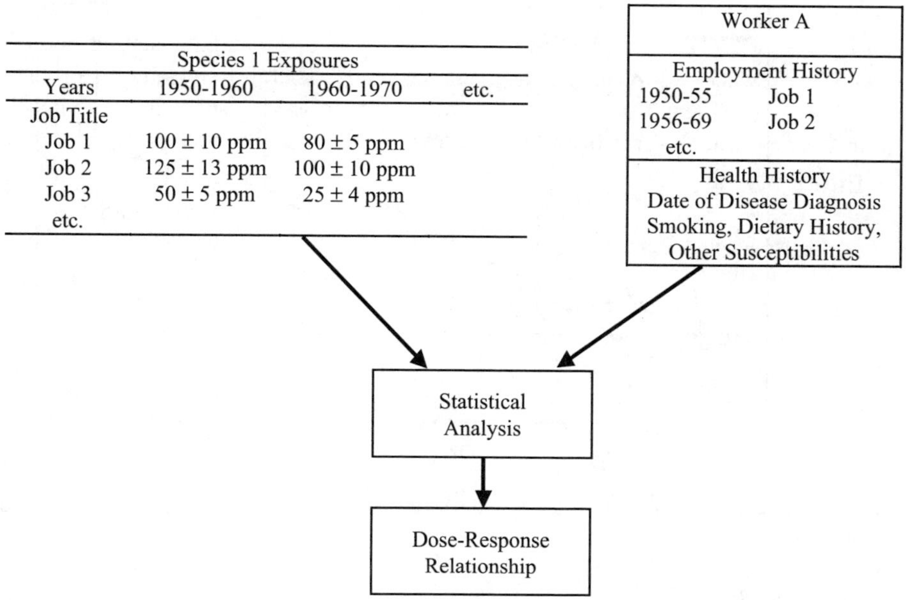

FIGURE 18.1 Using exposure histories in epidemiological studies.

health effects. Therefore, the calculation of a dose using a model similar to Equation 18.1, although most desirable, is often not feasible. In many cases, surrogates for the dose have been used, and these get progressively cruder as the available information gets more sparse. As mentioned earlier, cumulative exposures, $\int_0^T E(t)dt$, have been used when the pharmacokinetics of the contaminant are not understood. When exposure data are also sparse, cumulative exposure surrogates such as the duration of employment in an industry are used, i.e., $\int_0^T dt$. Simple categorization of jobs as exposed vs. nonexposed, or semiquantitative estimates such as categorizing high, moderate, or low exposures, have also been used. These surrogates do not allow for the quantitative evaluation of health risks.

In Chapter 16, the effects of measurement error on the dose–response relationship was described. Whereas classical (random) errors tend to attenuate the slope of the dose–response curve, Berkson errors increase the variance in the slope. Using a surrogate will bias the relationship between the dose and effect. Figure 18.2 shows these various effects. The solid line shows the true (but unknown) relationship between the dose and health effect. If a study has only random errors, the observed slope of the dose–response curve is less than the true slope. If a study has only Berkson errors, the slope is not attenuated, but the error bars around the estimates are increased. Finally, if a study uses a biased estimate of dose with no random error, the slope is unchanged, but the intercept is shifted. As mentioned in Chapter 16, most epidemiological studies have all three types of errors.

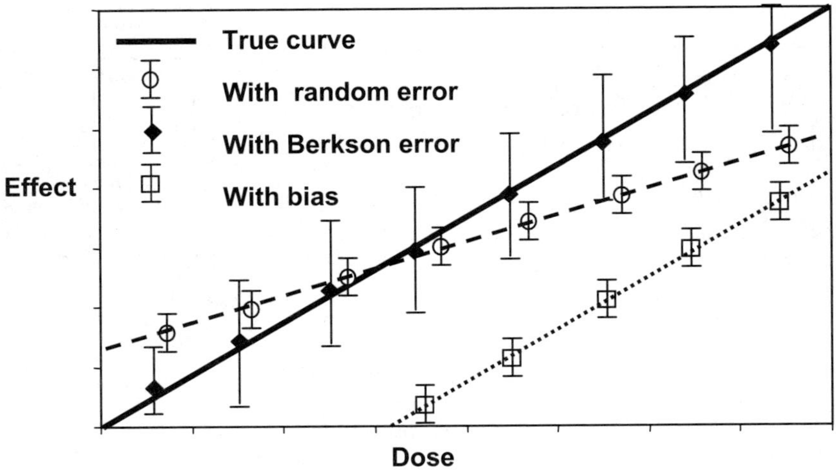

FIGURE 18.2 Effects of random and Berson errors and bias on a hypothetical dose–response relationship.

18.2.3 Sparse Data

The process of reconstructing exposure over long periods is fraught with uncertainties and subjective biases: changes in measurement criteria over time, changes in instruments and analysis methods, and changes in workplace practices, inventories, industrial processes, and plant-specific ventilation patterns, which may modify exposures. Measurements of personal exposures are, at best, temporally sporadic, and for many periods, not even available.

As an example, consider the data set for airborne nickel exposures obtained from one specific area and for one specific job title in a nickel smelter, shown in Table 18.1. Konimeter measurements of particle count (in units of particles per cubic centimeter or ppcc) were the norm in the early years; instantaneous measurements were obtained by drawing 5 ml of air from the breathing zones of the workers and impacting the particles onto an adhesive-coated glass slide. In the early 1970s, there was a move away from the count to a mass-concentration metric measured using a Hi-Vol area sampler. These gravimetric measurements used a sampling flow rate of 1400 to 3500 l/min for ~3 h. In the late 1970s, personal sampling over 8-h time-weighted average (TWA) assessed exposures to total nickel using 37-mm filters at a flow rate of 2 l/min, which were then analyzed by mass spectrometry. The most recent measurements for nickel aerosol (not shown in the table) are expressed in terms of the inhalable fraction of the aerosol, and the concentrations are reported for different chemical species of nickel. Thus, the exposure metric (particle number concentrations in particles per unit volume of air; mass concentration of overall dust, mg/m^3; and concentration of nickel), and the strategy and samplers used have changed over a period of several decades.

At the same time, Table 18.1 also illustrates the sparseness of the data set. The data shown are the arithmetic mean exposures together with the number of samples (in **bold**) and 95% confidence intervals (in *italics*). It is important to note that the

TABLE 18.1
Historical Mean Exposures for One Homogeneous Exposure Group of Workers in a Nickel Smelter

Period	Konimeter (ppcc)	Hi-Vol (mg of dust/m³)	Hi-Vol (mg of Ni/m³)	Personal (mg of dust/m³)	Personal (mg of Ni/m³)
1956–1963	959	—	—	—	—
	(24)				
	(765–1153)				
1964–1966	561	17	9.8	—	—
	(15)	**(1)**	**(1)**		
	(458–664)				
1967–1971	623	16.5	6.53	—	—
	(27)	**(2)**	**(2)**		
	(530–716)	*(0–98)*	*(0–55.8)*		
1972–1975	529	53.1	37.2	—	—
	(18)	**(27)**	**(11)**		
	(456–602)	*(6.9–99.3)*	*(11.9–62.4)*		
1976–1979	—	1.31	—	1.31	4.35
		(17)		**(11)**	**(11)**
		(0.79 –1.83)		*(0–27.8)*	*(0–10.4)*

Note: Bold parenthetical numbers indicate the number of samples, and italics indicate the 95% confidence intervals for the data reported

original raw measurements are no longer available and that only such summary data are available. Thus, over 7 years from 1964 to 1971, there are only 3 Hi-Vol measurements. The very small number of measurements also points out the inconsistencies in the data set. For example, the trends in the mean values of the konimeter measurements are not the same as the trends in the Hi-Vol measurements.

For an epidemiological study, all these different measurements and metrics need to be converted to a single, truly health-related index. Exposures to airborne nickel have been linked to sinus, nasal, and lung cancer. Thus, the inhalable fraction, defining all particles that can enter the body through the nose and/or mouth during breathing, is the most appropriate exposure metric. Therefore, it is necessary to obtain conversion factors to convert all these measurements into inhalable nickel concentration. These are typically obtained from side-by-side comparisons of these instruments in various environments that have very specific aerosol size distributions. Although it may be possible to obtain the instruments to carry out such experiments, recreating the process that created a specific aerosol size distribution may be quite problematic. Thus, there will be considerable uncertainty in the conversion factors as well. Additionally, in many instances, there may not be a direct conversion factor from one type of measurement to the modern exposure metric.

For example, in the case of nickel, there is no conversion factor between konimeter counts and the inhalable-mass concentration. Therefore, the konimeter particle counts obtained in the breathing zone of the worker at a given workstation were first converted to a personal respirable-mass concentration value. Respirable-mass concentration values were then converted to a personal inhalable-mass concentration value. Side-by-side comparisons of instantaneous konimeter measurements and real-time, 1-min average respirable-aerosol concentrations measured by a GCA respirable-dust monitor (Marple and Rubow, 1978) were performed at 3 different times in 12 separate locations in the nickel industry during the period 1976 to 1977. An average conversion factor of 0.0021 mg m^{-3}/ppcc, with lower and upper bounds of 0.00059 and 0.0063 mg m^{-3}/ppcc, was obtained from a linear regression fit to the data. This is comparable to conversion factors of between 0.0002 mg m^{-3}/ppcc to 0.003 mg m^{-3}/ppcc obtained by Verma et al. (1989) for hard-rock miners in Ontario. Conversion factors for the ratio of respirable dust to personal inhalable dust were obtained from measurements of particle size distributions using a personal cascade impactor (Tsai, 1995). From these distributions the respirable and inhalable masses were determined, and an average ratio of respirable to inhalable of 0.1 was obtained with a standard deviation of 0.02. The two conversion factors, with their associated uncertainties, were then used multiplicatively to obtain the conversion factor for konimeter readings to inhalable-mass concentration. The uncertainty in the overall conversion factor can be obtained by a Monte Carlo simulation procedure, as described in Chapter 17.

Due to these uncertainties and constraints, it is important to develop a systematic framework to estimate historical levels of exposure over a time span that has epidemiological significance, and analyze assumptions built into these estimates.

18.2.4 Exposure Variability

Due to the sparseness of available exposure-monitoring data, it becomes necessary to classify the workers who have similar exposures into groups called similar exposure groups or SEGs. As discussed extensively in Chapter 15 and Chapter 16, an important assumption in such a classification is that the workers within each SEG have similar exposure distributions; specifically, that each worker's exposure profile is very similar to every other worker. In many retrospective exposure assessment studies, this classification is based primarily on shared characteristics. Corn and Esmen (1979) proposed a classification based on work similarity (similar profiles of job tasks), similarity of hazardous agents (similar chemicals to which they are exposed), and environmental similarity (ventilation characteristics, processes, etc.). Such a classification assumes that the variability in exposure is primarily due to within-worker variability. However, if individual workers have exposures that are significantly different (high between-worker variability), then the differences in individual work practices in performing the jobs and tasks are driving the exposure variability. In such a case, the classification scheme based on observed workplace and work-practice similarities may not be able to detect these differences. Thus, workers in two different SEGs may have overlapping exposure distributions that, in turn, may cause misclassification of exposures. This may cause errors in the relationship between exposures and health effects. As we have discussed in the previous chapters, determining the within- and between-worker components of variability requires multiple measurements of exposure from each worker in an SEG. As Table 18.1 illustrated, replicate measurements are not available in historical data sets. Without replicate data, estimates of the components of variability need to be obtained from smaller pilot studies or interviews of veteran workers about variability in the task compositions of job titles.

18.2.5 Imputation of Missing Values by Interpolation and Extrapolation

Once the exposure data matrix is generated from the available exposure data for specific job categories and years, the missing cells need to be estimated. The missing data can be estimated using various imputation methods. For example, for a job category with data missing for certain years, simple linear interpolation can be used. The same approach can be used to linearly extrapolate from the last available data point to all previous or successive years.

Rice et al. (1997) used imputed marginal means calculated using a stepwise procedure, starting from a baseline of available measurements on industry/company/site/job. Next, it was assumed that, within a given industry and company, the same job across multiple sites had similar exposures. From this assumption, a marginal median of the measurements across all sites for a particular industry/company/job was computed. This allowed some additional missing cells to be estimated. Next, the following were computed in sequence and, at each step, accounted for some more missing data: (1) marginal medians of the measurements across all sites/jobs for a particular industry/company; (2) marginal medians of the measurements across all company/sites for a particular industry/job; (3) marginal medians of the measurements across all companies/sites/jobs for a particular industry; and finally (4) marginal medians of the measurements across all companies/sites/jobs for the usual industry. Rice et al. (1997) found that the highest risk estimates resulted from the most complete data set. In the partial data sets, there was nondifferential misclassification that resulted in lower risk estimates. It is clear that missing data significantly affect the resultant dose–response relationship.

A more sophisticated approach using statistical modeling has also been proposed, in which the dimensions of the exposure data matrix are the explanatory variables, and the exposure estimate is the dependent variable. For example, Hallock et al. (1994) used a linear model and carried out an analysis of variance (ANOVA) to evaluate the effects of time period, machining operation, machining fluid, plant, and other variables on machining-fluid concentration. The model has the simple form:

$$Y_{ijklm} = \alpha + \sum_i \beta_i T_i + \sum_j \beta_j \, Operation_j + \sum_k \beta_k \, Fluid_k + \sum_l \beta_l \, Plant_l + \varepsilon_m \tag{18.2}$$

Here, T_i denotes the time periods, $Operation_j$ the various machining operations, $Fluid_k$ the various machining fluids, $Plant_l$ the various plants, and ε_m the residual error. The parameter estimates (βs) obtained from the ANOVA were used to estimate concentrations for operations, fluids, and plants for which no sampling data were available. Because the parameters are estimated by linear least-squares regression, more data points than variables are needed. Other examples of such statistical modeling approaches for exposure data matrices are provided by Seixas and Checkoway (1995).

Hornung et al. (1994) have developed statistical models in which the explanatory variables are exposure determinants such as year, job, department, and type of product, as well as engineering, administrative, and process controls of various types. The dependent variable is the exposure level. The model was developed using one half of the available data set and then used to predict the other half. The predictions were finally compared with the actual data in a validation step.

18.2.6 Using Knowledge of Exposure Modifiers

When there is a lack of available exposure data over time, other sources of information regarding the workplace may aid exposure reconstruction. Esmen (1979) proposed a method to estimate historical exposures by making adjustments to current data. These adjustments or extrapolations are based on changes in the process, physical parameters of the agent, and use of personal protective devices. However, subjective judgments would strongly influence these adjustments. Schneider and colleagues identified *universal exposure modifiers* that mediate exposure in all workplaces (Schneider et al., 1991). These exposure modifiers can be used as input parameters to a deterministic exposure model, and historic exposure data can be used to adjust the model parameters.

These modifiers are: changes in the industrial process (e.g., change in smelting temperature, ore feed composition, etc.), installation of pollution control equipment in the plant, changes in ventilation patterns, changes in work practices, and use of personal protective equipment. When used to represent a change in exposure preceding a period for which exposure measurements are available, exposure modifiers may be assigned numerical values that take the following form (which differs slightly from the formulation of Schneider et al., 1991):

$$\text{Modifier} = \left(\frac{\text{Exposure before modification}}{\text{Exposure after modification}} \right) \tag{18.3}$$

These modifiers can be generated using explicit models available in the literature. The models will contain a number of parameters whose historical values are known with varying levels of uncertainty. Expert judgment will be used to estimate the parameter values and explicate the uncertainties.

Figure 18.3 shows the conceptual task at hand. The starting point is the determination of E_{ref}, the reference measurement of current exposures. Using this as an anchoring point, one can determine the exposure modifier for each point of interest, $M_i(t)$, that modifies the exposure with reference to current measurement.

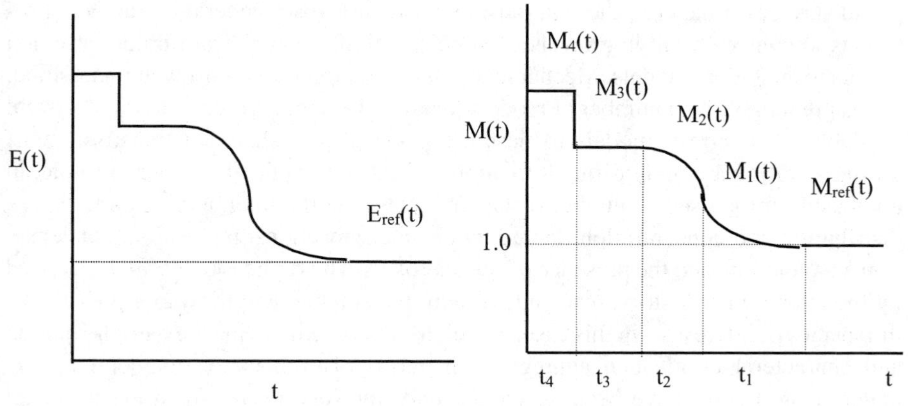

FIGURE 18.3 Obtaining exposure modifiers and actual exposures over past time periods.

18.2.7 Exposure Models

In order to use exposure modifiers, it is necessary to have an understanding of exposure models with a clear and well-defined rationale and explicit assumptions. It is useful to start with a broad conceptualization of the worker exposure mechanism. For example, for an aerosol exposure, the paradigm is as follows:

1. There is a source of the contaminant aerosol. The source output strength depends on the process and plant throughput.
2. There is a mechanism by which the aerosol is dispersed throughout the workplace. The parameters of interest are the rates of ventilation and recirculation.
3. Exposure for a given worker is related to the fraction of time that the worker spends in each location (microenvironment) within the workplace. This is related to work schedules and practices.

There are a number of exposure models available in the literature, and some of the simpler ones were discussed in Chapter 17. Each model contains a number of input parameters. Changes in plant conditions (i.e., modifiers) will affect input parameters, thereby changing the outputs of these models. There can be sudden step changes in these modifiers (e.g., when a process is moved to a new plant location over a short time period) or gradual changes (e.g., a change in feedstock quality over several years). Other factors that may affect estimates of past exposures include such changes as the introduction of respiratory protection equipment and operational issues such as work stoppages.

18.2.7.1 Contaminant Generation Models

Contaminant generation rates for a limited number of processes are known, with varying levels of sophistication, ranging from crude emission factors to detailed analytical models. There are several approaches to modeling vapor generation from liquid surfaces. Likewise, the relationship between aerosol generation rate and process is known with varying levels of sophistication, ranging from crude emission factors to analytical models. Mechanical dust generation is the most well understood, and is predictable by a number of models (cited earlier) with the easy-to-use software available. In contrast, models to describe physical and chemical transformations during smelting are more difficult to apply to real-life applications. For example, in combustion processes, a number of factors determine the final aerosol particle size distribution and concentration, including chemical reactions, nucleation, condensation, coagulation, and the presence of seed aerosols. These phenomena are influenced by the temperature history, residence time in the smelter, and the vapor pressure of the species of interest — in this case, nickel. Models that describe the basic formation and characteristics of such aggregates, in terms of combustion temperature and material properties, have been developed only for very well-defined experimental situations. In contrast, a number of studies have looked at dust generation during the handling of bulk solid and aggregated material (BOHS, 1985, 1988; Cowherd et al., 1989; Castor and Gray, 1992; Chambers, 1992; Heitbrink et al., 1992). Plinke et al. (1991; 1994a; 1994b; 1995) modeled dust generation as an interaction between external forces that separate particles and interparticle binding forces. They empirically predicted the mass of dust generated as a function of mass of bulk material, material composition (described by its melting temperature and particle density), moisture content, particle size distribution, and some parameter related to the power input to the system (such as the height from which bulk material is dropped and the impact area).

18.2.7.2 Ventilation Box Models

After the dust becomes airborne, the room ventilation or local exhaust ventilation disperses the aerosol in the environment. Chapter 17 describes several models, including the one-box and two-box models for vapors and aerosols. For example, the steady state equilibrium concentration of aerosol in a well-mixed room is given by

$$\mathrm{C}_{\mathrm{equil}} = \frac{G}{V_s A + K Q_{vent} + R} \tag{18.4}$$

Depending on the assumptions made about ventilation rates, mixing efficiency, and inclusion of removal mechanisms other than sedimentation, a number of models can be folded into this framework.

18.2.7.3 Worker Time–Activity Models

The worker's personal exposure can be modeled using the concentrations experienced during different tasks and the times spent in performing those tasks. A time–activity model can take the general form:

$$E_i = \sum_{j=1}^{N} C_j t_{ij} \tag{18.5}$$

where E_i is the time-weighted integrated exposure for worker i over the specified time period for a given task; C_j is the pollutant concentration associated with task j or in microenvironment (work area) j; t_{ij} is the total time spent by worker i in task or microenvironment j; and N is the total number of tasks/microenvironments that the worker moves through. Esmen (1979) suggested a very useful method of using Occupational Titles (*OT*) to obtain the fractions of time spent in a particular microenvironment. Briefly, the idea is to express each *OT* as a vector function with time-dependent Uniform Tasks (UT_i). Then, X_i is the estimate of the fraction of time spent by a worker in a given *OT* performing a specific UT_i. Therefore,

$$OT = [X_1\ X_2 \ldots X_N]$$

and

$$\sum_{j=1}^{N} X_j = 1, \text{ where } 0 \leq X_j \leq 1. \tag{18.6}$$

This model provides a useful mechanism by which changes in job descriptions and tasks associated with jobs get reflected in changes in personal exposures over time.

If historical information on the time-fraction composition of *OT* classes is available, then it is straightforward to estimate exposures using Equation 18.4 and Equation 18.5, provided the exposure concentration associated with each uniform task (*UT*) is known. If the historical composition of each *OT* is unknown, then the X_j's can be inferred from the current composition of the *OT*, and interviews of veterans and "old-timers" at the plant, with additional assessments based on plant history.

18.2.8 Leveraging All Relevant Information — Bayesian Methods

It is clear from the above discussion that, although many sources of information exist that may be helpful in reconstructing historical exposures, no one source by itself will be sufficient. Retrospective exposure reconstruction based solely on sparse historical measurements leads to estimates with such large uncertainties as to be useless for developing quantitative dose–response relationships for epidemiology. Additional inputs are needed in order to estimate exposures as a function of time from relatively sparse discrete measurements. These additional inputs can take the form of expert judgments from professionals with relevant experience and insights, or outputs from exposure models, or some combination of the two. A Bayesian probabilistic framework was first proposed by Ramachandran and Vincent (1999) for synthesizing expert judgment, historical information about workplace conditions, and incomplete or sparse measurements, in order to determine exposure as a function of time and place. The output from this procedure is an exposure matrix by time and task group. The uniqueness of this approach is that exposures are represented as probability distributions instead of averages. Such an exposure matrix can then be used directly in epidemiological studies. This approach has the advantage of explicitly accounting for the relevant uncertainties and yields a probability distribution of the exposure history. That is, for each point in time in a given workplace, the exposure is represented as a probability distribution. Such an approach necessarily draws on findings from a wide variety of fields: engineering knowledge of the factors affecting the generation and dispersion of contaminants, job–task patterns, uncertainty analysis, psychology of expert judgment elicitation, and decision making.

In the Bayesian view, a measurement process serves to refine previous knowledge of physical parameters by adjusting their probability distributions. It is thus based on inductive reasoning. Most industrial hygienists are Bayesian practitioners (even if unknowingly and informally) when they make initial educated guesses about exposures in a workplace (even if they are crude estimates of high vs. low exposures), which are subsequently refined by the actual measurements of exposures. The Bayesian framework formalizes this commonsense approach to exposure assessment. If the physical quantity of interest is represented by f and the measured data are represented by m, then the Bayesian expression for the updated probability distribution of f is

$$P_{post}(f/m) = \frac{P_0(f)\,P_L(m/f)}{P(m)} \tag{18.7}$$

where $P_0(f)$ is the probability distribution of f prior to making any measurements (the "prior"); $P_L(m/f)$ is the likelihood that, given the true value f, the measurement m is observed; P(m) is the probability that the measurement m is observed; and $P_{post}(f/m)$ is the updated probability that the physical quantity of interest is f, given that measurements m are observed (the "posterior").

The above framework is applicable to a situation in which subjective inputs, such as expert judgments about the probability distribution of a particular parameter (such as aerosol concentration under specified plant-operating conditions), are to be synthesized with objective measurements of the same parameter. The updated probability will provide a better estimate (i.e., narrower probability distribution) of the parameter of interest than either the subjective prior probability provided by the experts or the objective — but sporadic and incomplete — measurements with wide error bars. In order to use Equation 18.7, the likelihood function, $P_L(m/f)$, needs to be estimated using the variance in exposures for the worker population due to environmental and analytical variability as well as systematic errors. A likelihood function for the actual historical measurements is evaluated using an assumed variance in the measurements. Because exposures are usually distributed lognormally, the likelihood function is given by

$$P_L(M/f) = \frac{\exp\left(\frac{-1}{2(\ln\sigma_M)^2}(\ln M - \ln f)^2\right)}{\sqrt{2\pi}\ln\sigma_M} \tag{18.8}$$

where $P_L(M/f)$ is the probability that a measured exposure M is observed when the true exposure is f.

An estimate of the prior probability distributions, $P_0(f)$, of the parameter of interest (e.g., exposure of a worker cohort) needs to be obtained using expert judgment coupled with analytical models. The expert prior distributions are then refined using mean exposures from the data set to obtain the posterior probability distributions of exposure modifiers, $P_{post}(f/m)$.

Figure 18.4 provides a schematic of the Bayesian framework for reconstructing past exposures. The experts are provided with an information packet that contains historical process information, process throughput levels for each year, the dimensions of the workplace, ventilation records, task descriptions for each job category, and the amounts of time spent by each job category in different locations in the building. Based on this information, the experts provide subjective probability distributions for input parameters to an exposure model that predicts exposure concentrations. This constitutes the prior estimate of exposure. The prior distribution of exposure is refined or updated using the average measured exposure (from historical measurements) and its associated variance. Thus, we obtain the posterior probability distribution for building concentrations as well as concentrations at specific locations in the building. This is done using Bayes theorem.

The Bayesian framework was used to reconstruct past exposures to inhalable nickel aerosol in a smelting operation (Ramachandran, 2001). Results of this analysis were compared with those obtained using a more traditional methodology for retrospective exposure assessment, which uses only the sparse exposure monitoring data. Figure 18.5 shows an example of the output from this methodology for reconstructing nickel exposures.

The exposure estimates based only on the limited information provided by sparse measurements have substantial uncertainties associated with them. However, if this information is supplemented with expert inputs that are informed by knowledge of historical conditions at the smelter, the uncertainties are considerably reduced.

18.2.9 Using Expert Judgment along with Deterministic Models

When insufficient exposure data are available to assess risk by conventional occupational hygiene methods, professional occupational hygienists routinely interpret the available information by informally using their own expert judgment. It is claimed that this invokes that part of occupational hygiene often referred to as art.

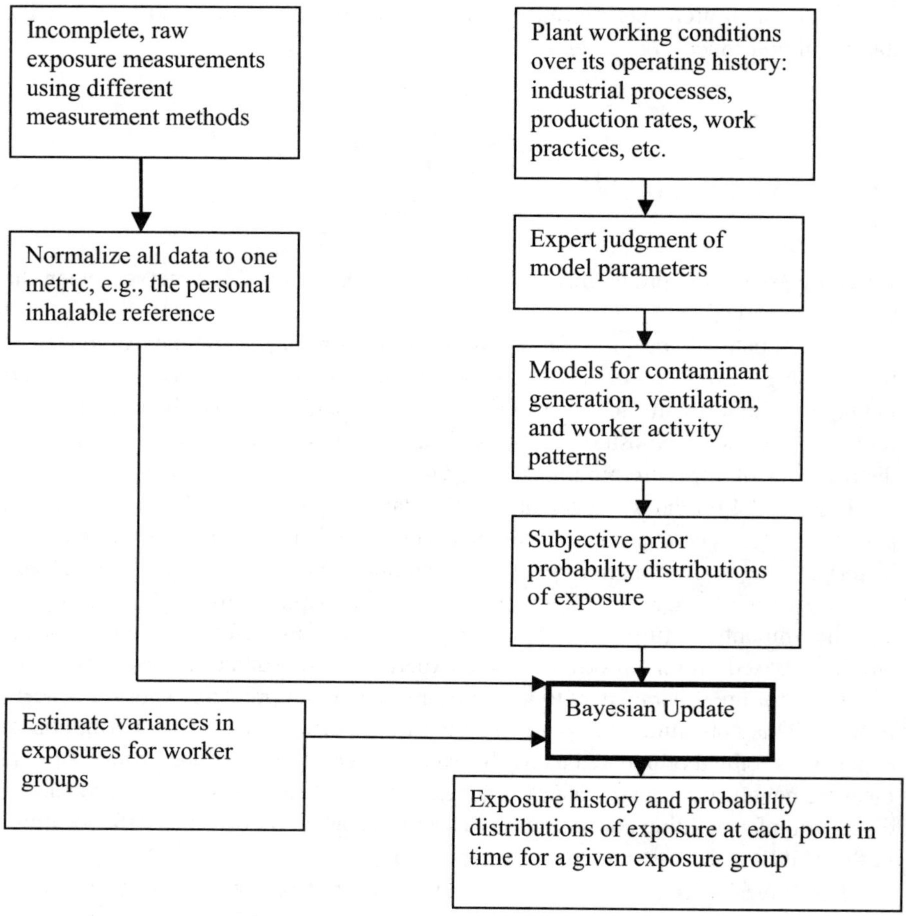

FIGURE 18.4 Bayesian methodology for retrospective exposure assessment.

Although, in the past, this has been regarded as something that is intangible and arising from their professional experiences, occupational hygiene researchers are beginning to take advantage of a formal body of methodology known as *expert judgment science*, which has worked well in other fields (e.g., Kromhout et al., 1987; Hawkins and Evans, 1989; Post et al., 1991; Cherrie and Schneider, 1999; Ramachandran and Vincent, 1999; Ramachandran, 2001).

As stated earlier, expert judgments can be used to determine prior probability distributions, $P_0(f)$, of the exposure. These judgments, by their very nature, are subjective. One way to determine $P_0(f)$ is to directly elicit the subjective probabilities of different values of past exposures. However, even a subjective assessment of past exposure is a complex decision, resting on a particular rationale and a hierarchy of assumptions. In view of this, it is better to disaggregate the problem, allowing expert judgment on its individual aspects. Morgan and Henrion (1990) observe that the decomposition of judgments into a series of conditional probability judgments, later combined, tended to produce judgments closer to the truth than direct assessments

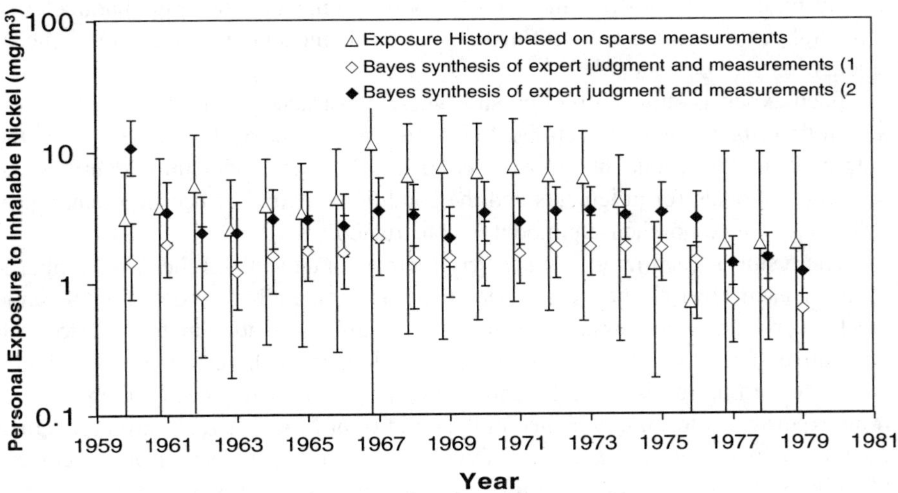

FIGURE 18.5 Comparison of exposure reconstructions using sparse measurements only with exposure reconstruction using Bayesian synthesis of expert judgments, deterministic exposure models, and historical measurements. Two experts were used in this instance. Note the smaller error bars for the Bayesian method.

of overall probability. This disaggregation is achieved by modeling each individual aspect of the problem.

As described in previous subsections, the determination of the exposure modifiers, $M(t_{past})$, is essentially the creation of models to estimate exposure history. Three broad classes of models have been identified: contaminant generation, ventilation, and time–activity models. Each of these models uses a number of parameters, which represent the next level of disaggregation. Some of these parameters may be the products of a third tier of models or are determined from historical records with some degree of uncertainty. Uncertainties in the model structure may arise due to scientific uncertainties about how each of the above mechanisms changes exposure. Characterization of this uncertainty must rely on subjective expert judgment.

For the nickel smelter example, the experts were provided with relevant plant records that included process information and production reports, ore throughput, physical dimensions of the workplace, ventilation records, task descriptions of each occupational title, personnel and safety records that contained historical lists of standard operating procedures, and results of interviews with veteran plant workers who possessed historical knowledge of plant conditions. They were also provided information about current estimates of exposure based on the personal inhalable measurements. Based on this information, the experts were asked to provide subjective probability distributions for each parameter for each time period of interest. The parameters and their associated uncertainties were then propagated through the models described above, along with expert-specified models, if any, to obtain probability distributions for exposures and exposure modifiers. Thus, the result was a distribution of exposure estimates for each point in time, weighted by their likelihood of being correct, as judged by experts. The example provided at the end of Chapter

17 and Figure 17.8 illustrate the use of expert judgments about each parameter of a general ventilation model to estimate the airborne nickel concentration in a nickel smelter.

Each expert is shown a preliminary model constructed using the exposure paradigm described in earlier sections. Each input parameter of this model can be the output of another model if the experts so decide. The model thus identifies the scientific rationale for judgments and the conditional nature of decision making. In this manner, a comprehensive model is constructed.

The result of each interview is a set of expert judgments on the relative plausibility of each level of the tree. Where there are contending models for the same mechanism, the expert assigns probability weights that add up to 1.00 to each alternative. These weights will reflect the confidence of the expert in a particular model, according to his or her scientific judgment. For example, in the above tree, if an expert has a lot of confidence in the validity of Model A for ventilation, some confidence in Model B, and none at all in Model C, this might result in an assignment of weights of 0.8, 0.2, and 0.0 for the three models, respectively. For each parameter of interest, a continuous subjective probability distribution is obtained that reflects the expert's state of belief. A series of questions are asked to establish several points (percentiles) on the distribution. The expert is asked to give reasons for his or her answers, while the interviewer questions the expert's judgment at every step. This procedure is normally adopted to combat overconfidence, which is a common trait observed in experts.

Recruitment of qualified professionals, practitioners, and researchers to interpret the data is crucial. The criteria for choosing experts include their level of relevant work experience in the industry, substantive contributions to the scientific literature, status in the scientific community (e.g., membership of editorial committees of key journals, membership of national or international scientific committees and advisory boards, etc.), and peer nomination. Another factor that should be considered in assembling the team is to provide for variety and balance of institutional perspectives by including experts from both industry and academia, and other stakeholders in the process.

18.2.10 Quality of Expert Judgment

The quality of expert judgment depends on (1) substantive expertise, referring to the knowledge that an expert has about the quantity of interest, and (2) normative expertise, referring to the skill in expressing beliefs in probabilistic terms, also known as calibration. Normative expertise or calibration is a measure of the accuracy of the expert judgment. There are two components to evaluating calibration: (1) knowledge, i.e., the accuracy of the experts' estimates of the quantities of interest, and (2) self-knowledge, i.e., the accuracy of the experts' estimates of the uncertainty in their estimate of the quantities of interest.

Kromhout et al. (1987) studied the qualitative estimation of task exposures by occupational hygienists, supervisors, and workers at a number of plants. Subjects were asked to rate exposure for 97 tasks in 5 plants, using a 4-point scale ranging from no exposure to high exposure. The authors found that the there was a significant correlation between the ratings and the measured mean exposures. They recommended that a combination of qualitative, subjective judgments and actual measurements might lead to better exposure estimates. It was effectively a Bayesian approach, although not in a formal sense.

Hawkins and Evans (1989) examined the ability of 24 occupational hygienists to estimate the distribution of exposures for a single process using toluene, based on experience and professional judgment. They provided estimates of the mean, median, range, and 90th percentile exposures, first using only qualitative information about the process and then using limited historical exposure data. This distribution was next compared with an empirical distribution determined from 134 recent exposure measurements collected from the process. The authors concluded that the experts were able to better estimate the 90th percentile than the median and that their accuracy improved substantially when presented with limited historical data.

Macaluso et al. (1993) used 5 experts to rate exposures in 1 of 6 exposure categories for 695 department–job–title–year combinations. The authors observed that for the low-exposure categories there could be considerable disagreement between experts, and cautioned against using expert judgments when exposures are low. They did not examine the causes of the disagreements, but indicated that such a study should be done.

Cock et al. (1996) studied exposure assessment by experts, using 15 experts to rank 14 fruit growing/pesticide application tasks with respect to potential dermal and respiratory exposure. They measured interexpert agreement using both Cohen's kappa statistic and an intraclass correlation coefficient determined using ANOVA. Clear differences between the experts were found in the exposure ratings, which were correlated with their level of expertise. A statistically significant relationship was found between the exposure rankings and actual measured exposures.

The above studies suggest that professional industrial hygienists are in fact well-calibrated and can indeed provide good estimates of exposures for retrospective epidemiological studies.

18.2.11 Validation of Retrospective Exposure Assessment Estimates

Validation of retrospective exposure assessments to ensure that the results are close to the true values always poses a significant problem. One method that has been proposed is to use the technique to predict current exposures for which, presumably, complete information is available (Ramachandran and Vincent, 1999). The limitation of this method is that expert judgment is better at predicting recent exposures than at predicting exposures that occurred several decades ago. Thus, success of any method in predicting current exposures should not be taken as a validation of its prediction of past exposures. Cherrie and Schneider (1999) used the correlation between estimated and measured values as a measure of validity, although they recognized the obvious limitation that the measured values were sparse and contained substantial errors. So, one might have a situation in which all the expert posterior values could fall within the confidence limits placed around the measurements merely because the measurements had very wide uncertainty. Another measure of validation is the degree of agreement between the experts. In this case, care needs to be taken to ensure that there is no bias because the experts come from similar backgrounds.

Given the lack of objective measures of validity, the only reasonable alternative is to invoke the rationality of the methodology. The use of a physical model provides a rational framework for predicting exposures. Although the inputs to these models are subjective probability distributions, they are anchored in actual historical plant information. Thus, an argument could be made that, if one accepts that the physical model chosen is appropriate and the choices for input parameters are reasonable, then one logically has to also accept the results of the rational procedure described earlier.

18.3 DOSE ESTIMATION

Whereas the previous section described methods for estimating exposure as a function of time, i.e., $E(t)$, as Equation 18.1 shows, two more quantities needing estimation to calculate dose are the time-dependent retention of the contaminant in the body, $R(t)$, and the time-dependent potency of the contaminant, $G(t)$.

18.3.1 Estimating *R(t)*

Every contaminant that the human body is exposed to may be taken up by the body. The contaminant then may or may not undergo various metabolic transformations. Ultimately, some of the contaminant or its transformed by-products will be retained in the body, whereas the rest will be eliminated. The toxicological literature describes the process by which contaminants are disposed of in the body. Here, respiratory tract deposition and retention of insoluble mineral dust (e.g., nickel oxide) will be described as examples of this process. A number of approaches are available for modeling the respiratory tract deposition of particles, some of which were described in Chapter 11. The most comprehensive model is the ICRP lung dosimetry model (ICRP, 1994), which provides deposition estimates in every airway generation based on detailed morphometric data about the respiratory tract. The model takes into account the physical mechanisms of diffusion, impaction, and gravitational settling, and provides good agreement with a broad range of experimental data.

Other models, such as the one by Heyder et al. (1986), also described in Chapter 11, are based on extensive experimental data and can be used to calculate the efficiencies of regional deposition in the human respiratory tract for particles of any aerodynamic size inhaled via any breathing pattern through the mouth or nose. Their models can be used to calculate the efficiency of deposition in the extrathoracic, tracheobronchial, and alveolar regions for nose and mouth breathing corresponding approximately to "at rest" (7.5 breaths per min, 1 l per breath) and "moderate work" (15 breaths per min, 1.5 l per breath). The Heyder et al. model includes considerations of the tidal volume of air inspired; the volumes of the extrathoracic, bronchial, and respiratory dead space regions; as well as the particle residence times for the different regions.

The clearance of deposited quartz particles depends primarily on the ability of the alveolar macrophages (AMs) to detect, phagocytoze, and transport particles to the mucociliary escalator, where they are eliminated from the lung. However, the ability of the AMs to remove particles from the alveoli becomes impaired at high-particulate lung burdens — a condition described as "overload" (Bolton et al., 1983; Morrow, 1988). This depression in the clearance rate of particles due to AM overload leads to increased retention and accumulation of particles in the lung; the AMs die and release particles into the pulmonary interstitium along with acute inflammatory mediators (Tran et al., 1995). More AMs are recruited if the inhaled quartz is not removed, and these AMs, in turn, also undergo necrosis and release more particles into the interstitium. It is believed that this cyclic behavior produces chronic inflammation and, ultimately, clinical symptoms of fibrosis.

A similar process of altered particle-retention kinetics caused by depressed AM clearance has also been seen in a number of studies with other particles such as diesel particulate matter (with elemental carbon being the relevant component of DPM) and nickel compounds (Morrow et al., 1991; Muhle et al., 1990; Mauderly et al., 1994; Bailey et al., 1982; Hsieh et al., 1999a, 1999b). Morrow (1988) proposed that it is the volumetric loading of the AM which ultimately affects their clearance function, and that a phagocytozed particulate lung burden of 6% of the normal AM volume is critical for the onset of overload. This corresponds to a volumetric lung burden of ~1 to 3 μl/g of lung tissue or ~1 to 3 mg/g of lung tissue, and is independent of the type of particle.

More cytotoxic particles such as crystalline silica also affect clearance rates, but at much lower lung burdens (Oberdörster, 1995). For mixed exposures to dusts of different toxicities, the situation is more complicated, with some studies suggesting an increase in the clearance half times for the less toxic material (McMillan et al., 1989).

Over the years, various particle deposition models have been proposed for the kinetics of deposition and retention of dust in the lung to predict the accumulation of lung burden due to chronic exposures to mineral dusts. Early ideas in this regard assumed that, given a constant level of exposure, the lung burden would reach a steady state value representing an equilibrium between the mass being deposited and cleared. In this early model, the lung was represented by three compartments, described as *fast*-clearing, *medium*-clearing, and *slow*-clearing. The fast-clearance compartment was related to the ciliary clearance process in the tracheobronchial region, whereas the medium and slow compartments were related to macrophage clearance in the interstitium. Each of the compartments followed linear kinetics, so that the instantaneous rate at which particulate matter was removed from a compartment was directly proportional to the mass present in that compartment. However, experiments using laboratory rats showed that, after an initial nonlinear phase, the lung burden increased steadily with time (see Figure 18.6).

Based on these findings, Vincent et al. (1987) proposed an additional *sequestration* compartment from which particles are not cleared at all, but sequestered in the pulmonary interstitium. The model equations for lung burden as a function of time predict quite well the experimental data for low-toxicity insoluble dust exposures (e.g., coal dust).

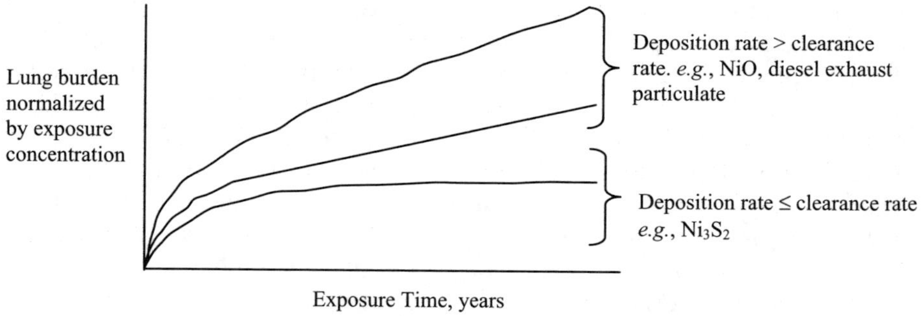

FIGURE 18.6 Lung burden as a function of exposure time, indicating the existence of a overload threshold. (Based on Oberdörster, G., 1995, Lung particle overload: implications for occupational exposures to particles, *Regul. Toxicol. Pharmacol.*, 27: 123–135.)

Hsieh et al. (1999b, 1999c) used bioassay data from inhalation studies in rats to develop a mathematical model of Ni-compound deposition and retention in the alveolar region of the rat lung. The model considered the removal of several deposited Ni compounds from alveoli by macrophage clearance and dissolution. NiO particles are poorly soluble in water, and their removal is controlled by macrophage clearance, whereas $NiSO_4$ is highly soluble and is cleared by dissolution. For the moderately soluble Ni_3S_2, both mechanisms are responsible for clearance. The clearance rate coefficients for NiO and $NiSO_4$ decreased with increasing lung burden, whereas the clearance rate coefficient for Ni_3S_2 increased with increasing lung burden (see Figure 18.6).

In the Hsieh et al. (1999b, 1999c) model, the alveolar region of the lung was considered as a single compartment that was used to describe the buildup of the each Ni compound, using kinetic equations of the form

$$\frac{dM}{dt} = \dot{r} - \lambda M \tag{18.9}$$

where M is the mass burden of each Ni compound, $\dot{r}$ the deposition rate of that Ni compound, and λ the total alveolar clearance rate coefficient of the Ni compound over all clearance pathways. The values of λ obtained from the rat studies were scaled up for predicting lung burdens in humans, accounting for differences in lung weight, minute ventilation, tidal volume, and differential regional deposition efficiencies of inhaled particles in rat and human lungs.

From their studies, Hsieh et al. (1999b, 1999c) determined that the rate of increase in lung burden for NiO is 2.7 (μg/mg m^{-3})/d. This value can be used for estimating human lung burdens for oxidic nickel, after appropriate scaling, as described in the next section.

However, for Ni_3S_2, the retention kinetics are different; the lung burden reaches an equilibrium value of 40 to 50 (μg/mg m^{-3}) and then does not increase with time (Hsieh et al., 1999b). In contrast, soluble nickel is cleared very quickly from the lungs by dissolution and is not retained at all.

The predictions of the dust retention models can be used to estimate lung burden of each compound as a function of time. These predictions are, of course, for the rat lung. Thus, the rate of accumulation of oxidic, sulfidic, and soluble nickel can be obtained separately in the rat lung. This can be extrapolated to human exposures by appropriately scaling the rat and human breathing rates, as well as the lung burden per unit mass of lung tissue. The following simple example illustrates the approach. These calculations are based on the method proposed by Vincent (1995).

Let us assume that the output of the exposure reconstruction procedure, described earlier, yielded the following exposure history for oxidic nickel for a particular worker who retired in 2000. We will neglect the associated uncertainties for the purpose of this example.

1950–1960	8 mg/m^3
1960–1970	4 mg/m^3
1970–1980	1 mg/m^3
1980–1990	0.4 mg/m^3
1990–2000	0.1 mg/m^3

We will assume that the worker worked for 5 d/week, 48 weeks/year; that the breathing rate for the worker is 20 l/min, whereas that for the rat is 0.1 l/min; and that the human lung weighs 1 kg, whereas the rat lung weighs 2 g.

Number of days worked in each 10 year period = $10 \times 48 \times 5 = 2400$ d.

Let us also assume that the slope of the lung burden graph for NiO is 2.7 μg/mg m^{-3} per day of exposure. Scaling the data for a human, the accumulation rate for the worker will be $2.7 \times (20/0.1) = 540$ μg/mg m^{-3} per day of exposure. Therefore, the cumulative lung burden for the first 10-year period (1950 to 1960) is equal to (8 mg/m^3) × (2400 d) × (540 μg/mg m^{-3}/d) = 10,370 mg, or a tissue burden of 10.3 mg/g^{-1}. Thus, the total amount of dust retained in the lungs and the tissue burden for each time interval are:

Year	Dust Retained	Tissue Burden
1950–1960	10,370 mg	10.37 mg/g^{-1}
1960–1970	5,185 mg	5.18 mg/g^{-1}
1970–1980	1,296 mg	1.29 mg/g^{-1}
1980–1990	518 mg	0.52 mg/g^{-1}
1990–2000	129 mg	0.13 mg/g^{-1}
Total	17.58 g	

The total lung burden in 2000 was 17.58 g. Because overload occurs at a tissue burden of ~1 mg/g, this would have occurred within the first decade of the worker's employment history. Thus, our dose metric for oxidic Ni is the cumulative dust retained in the lung (17.58 g).

18.3.2 ESTIMATING *G(t)*

Although the parameter $G(t)$ is just as important, it is more difficult to quantify. This parameter reflects the toxic effect transmitted to the body as a function of time. Some early progress in this regard was made by linking the kinetic behavior of lung burden and cell response based on the cell lavage studies by Donaldson et al. (1988). The cell response was taken to be a measure of $G(t)$. From the results of inhalation experiments with rats for relatively innocuous titanium dioxide and relatively harmful quartz, they found that for TiO_2, $G(t)$ reaches a maximum soon after the particle contacts the lung and then quickly decays, whereas for quartz, $G(t)$ is high initially and remains so. However, no such effects have been studied in humans.

The simplest models used in epidemiological studies calculate dose as the cumulative exposure in which each exposure is equally weighted in terms of its potency, and they ignore clearance. Consider a hypothetical exposure history over a 5-year period as shown in the following table:

1995–1996	5 mg/m^3
1996–1997	4 mg/m^3
1997–1998	3 mg/m^3
1998–1999	2 mg/m^3
1999–2000	1 mg/m^3

Then the simple model yields a cumulative exposure after T years given by

$$Cumulative(T) = \sum_{i=1}^{n} C_i \, t_i \tag{18.10}$$

$$Cumulative(5) = 5 \times 1 + 4 \times 1 + 3 \times 1 + 2 \times 1 + 1 \times 1 = 15 \ \text{mg/m}^3 \text{ years.}$$

However, it is reasonable to expect that the deposited particles that stay a long time in the lung from earlier exposures have a greater impact on health outcome than particles deposited more recently (Jahr, 1974). Thus, for insoluble particles, greater weight needs to be given to the effect of earlier exposures. One implementation of this has been to use the following weighting scheme:

$$Cumulative(T) = \sum_{i=1}^{n} C_i \left[T - \frac{1}{2}(t_i - t_{i+1}) \right] \quad (18.11)$$

For the same exposure history, this would yield a cumulative exposure of

$$\begin{aligned} Cumulative(5) &= 5\times(5-0.5)+4\times(5-1.5)+3\times(5-2.5)+ \\ &\quad 2\times(5-3.5)+1\times(5-4.5) \\ &= 47.5\ \text{mg/m}^3\text{years} \end{aligned}$$

Thus, Equation 18.10 and Equation 18.11 lead to very different cumulative exposures, and there is some evidence in the literature to suggest that Equation 18.11 better reflects the biology. Seixas et al. (1993) have described a simple and flexible statistical model that uses an exposure metric which accounts for the time between exposure and measurement of outcome. In this manner, exposure histories can be used in conjunction with pharmacokinetic and pharmacodynamic models to obtain better estimates of biologically relevant doses to organs or tissues.

18.4 CONCLUDING REMARKS

The problem of dose reconstruction for epidemiological purposes is one of the most challenging issues to confront occupational hygienists. It involves solving the problems of historical exposure reconstruction in the face of sparse data and changing occupational environments and instrumentation. It requires a fairly deep knowledge of exposure variability, the instrumentation used to obtain the exposure data, and the appropriate health-relevant metric of exposure. It also requires a knowledge of exposure modeling, the proper use of professional or expert judgment and its elicitation, the toxicokinetics of the contaminant, and the dynamical process of the effects of the contaminant. The Bayesian statistical framework presented in this chapter allows for a synthesis of these disparate pieces of information in a logically coherent manner. It is clear that this problem is one that truly demands all the resources a well-trained occupational hygienist can bring to bear on it.

REFERENCES

ACGIH (1999), *Bioaerosols: Assessment and Control*, Macher, J., Ed., ACGIH, Cincinnati, OH.

ACGIH (2004), 2004 TLVs and BEIs, Cincinnati, OH.

Adamson, A.W. (1973), *A Textbook of Physical Chemistry,* Academic Press, New York.

Aizenberg, V., Grinshpun, S.A., Willeke, K., Smith J., and Baron P.A. (2000), Performance characteristics of the button personal inhalable sampler, *Am. Ind. Hyg. Assoc. J.*, 61: 398–404.

American Society of Testing and Materials (ASTM) (2000), *ASTM standard practice for controlling and characterizing errors in weighing collected aerosols* (ASTM D 6552), ASTM.

Armstrong, B.G. (1990), The effects of measurement errors on relative risk regressions, *Am. J. Epidemiol.*, 132: 1176–1184.

Bailey, M.R., Fry, R.A., and James, A.C. (1982), Long term clearance kinetics of insoluble particles from the human lung, *Ann. Occup. Hyg.*, 26: 273–290.

Baldwin, P. and Maynard, A. (1998), A survey of wind speeds in indoor workplaces, *Ann. Occup. Hyg.*, 42: 303–313.

Baron, P. and John, W. (1999), Sampling for thoracic aerosol, in *Particle Size Selective Sampling for Particulate Air Contaminants*, Vincent, J.H., Ed., ACGIH, Cincinnati, OH.

Baron, P.A. (1986), Calibration and use of the APS (APS 3300), *Aerosol Sci. Technol.*, 5: 55–69.

Bartley, D.L. (2001). Definition and assessment of sampling and analytical accuracy. *Ann Occup. Hyp.*, 45: 357–364.

Bolton, R.E., Vincent, J.H., Jones, A.D., Addison, J., and Beckett, S.T. (1983), An overload hypothesis for pulmonary clearance of UICC amosite fibres inhaled by rats, *Br. J. Ind. Med.*, 40: 264–272.

British Occupational Hygiene Society (BOHS) (1985), *Dustiness Estimation Methods for Dry Materials*, BOHS Technology Committee Working Group on Dustiness Estimation, Technical Guide No. 4, Science Reviews, Northwood, Middlesex, U.K.

British Occupational Hygiene Society (BOHS) (1988), Progress in dustiness estimation: methods for dry materials, *Ann. Occup. Hyg.*, 32: 535–556.

Brunekreef, B., Noy, D., and Clausing, P. (1987), Variability of exposure measurements in environmental epidemiology, *Am. J. Epidemiol.*, 125: 892–898.

Buringh, E. and Lanting, R. (1991), Exposure variability in the workplace: its implications for the assessment of compliance, *Am. Ind. Hyg. Assoc. J.*, 52: 6–13.

Burstyn, I. and Teschke, K. (1999), Studying the determinants of exposure: a review of methods, *Am. Ind. Hyg. Assoc. J.*, 60: 57–72.

Castleman, B.I. and Ziem, G.E. (1988), Corporate influence on threshold limit values, *Am. J. Ind. Med.*, 13: 531–559.

Castor, W. and Gray, A. (1992), Evaluating the dustiness of powders, *Powder Handling Processes*, 2: 145–148.

CEN (Comité Européen de Normalisation) (1995), *Workplace atmospheres — Guidance for the assessment of exposure by inhalation of chemical agents for comparison with limit values and measurement strategy*, European Standard EN 689, effective no later than August 1995 (English version).

Chambers, A.J. (1992), Assessment of alumina dustiness, *Powder Handling Processes*, 4: 47–52.

Chan, T.L. and Lippmann, M. (1980). Experimental measurements and empirical modelling of the regional depostion of inhaled particles in humans, *Am. Ind. Hyg. Assoc. J.*, pp. 399–409.

Chen, B.T., Cheng, Y.S., and Yeh, H.C. (1985), Performance of a TSI aerodynamic particle sizer, *Aerosol Sci. Technol.*, 4: 89–97.

Chen, B.T. and Crow, D.J. (1986), Use of an aerodynamic particle sizer as a real-time monitor in generation of ideal solid aerosols, *J. Aerosal Sci.,* 17: 963–972.

Chen, B.T., Cheng, Y.S., and Yeh, H.C. (1985), An experimental approach to studying particle density effects in the TSI aerodynamic particle sizer (3300), *J. Aerosal Sci.,* 20: 1489–1492.

Cherrie, J.W. and Schneider, T. (1999), Validation of a new method for structured subjective assessment of past concentrations, *Ann. Occup. Hyg.***,** 43: 235–245.

Cochran, W.G. (1968), Errors of measurement in statistics, *Technometrics*, 10: 637–666.

Cock, J., Kromhout, H., Heederik, D., and Burema, J. (1996), Experts' subjective assessment of pesticide exposure in fruit growing, *Scand. J. Work. Environ. Health,* 22: 425–432.

Corn, M. and Esmen, N.E. (1979), Workplace exposure zones for classification of employee exposures to physical and chemical agents, *Am. Ind. Hyg. Assoc. J.*, 40: 47–57.

Cowherd, C., Grelinger, M.A., Englehart, P.J., Kent, R.F., and Wong, K.F. (1989), An apparatus and methodology for predicting the dustiness of materials, *Am. Ind. Hyg. Assoc. J.*, 50: 123–130.

Crane, R.I. and Evans, R.L. (1977), Inertial deposition of particles in a bent pipe, *J. Aerosal Sci.,* 8: 161–170.

Donaldson, K., Bolton, R.E., Brown, D.M. et al. (1988), *Studies on the cellular response in lung tissue to the inhalation of mineral dust*, Edinburgh: Institute of Occupational Medicine, IOM report TM/88/01.

Donaldson, K., Stone, V., Seaton A., and MacNee, W. (2001), Ambient particle inhalation and the cardiovascular system: potential mechanisms, *Environ. Health Perspect.,* 109: 523–527.

Dunkhorst, W., Lodding, H., and Koch, W. (1995), A new personal monitor for real-time measurement of the inspirable, the thoracic, and the respirable fraction of airborne dust, *J. Aerosal Sci.,* 26: S107–S108.

Durham, M.D. and Lundgren, D.A. (1980), Evaluation of aerosol aspiration efficiency as a function of Stokes' number, velocity ratio and nozzle angle, *J. Aerosal Sci.,* 11: 179–188.

EASE (1997), The EASE model: a system for the estimation and assessment of substance exposure, Version 2 for Windows, Developed by HSE with AIAI, Edinburgh, U.K.

Esmen, N. (1979), Retrospective industrial hygiene surveys, *Am. Ind. Hyg. Assoc. J.*, 40: 58–65.

Fabries, J.F., Gorner, P., and Wrobel, R. (1989), A new air sampling instrument for the assessment of the thoracic fraction of an aerosol, *J. Aerosal Sci.,* 20: 1589–1592.

Figliola, R.S. and Beasley, D.E. (1995), *Theory and Design for Mechanical Measurements*, 2nd ed., John Wiley & Sons, New York.

Friedlander, S.K. (1977), *Smoke, Dust, and Haze*, John Wiley & Sons, New York.

Gardiner, K. (1995), Sampling strategies (chap. 17), in *Occupational Hygiene*, Harrington, J.M. and Gardiner, K., Eds., Blackwell Scientific, Oxford.

Gibson, H., Vincent J.H., and Mark D. (1987), A personal inspirable aerosol spectrometer for applications in occupational hygiene research, *Ann. Occup. Hyg.*, 31(4A): 463–479.

Grinshpun, S., Willeke, K., and Kalatoor, S. (1993), A general equation for aerosol aspiration by thin-walled sampling probes from calm and moving air, *Atmos. Environ.*, 27A: 1459–1470.

Hallock, M.F., Smith, T.J., Woskie, S.R., and Hammond, S.K. (1994), Estimation of historical exposures to machining fluids in the automotive industry, *Am. J. Ind. Med.*, 26: 621–634.

Hansson, S.O. (1998), *Setting the Limit: Occupational Health Standards and the Limits of Science*, Oxford University Press, Oxford.

Hawkins, N.C. and Evans, J.S. (1989), Subjective estimation of toluene exposures: a calibration study of industrial hygienists, *Applied Industrial Hygiene*, 4: 61–68.

Heederik, D. and Attfield, M. (2000), Characterization of dust exposure for the study of chronic occupational lung disease: a comparison of different exposure assessment strategies, *Am. J. Epidemiol.*, 151: 982–990.

Heitbrink, W.A., Baron, P.A., and Willeke, K. (1992), An investigation of dust generation by free falling powders, *Am. Ind. Hyg. Assoc. J.*, 53: 617–624.

Hewett, P. (1995), Sample size formulae for estimating the true arithmetic or geometric mean of lognormal exposure distributions, *Am. Ind. Hyg. Assoc. J.*, 56: 219–225.

Hewett, P. (1998a), Letter to the editor — comments relating to Lyles, Kupper, and Rappaport: a lognormal distribution-based exposure assessment method for unbalanced data, *Ann. Occup. Hyg.*, 42: 413–417.

Hewett, P. (1998b), Rejoinder to the response by Lyles, Kupper, and Rappaport, *Ann. Occup. Hyg.*, 42: 420–421.

Hewett, P. (2001), Misinterpretation and misuse of exposure limits, *Appl. Occup. Environ. Hyg.*, 16: 251–256.

Hewett, P. (2003), A model for designing a performance-based exposure assessment strategy, Technical Report No. 03-03, Exposure Assessment Solutions.

Hewett, P. and Ganser, G.H. (1997), Simple procedures for calculating confidence intervals around the sample mean and exceedance fraction derived from lognormally distributed data. *Appl. Occup. Environ. Hyg.*, 12: 132–142.

Heyder, J. and Gebhart, J. (1977), Gravitational deposition of particles from laminar aerosol flow through inclined circular tubes, *J. Aerosal Sci.,* 8: 289–295.

Heyder, J., Gebhart, J., Rudolf, G., Schiller, C.F., and Stahlhofen, W. (1986), Deposition of particles in the human respiratory tract in the size range 0.005–15 μm, *J. Aerosal Sci.,* 17: 811–825.

Hinds, W.C. (1999), *Aerosol Technology: Properties, Behavior, and Measurement of Airborne Particles,* 2nd ed. John Wiley & Sons, New York.

Holman, J.P. (1972), *Heat Transfer*, McGraw-Hill, New York.

Hornung, R.W., Greife, A.L., Stayner, L.T., Steenland, N.K., Herrick, R.F., Eliott, L.J., Ringenburg, V.L., and Morawetz, J. (1994), Statistical model for prediction of retrospective exposure to ethylene oxide in an occupational mortality study, *Am. J. Ind. Med.*, 25: 825–836.

Hsieh, T. H., Yu, C. P., and Oberdörster, G. (1999c), Modeling of deposition and clearance of inhaled Ni compounds in the human lung, *Regul. Toxicol. Pharmacol.,* 30: 18–28.

Hsieh, T.H., Yu, C.P., and Oberdorster, G. (1999b), A dosimetry model of nickel compounds in the rat lung, *Inhal. Toxicol.*, 11(3): 229–248.

Hsieh, T.H., Yu, C.P., and Oberdorster, G. (1999a), Deposition and clearance models of Ni compounds in the mouse lung and comparisons with the rat models, *Aerosol Sci. Technol.*, 31(5): 358–372.

Hurley, J.F., Burns, J., Copeland, L., Dodgson, J., Jacobson, M. (1982). Coalworkers simple pneumoconiosis and exposure to dust at 10 British coal mines. *Br. J. Ind. Med.*, 39: 120–127.

Hurley, J.F., Alexander, W.P., Hazeldine, D.J., Jocobsen, M., Maclaren, W.M. (1987). Exposure to respirable coalmine dust and incidence of progresive massive fibrosis. *Br. J. Ind.* Md. 44: 661–672.

International Commission on Radiological Protection (ICRP) (1975), *Reference Man*, ICRP Publication 23, Pergamon, Elmsford, NY, pp. 122–124.

International Commission on Radiological Protection (1994), *Human Respiratory Tract Model for Radiological Protection*, ICRP Publication 66, Elsevier Science, Tarrytown, NY.

ISO (1993), *Guide to the Expression of Uncertainty*, International Organization for Standardization, Geneva.

Jahr, J. (1974), Dose-response basis for setting a quartz threshold limit value, *Arch. Environ. Health*, 29: 338–340.

Jayasekera, P.N. and Davies, C.N. (1980), Aspiration below wind velocity of aerosols with sharp-edged nozzles facing the wind, *J. Aerosal Sci.*, 11: 535–4 .

Jayjock, M.A. (1997), Uncertainty analysis in the estimation of exposure, *Am. Ind. Hyg. Assoc. J.*, 58: 380–382.

Kennedy, E.R., Fischbach, T.J., Song, R., Eller, P., and Shulman, S.A. (1995), *Guidelines for Air Sampling and Analytical Method Development and Evaluation*, DHHS (NIOSH) Publication No. 95-117, Cincinnati,OH.

Kenny, L.C., Aitkens, R., Chalmers, C., Fabries, J.F., Gonzalez-Fernandes, E., Kromhout, H., Liden, G., Mark, D., Riediger, G., and Prodi, V. (1997), A collaborative European study of personal inhalable aerosol sampler performance, *Ann. Occup. Hyg.*, 41: 135–153.

Kerker, M. (1969), *The Scattering of Light and Other Electromagnetic Radiation*, Academic Press, New York.

Kromhout, H., Oostendorp, Y., Heederik, D., and Boleij, J.S.M. (1987), Agreement between qualitative exposure estimates and quantitative exposure measurements, *Am. J. Ind. Med.*, 12: 551–562.

Kromhout, H., Symanski, E., and Rappaport, S.M. (1993), A comprehensive evaluation of within- and between-worker components of occupational exposures to chemical agents, *Ann. Occup. Hyg.*, 37: 253–270.

Lee, K.W. and Liu, B.Y.H. (1982), Theoretical study of aerosol filtration by fibrous filters, *Aerosol Sci. Technol.*, 1: 147–161.

Lee, K.W. and Ramamurthi, M. (1993), Filter collection, in *Aerosol Measurement: Principles, Techniques, and Applications*, Willeke, K. and Baron, P.A., Eds., Van Nostrand Reinhold, New York.

Leidel, N.A., Busch, K.A., and Lynch, J.R. (1977), Occupational Exposure Sampling Strategy Manual, National Institute for Occupational Safety and Health (NIOSH) Publication No. 77–173 (available from the National Technical Information Service (NTIS) Publication No. PB274792).

Levin, L.S., Rice, C.H., Lemasters, G.K., Lockey, J.E., and Medvedovic, M. (2000), What is the potential measurement error in occupational exposure studies? *J. Air Waste Manage. Assoc.*, 50: 941–947.

Lippmann, M. (1977), Regional deposition of particles in the human respiratory tract, in *Handbook of Physiology, Section 9, Reactions to Environmental Agents,* Lee, D.H.K., Falk, H.L., and Murphy, S.D., Eds., American Physiological Society, Bethesda, MD, pp. 213–232.

Liu, B.Y.H. and Agarwal, J.K. (1974), Experimental observation of aerosol deposition in turbulent flow, *J. Aerosal Sci.,* 5: 145–155.

Lyles, R.H., Kupper, L.L., and Rappaport, S.M. (1997), A lognormal distribution-based exposure assessment method for unbalanced data, *Ann. Occup. Hyg.*, 41: 63–76.

Lynch, J.R. (1994), Measurement of worker exposure, in *Patty's Industrial Hygiene and Toxicology*, 3rd ed., Vol. 3, Part A. Harris, R.L., Cralley, L.J., and Cralley, L.V., Eds., John Wiley & Sons, New York.

Macaluso, M., Delzell, E., Rose, V., Perkins, J., and Oestenstad, K. (1993), Inter-rate agreement in the assessment of solvent exposure at a car assembly plant, *Am. Ind. Hyg. Assoc. J.*, 54: 351–359.

Mark, D. and Vincent, J.H. (1986), A new personal sampler for airborne total dust in workplaces, *Ann. Occup. Hyg.*, 30: 89–120.

Marple, V.A. and Rubow, K.L. (1978), An evaluation of the GCA respirable dust monitor 101–1, *Am. Ind. Hyg. Assoc. J.*, 39: 17–25.

Marple, V.A. and Rubow, K.L. (1983), Impactors for respirable dust sampling, in *Aerosols in the Mining and Industrial Work Environments*, Marple, V.A. and Liu, B.Y.H., Eds., Ann Arbor Science, MI, chap. 60.

Mauderly, J.L., Snipes, M.B., Barr, E.B., Belinsky, S.A. et al. (1994), Pulmonary toxicity of inhaled diesel exhaust and carbon black in chronically exposed rats, HEI Research Report, 68.

Maynard, A.D. (1999), Measurement of aerosol penetration through six personal thoracic samplers under calm air conditions, *J. Aerosal Sci.,* 30(9): 1227–1242.

McMillan, C.H., Jones, A.D., Vincent, J.H., Johnston, A.M., Douglas, A.N., and Cowie, H. (1989), Accumulation of mixed mineral dusts in the lungs of rats during chronic inhalation exposure, *Environ. Res.*, 48: 218–237.

Moelwyn-Hughes, E.A. (1957), *Physical Chemistry,* Pergamon, New York.

Morgan, M.G. and Henrion, M. (1990), *Uncertainty: A Guide to Dealing with Uncertainty in Quantitative Risk and Policy Analysis*, Cambridge University Press, New York.

Morrow, P.E., Muhle, H., and Mermestein, R. (1991), Chronic inhalation study findings as a basis for proposing a new occupational dust exposure limit, *J. American Coll. Toxicology,* 10: 279–290.

Morrow, P.E. (1988), Possible mechanisms to explain dust overloading of the lungs, *Fundam. Appl. Toxicology,* 10: 369–384.

Muhle, H., Creutzenberg, O., Fuhst, R., Koch, W., Mohr, U., Takenaka, S., Morrow, P.E. et al. (1990), Dust overloading of lungs: investigations of various materials, species differences and irreversibility of effects, *J. Aerosol Med.,* 3(Suppl. 1): S111–S128.

Mulhausen, J.R. and Damiano, J. (1998), *A Strategy for Assessing and Managing Occupational Exposures*, 2nd ed., AIHA Press.

National Academy of Sciences (1991), *Human Exposure Assessment for Airborne Pollutants: Advances and Opportunities,* National Academy Press, Washington, D.C.

Nicas, M. (1996), Estimating exposure intensity in an imperfectly mixed room, *Am. Ind. Hyg. Assoc. J.,* 57: 542–550.

Nicas, M. (2000), Two-zone model, chap. 8, in *Mathematical Models for Estimating Occupational Exposures to Chemicals***.** Keil, C.B., Ed., AIHA Press, Fairfax, VA.

Nicas, M. and Jayjock, M. (2002), Uncertainty in exposure estimates made by modeling versus monitoring, *Am. Ind. Hyg. Assoc. J.*, 63: 275–283.

Nicas, M., Simmons, B.P., and Spear, R.C. (1991), Environmental versus analytical variability in exposure measurements, *Am. Ind. Hyg. Assoc. J.*, 52: 553–557.

NIOSH (1994), *Manual of Analytical Methods*, Eller, P., Ed., 4th ed., U.S. Department of Health and Human Services.

Oberdörster, G. (1995), Lung particle overload: implications for occupational exposures to particles, *Regul. Toxicol. Pharmacol.*, 27: 123–135.

Okazaki, K. and Willeke, K. (1987a), Transmission and deposition behavior of aerosols in sampling inlets, *Aerosol Sci. Technol.*, 7: 275–283.

Okazaki, K., Wiener, R.W., and Willeke, K. (1987b), The combined effect of aspiration and transmission on aerosol sampling accuracy for horizontal isoaxial sampling, *Atmos. Environ.*, 21: 1181–1185.

Okazaki, K., Wiener, R.W., and Willeke, K. (1987c), Isoaxial sampling: nondimensional representation of overall sampling efficiency, *Environ. Sci. Technol.*, 21: 178–182.

Okazaki, K., Wiener, R.W., and Willeke, K. (1987d), Nonisoaxial aerosol sampling: mechanisms controlling the overall sampling efficiency, *Environ. Sci. Technol.*, 21: 183–187.

OSHA (Occupational Safety and Health Administration) (2001), Appendix B to the formaldehyde standard, Code of Federal Regulations 29, Part 1910.1048.

OSHA (Occupational Safety and Health Administration) (2002), 29 CFR 1910.1000 Subpart Z Toxic and Hazardous Substances, Tables Z-1, Z-2, and Z-3.

Plinke, M., Leith, D., Boundy, M.G., and Löffler, F. (1995), Dust generation from handling powders in industry, *Am. Ind. Hyg. Assoc. J.*, 56: 251–257.

Plinke, M., Leith, D., Goodman, R.G., and Löffler, F. (1994b), Particle separation mechanisms in flow of granular materials, *Part. Sci. Technol.*, 12: 71–87.

Plinke, M., Leith, D., Hathaway, R., and Löffler, F. (1994a), Cohesion in granular materials, *Bulk Solids Handling*, 14: 101–106.

Plinke, M., Leith, D., Holstein, D., and Boundy, M.G. (1991), Experimental examination of factors that affect dust generation, *Am. Ind. Hyg. Assoc. J.*, 52: 521–528.

Post, W., Kromhout, H., Heederik, D., Noy, D., and Duijzentkunst, R.S. (1991), Semiquantitative estimates of exposure to methylene chloride and styrene: The influence of quantitative exposure data, *Appl. Occup. Environ. Hyg.*, 6: 197–204.

Pui, D.Y.H., Romay-Novas, F., and Liu, B.Y.H. (1987), Experimental study of particle deposition in bends of circular cross-section, *Aerosol Sci. Technol.*, 7: 301–315.

Raabe, O.G., and Stuart, B.O. (1999), Sampling criteria for the thoracic and respirable fractions, in *Particle Size Selective Sampling for Particulate Air Contaminants*, Vincent, J.H., Ed., ACGIH, Cincinnati, OH.

Ramachandran, G. (2001), Retrospective exposure assessment using Bayesian methods, *Ann. Occup. Hyg.*, 45(8): 651–667.

Ramachandran, G. and Vincent, J.H. (1999), A Bayesian approach to retrospective exposure assessment, *Appl. Occup. Environ. Hyg.*, 14(8): 547–557.

Ramachandran, G., Adgate, J.L., Pratt, G.C., Hill, N., Bock, D., and Sexton, K. (2000), Comparison of short-term variations (15-minute averages) in outdoor and indoor $PM_{2.5}$ concentrations, *J. Air Waste Manage. Assoc.*, 50: 1157–1166.

Ramachandran, G., Adgate, J.L., Pratt, G.C., and Sexton, K. (2003), Characterizing indoor and outdoor 15-minute average $PM_{2.5}$ concentrations in urban neighborhoods, *Aerosol Sci. Technol.*, 37: 33–45.

Rappaport, S.M. (1984), The rules of the game: an analysis of OSHA's enforcement strategy, *Am. J. Ind. Med.*, 6: 291–303.

Rappaport, S.M. (1991), Assessment of long-term exposures to toxic substances in air — review, *Ann. Occup. Hyg.*, 35: 61–121.

Rappaport, S.M. (1994), Interpreting levels of exposure to chemical agents, in *Patty's Industrial Hygiene and Toxicology*, 3rd ed., Vol. 3, Part A, Harris, R.L., Cralley, L.J., and Cralley, L.V. Eds., John Wiley & Sons, New York.

Rappaport, S.M., Kromhout, H., Symanski, E. (1993), Variation of exposure between workers in homogeneous exposure groups, *Am. Ind. Hyg. Assoc. J.*, 54: 654–662.

Rappaport, S.M., Kupper, L.L., Lyles, R.H. (1998a), Response to letter to the editor by Hewett, *Ann. Occup. Hyg.*, 42: 417–420.

Rappaport, S.M., Kupper, L.L., Lyles, R.H. (1998b), Rejoinder to the rejoinder by Hewett, *Ann. Occup. Hyg.*, 42: 421–422.

Rappaport, S.M., Lyles, R.H., and Kupper, L.L. (1995), An exposure assessment strategy accounting for within- and between-worker sources of variability. *Ann. Occup. Hyg.*, 39: 469–495.

Reist, P.C. (1993), *Aerosol Science and Technology,* McGraw-Hill, New York.

Rice, C., Checkoway, H., Dosemici, M., Stewart, P., and Blair, A. (1997), Effects of exposure estimation procedures on the evaluation of exposure response relationships for silicosis, *Ann. Occup. Hyg.*, 41: 485–490.

Roach, S.A. and Rappaport, S.M. (1990), But they are not thresholds: a critical analysis of the documentation of threshold limit values, *Am. J. Ind. Med.*, 17: 727–753.

Rubow, K. L.,. Marple, V.A., Olin, J., and McCawley, M.A. (1987), A personal cascade impactor: design, evaluation, and calibration, *Am. Ind. Hyg. Assoc. J.*, 48(6): 532–538.

Schlichting, H. (1968), *Boundary Layer Theory,* 6th ed., McGraw-Hill, New York.

Schneider, T., Jørgensen, O., and Lauersen, B. (1991), Evaluation of exposure information, *Appl. Occup. Environ. Hyg.*, 6: 475–481.

Seixas, N.S. and Checkoway, H. (1995), Exposure assessment in industry specific retrospective occupational epidemiology studies, *Occup. Environ. Med.*, 52: 625–633.

Seixas, N.S., Robins, T.G., and Becker, M. (1993), A novel approach to the characterization of cumulative exposure for the study of chronic occupational disease, *Am. J. Epidemiol.*, 137: 463–471.

Sexton, K., Callahan, M.A., and Bryan, E.F. (1995), Estimating exposure and dose to characterize health risks: the role of human tissue monitoring in exposure assessment, *Environ. Health Perspect.* (Suppl. 3): 13–30.

Skoog, D.A. (1985), *Principles of Instrumental Analysis,* 3rd ed., Saunders College Publishing, Philadelphia.

Spear, R.C., Selvin, S., and Francis, M. (1986), The influence of averaging time on the distribution of exposures, *Am. Ind. Hyg. Assoc. J.*, 47: 365–368.

Sreenath, A., Ramachandran, G., and Vincent, J.H. (1997), Experimental investigations into the nature of airflows near bluff bodies with aspiration, with implications to aerosol sampling, *Atmos. Environ.,* 31: 2349–2359.

Sreenath, A., Ramachandran, G., and Vincent, J.H. (1999), Experimental measurements and development of improved physical models for aerosol sampler aspiration efficiency, *Appl. Occup. Environ. Hyg.*, 14, 624–631.

Sreenath, A., Ramachandran, G., and Vincent, J.H. (2001), Experimental study of particle losses close to the entry of thin-walled sampling probes at varying angles to the wind, *Aerosol Sci. Technol.*, 35: 767–778.

Sreenath, A., Ramachandran, G., and Vincent, J.H. (2002), Aspiration characteristics of idealized blunt aerosol samplers at large angles to the wind, *J. Aerosal Sci.,* 33: 81–881.

Stahlhefen, W., Gebhart, J., and Heyder, J. (1980). Experimental determination of the regional deposition of aerosol particles in the human respiratory tract. *Am. Ind. Hyp. Assoc. J.,* 41: 385–398.

Stancliffe, J.D. and Kenny, L.C. (1997), Sampling characteristics of modified personal inhalable sampler inlets, *J. Aerosal Sci.,* 25(S1): S601.

Taylor, J.R. (1997). *An Introduction to Error Analysis*. 2nd ed. University Science Books, Sausalito, California.

Tran, C.L., Jones, A.D., and Donaldson, K. (1995), Mathematical model of phagocytosis and inflammation after the inhalation of quartz at different concentrations, *Scand. J. Work Environ. Health*, 21(Suppl. 2): 50–54.

Tsai, P.J. (1995), Health-related aerosol exposures of the nickel industry workers, Ph.D. Thesis, University of Minnesota.

Tuggle, R.M. (1981), The NIOSH decision scheme, *Am. Ind. Hyg. Assoc. J.*, 42: 493–498.

Verma, D.K., Sebestyen, A., Julian, J.A., Muir, D.C.F., Schmidt, H., Bernolz, C.D., and Shannon, H.S. (1989), Silica exposures and silicosis among Ontario hard rock miners: II exposure estimates, *Am. J. Ind. Med.*, 16: 13–28.

Vicent, J.H. (1989). Aerosol Sampling: Science and Practice. John Wiley and Sons.

Vincent, J.H. (1995), *Aerosol Science for Industrial Hygienists*, Pergamon, Elsevier Science, New York.

Vincent, J.H. (1999), Sampling criteria for the inhalable fraction, in *Particle Size Selective Sampling for Particulate Air Contaminants*, Vincent, J.H., Ed., ACGIH, Cincinnati, OH.

Vincent, J.H., Aitken, R.J., and Mark, D. (1993), Porous plastic foam filtration media: penetration characteristics and applications in particle size selective sampling, *J. Aerosal Sci.,* 24: 929–944.

Vincent, J.H. and Donaldson, K. (1990), A dosimetric approach for relating the biological response of the lung to the accumulation of inhaled mineral dust, *Br. J. Ind. Med.*, 47: 302–307.

Vincent, J.H., Jones, A.D., Johnston, A.M., McMillan, C., Bolton, R.E., and Cowie, H. (1987), Accumulation of inhaled mineral dust in the lung and associated lymph nodes: implications for exposure and dose in occupational lung disease, *Ann. Occup. Hyg.*, 31: 375–393.

Vincent, J.H., Mark, D., Jones, A.D., and Donaldson, K. (1988), A rationale for assessing exposure-dose-response relationships for occupational dust-related lung disease, *Proceedings of the 7th International Conference on the Pneumoconiosis* (Pittsburgh), Public Health Service Publication, pp. 151–157.

Volckens, J. and Leith, D. (2002a), Electrostatic sampler for semivolatile aerosols: chemical artifacts, *Environ. Sci. Technol.,* 36: 4608–4612.

Volckens, J. and Leith, D. (2002b), Filters and electrostatic samplers for semivolatile aerosols: physical artifacts, *Environ. Sci. Technol.,* 36: 4613–4617.

Volckens, J., Boundy, M., Leith, D., and Hands, D. (1999), Oil mist concentration: a comparison of sampling methods, *Am. Ind. Hyg. Assoc. J.,* 60: 684–689.

Wang, H. and John, W. (1987), Density correction for the aerodynamic particle sizer, *Aerosol Sci. Technol.,* 6: 191–198.

Wegman, D.H., Eisen, E.A., Woskie, S.R., and Hu, X. (1992), Measuring exposure for the epidemiologic study of acute effects, *Am. J. Ind. Med.,* 21: 77–89.

White, F.M. (1986), *Fluid Mechanics,* 2nd ed., McGraw-Hill, New York.

Williams, K., Fairchild, C., and Jaklevic, J. (1993). Dynamic mass measurement techniques, in *Aerosol Measurement: Principles, Techniques, and Applications*, Willeke, K. and Baron, P.A., Eds., pp. 296–312.

Zeger, S.L., Thomas, D., Dominici, F., Samet, J.M., Schwartz, J., Dockery, D., and Cohen, A. (2000), Exposure measurement error in time-series studies of air pollution: concepts and consequences, *Environ. Health Perspect.,* 108: 419–426.

Index

A

B

P

Q

R

S

T

U

V